MANUAL OF NUTRITION AND DIET THERAPY

MANUAL OF NUTRITION AND DIET THERAPY

UNIVERSITY HOSPITAL
UNIVERSITY OF MICHIGAN
Ann Arbor, Michigan

EDITED BY
Norma Jean Grills, R.D., M.S.
Marcia Vermaire Bosscher, R.D., M.P.H.

WITH 33 CONTRIBUTORS

MACMILLAN PUBLISHING CO., INC.
New York

COLLIER MACMILLAN PUBLISHERS
London

PRINTED IN THE UNITED STATES OF AMERICA

Macmillan Publishing Co., Inc.
866 Third Avenue, New York, New York 10022

Collier Macmillan Canada, Ltd.

Library of Congress Cataloging in Publication Data

Michigan. University. Hospital.
Manual of nutrition and diet therapy.

Includes index.
1. Diet therapy. 2. Nutrition. I. Grills, Norma Jean. II. Bosscher, Marcia Vermaire. III. Title. [DNLM: 1. Diet therapy. 2. Nutrition. WB 400 U645d]
RM216.M483 1981 615.8'54 80-24598
ISBN 0-02-347280-4

Printing: 1 2 3 4 5 6 7 8 Year: 1 2 3 4 5 6 7 8

This manual is dedicated to the memory of

Joyce Compomizzo Girz, R.D.

whose strength, courage, and compassion
challenges each of us
to reach our highest potential.

ACKNOWLEDGMENT

This 10th edition of the Manual of Nutrition and Diet Therapy of the University Hospital has been developed to meet the needs of the expanded role which clinical dietitians have accepted in the provision of modern health care. This manual reflects an upgrading of professional standards and has three major purposes:

- To present standards of practice consistent with the expanding data base and technological advancements of the field.
- To present the rationale for nutrition assessment and management for a wide variety of disorders and diseases being treated in hospitals and ambulatory care facilities.
- To serve as a nutrition text for dietitians and other health care professionals.

For at least 50 years a dict manual has been utilized in the department and throughout the clinical areas of University Hospital. The tenth edition represents the time, effort, and composite knowledge of the current clinical dietetic staff and the Dietary Advisory Committee, 1978 through 1980.

Sincere appreciation is extended to Norma J. Grills, Assistant Director, who conceived the present format. She served as the coordinator and as a writer. There were many factors involved in the development and the publication which required direct attention and guidance.

Marcia V. Bosscher served as an editor, and was the major researcher for this project. Her dedication, expertise, interest, and continuing attention to accuracy contributed in a major way to the success of this document.

Additionally, members of the Nutrition Advisory Committee offered valuable and untiring guidance, professional knowledge, and encouragement. Sincere gratitude and appreciation is expressed to each of them as they gave freely of their time throughout the development of this manual. The members were:

George E. Bacon, M.D., M.S.
Professor of Pediatrics and Communicable Diseases
Instructor in Pharmacology

David R. Bassett, M.D.
Associate Professor of Internal Medicine

Alma L. Bolles, B.S.N.
Head Nurse, Pediatrics

Kathryn M. Clark, B.S.N.
Head Nurse, Pediatrics

William W. Coon, M.D.
Professor of Surgery

Arthur B. French, M.D.
Professor of Internal Medicine

Wilma Geels, R.N., M.S.N.
Clinical Nurse Specialist, Otorhinolaryngology

Norma J. Grills, R.D., M.S.
Assistant Director, Dietetics

Acknowledgment

George H. Nolan, M.D., M.P.H.
Associate Professor of Obstetrics and Gynecology

Phyllis M. Patterson, R.N., M.S.
Clinical Nurse Specialist, Nursing Office

Sumer Pek, M.D.
Professor of Internal Medicine

Paul Stark, M.B.A.
Assistant Director, Ancillary Service

Richard H. Wheeler, III, M.D.
Assistant Professor of Internal Medicine

Without hospital administrative support, the hopes and dreams for this publication would not have become a reality. Paul Stark, then Assistant Director of University of Michigan Hospital, was the administrative officer for the Department of Dietetics. The Department is particularly appreciative of his support and leadership in launching this project and getting the action underway. The support of successive assistant directors, David L. White and Gary L. Calhoun, has enabled the Department to proceed with this publication. Each of them, as well as William H. Borton, Associate Director, has contributed their support and has shared our enthusiasm.

Royalty from this publication is earmarked for the continued development of this document. This is particularly appropriate with the rapid expansion of knowledge in the field of nutrition. There is continuing stimulation from the clinical dietitians, students, and other members of the health care team in addressing practices in health care. The contrasting of apparently conflicting approaches to nutrition management stimulates a markedly high degree of thought and discussion. It is sincerely hoped that this manual will stimulate a greater attempt to integrate the many values of both scientific and behavioral approaches to clinical practice.

Ethel A. Downey
Director
Department of Dietetics

FOREWORD

I am pleased to be able to comment on this important, new addition to the health care literature in the field of nutrition and diet therapy. Comparing it to the old-fashioned "Diet Manual" reminds one again that the field of nutrition has finally come of age.

The reader will find within these pages a complete and clearly explained text covering our current knowledge of the biochemistry, pathophysiology, and dietary sources of the known nutrient elements and their relationship to the life-long preservation of health as well as their importance in both the pathogenesis and management of specific diseases.

Several features of this work which I particularly like are:

There is an obvious sensitivity on the part of the authors to the fact that specific therapeutic diets may generate undesirable emotional or physical side effects which often can be minimized by appropriate attention. This problem is perhaps the single most important case of failure to achieve patient acceptance and compliance and is one too long neglected by many professionals.

The carefully prepared explanations of the scientific rationale for the use of therapeutic diets in the management of specific diseases provide a convenient resource for increased understanding by the prescriber and are useful in patient education as well.

The cited references are more than adequate for the most ardent student of nutrition. The suggested additional references for lay education are particularly welcome.

Whether you are a serious student of the relationship between nutrition and health or a lone practitioner seeking help with a specific therapeutic problem, I commend this work to you as a valuable desk-side reference.

David G. Dickinson, M.D.
Professor of Pediatrics and Communicable Diseases
University of Michigan Medical School
and
Chief of Clinical Affairs
University Hospital

PREFACE

Adequate nutritional status is recognized as an important component in the maintenance of health and the prevention and/or control of disease. Genetic, environmental, social, cultural, psychological, physiological, and biochemical factors influence the nutrient needs of individuals and their ability or capacity to ingest, absorb, utilize, or sythesize nutrients.

This manual provides the health care worker with information to be used in planning, implementing, and evaluating nutrition therapies designed to maintain an adequate nutritional status. Emphasis is directed toward individualization of the therapies.

Nutrition therapies described are appropriate for hospital or ambulatory care settings. In both settings the addition of a restrictive diet to other treatment modalities often increases anxiety and depression. When establishing nutrition therapies, both the client and the primary goal of treatment need to be considered. As few changes as possible from "normal" living patterns are generally more acceptable to the individual, including food intake patterns. If major changes are necessary, it is often possible to introduce them in phases, setting short-term achievable goals. Adherence to the nutrition therapies (diet prescriptions) may be increased by providing the individual with information about the necessity of the change and by identifying observable measurements of the effectiveness of the change.

To facilitate easy use of the material within this manual, the diets are identified by nutrient, method of administration, or disease. Combinations of the diets may be prescribed. Listed under each diet is the following information: indications for use, description, guidelines for nutritional management, nutrient adequacy, and references.

Indications for use include diseases or conditions ameliorated by the diet, symptoms of the disease that may respond to nutrition intervention, length of time for which the diet is required, and/or criteria for termination or relaxation of restrictions. Conditions that may have historically been treated by the diet or conditions that would contraindicate use of the diet are listed. The description is the rationale for the use of the diet, including a brief physiological and/or biochemical explanation as well as goals of the dietary treatment. Guidelines for nutritional management is the translation of dietary goals into practical guides for meal planning. When appropriate, extensive food lists or food exchange systems, step-by-step procedures for calculating the diet, or sample menus are included. Nutrient adequacy is based on the 1980 recommended dietary allowances. Nutrients that may be excessive or need supplementation are identified. A comprehensive list of references cited is included as are some references for the lay person.

Assisting in the development of this manual were many individuals without whose commitment and wide variety of experience and knowledge this manual would not be possible. We express our appreciation to all those who contributed and especially to members of the *Diet Manual* task force: Lynn Byl, Joyce Kerestes, Debra Lewandowski, Janet Rimar, Ann Twork, and Janet Valentine, who evaluated every diet for accuracy and clarity; Ruth Farquharson, who typed the majority of the final manuscript; and Irene Smith, office coordinator, who continued to work calmly and efficiently under the added confusion, pressures, and responsibilities of the last two years.

The editors
Norma J. Grills
Marcia V. Bosscher

CONTRIBUTORS

Herminia Tabotabo Azhar, R.D.
Head Dietitian, Adult Medicine-Surgery

Sharon M. Boyd, R.D., M.S.
Nutrition Specialist, Renal

Lynn N. Byl, R.D., M.S.
Ambulatory Care: Lipid, Hypertension, and Arthritis

Jane C. Chandler, R.D.
Pediatrics, Adolescents and Cardiovascular

Grace Huifeng Chen, R.D.
Adult Medicine-Surgery

Gloria Chua Tseng, R.D., M.S.
Adult Medicine-Surgery

Patricia A. Corvi, R.D.
Head Dietitian, Ambulatory Care

Jane M. Galant, M.S., R.D.
Nutrition Specialist, Pediatric Neurology

Joyce C. Girz, R.D.
Generalist

Margaret Healey Keehner, R.D.
Adult Medicine-Surgery, Oncology

Debra J. Hufstetler, R.D., M.P.H.
Adult Medicine-Surgery

Constance R. Hydrick, M.S., R.D.
Head Dietitian, Clinical Research Center

Meda J. Johnson, R.D.
Generalist

R. Natalie Kellogg, M.P.H., R.D.
Research

Joyce K. Kerestes, R.D.
Head Dietitian, Adult Medicine-Surgery

Connie L. Langkabel, R.D.
Adult Medicine-Surgery

Andrea J. Lasichak, R.D.
Adult Medicine, Diabetes

Debra A. Lewandowski, R.D.
Adult Medicine-Surgery

Grace Lim, R.D.
Generalist

Nelda M. Mercer, R.D., M.S.
Nutrition Specialist, Research

Linda D. Morris, R.D.
Generalist

Susan K. Raatz, R.D., M.S.
Nutrition Specialist, Psychiatry

Janet E. Rimar, R.D.
Research

Teresa W. Schmelzel
Dietitian Assistant

Denise A. Stys, R.D.
Adult Medicine-Surgery, Burn and Otorhinolaryngology

Christine M. Tiernan, M.P.H., R.D.
Pediatrics, Toddlers and Oncology

Elizabeth A. Tolley, R.D.
Adult Medicine

Judith E. Tomer, R.D.
Ambulatory Care, Internal Medicine

Ann M. Twork, R.D., M.S.
Renal

Janet A. Valentine, R.D., M.S.
Head Dietitian, Pediatrics and Obstetrics

Kathryn B. Van Sickle, R.D.
Pediatrics

Marianne Wolfe, R.D.
Generalist

Deborah M. Yonkoski, R.D.
Pediatrics, Infants

CONTENTS

TABLES

PART I
HIGH-RISK MANAGEMENT

PART II
BASIC

PART III
MODIFICATIONS IN CONSISTENCY

PART IV
FIBER MODIFICATIONS

PART V
ENERGY MODIFICATIONS

PART VI
PROTEIN MODIFICATIONS

PART VII
FAT MODIFICATIONS

PART IX
MINERAL MODIFICATIONS

PART X
FOOD SENSITIVITY

PART XI
MATERNAL

PART XII
INFANTS AND CHILDREN

PART XIII TEST

PART XIV OTHER

APPENDIX

FIGURES

PART X
FOOD SENSITIVITY

PART XI
MATERNAL

PART XII
INFANTS AND CHILDREN

PART I
High-Risk Management

1

Nutrition Assessment

INDICATIONS FOR USE

Nutrition assessment is indicated for hospitalized and ambulatory care individuals with one or more of the conditions identified in Table 1-1. These situations and/or diseases increase or decrease nutrient requirements and affect an individual's ability to ingest, absorb, utilize, synthesize, or store essential nutrients. They predispose to malnutrition.

DESCRIPTION

Upon admission, between 33% and 65% of all hospitalized patients are, to some degree, malnourished. Individuals with stays of two weeks or longer demonstrate deterioration in a number of nutrition assessment parameters. (1–8) Morbidity, mortality, and complications of the disease processes or surgical procedures are increased in malnourished individuals. Timely administration of appropriate nutrition therapies—oral, tube, parenteral, or combinations of the three—decreases complications, length of hospitalization, and mortality rates. (9–11)

Nutrition assessment may be limited or extensive. (9–16) The goals are to

- Identify individuals who require aggressive nutrition support to restore or maintain nutritional status.
- Identify nutrition therapies.
- Monitor efficacy of nutrition therapies.

A limited assessment may review only actual height and weight and recent changes in these measures or serum albumin and total lymphocyte count in conjunction with present disease state, treatment plans, and ability to ingest and absorb nutrients. An extensive assessment includes a detailed review of physical, medical, surgical, drug, and diet history in relationship to the present care plans, nutrient requirements, and probable nutrient intake. A more extensive assessment may also include appraisal of cell-mediated immunity and nitrogen balance. (13, 15) Extensive assessments may not be necessary or practical in all clinical settings.

Assessment of protein status is of primary importance. Deficits in protein compartments affect wound healing, enzyme synthesis, resistance to infection, and recovery rates. The protein compartments are somatic (skeletal muscle) and visceral (nonmuscle). Somatic proteins are basically measured by anthropometry (e.g., height, weight, triceps skinfold, midarm circumference, midarm muscle circumference, and creatinine–height index). Visceral proteins are measured by laboratory analysis (e.g., total lymphocyte count, albumin, total iron-binding capacity, and transferrin).

Values indicating somatic and/or visceral protein deficits identify individuals at risk or with marginal or overt malnutrition, failure-to-thrive, marasmus, kwashiorkor, or marasmus–kwashiorkor syndrome.

Failure to thrive (infants and young children) is characterized by substandard growth without overt clinical or biochemical signs. Weight is more affected than height.

Marasmus is characterized by wasting of somatic protein mass and subcutaneous fat reserves due to an inadequate intake of both protein and calories, although the protein–calorie ratio may be normal. Immune function may become depressed. Edema is usually not present. A child is usually underdeveloped in relation to age and an adult very thin. Hair may be dyspigmentated, thin, or easily pluckable.

Kwashiorkor is characterized by loss of visceral protein mass while somatic proteins may be maintained. Edema may mask muscle wasting. Hair changes are usually present in more severe cases, and apathy is present. Individuals of normal weight or overweight individuals with slightly decreased caloric intakes and inadequate protein intakes are usually victims.

Marasmus and kwashiorkor coexist in many malnourished individuals. Visceral proteins are rapidly depleted by catabolic stress and chronic illness, or injury causes atrophy of adipose and skeletal muscles and continual depression of normal nutrient intake. Deficits of other essential nutrients—vitamins, minerals, and trace elements—are usually high in the marasmus–kwashiorkor syndrome. This syndrome is the most life threatening and requires prompt and aggressive nutrition therapy for survival. (12, 17)

Deficits of other essential nutrients are recognized by physical signs. Table 1-2 lists some physical signs indicative or suggestive of malnutrition. Physical signs lack nutrient specificity and may be caused by nonnutritional environmental influences, disease conditions, or treatments. Most signs are not specific to one nutrient but are of a complex etiology. Nutrient-specific biochemical measures help to substantiate deficits. Table 1-3 lists functions, deficiency signs, toxicity potential, biochemical measures of status, and some common food sources of essential vitamins, minerals, and trace elements.

Table 1-4 is a nutrition assessment worksheet, and Tables 1-5, 1-6, 1-7, and 1-8 identify standards for evaluating adequacy of values. It is important to note that an abnormal value in one or more measures may not be indicative of malnutrition but of other conditions (e.g., state of hydration, excretion rates, or present nutrient intakes). However, an abnormal value of one measure may place the individual in the high-risk category.

GUIDELINES FOR NUTRITIONAL MANAGEMENT

Types of nutrition therapies recommended are dependent upon the individual's preadmission nutritional status, age, developmental and growth state, disease state, stress level, physical and psychological states, length of illness, and number of surgeries recently performed and/or planned as well as the functional ability of the individual's gastrointestinal tract. When the decision to feed is reached, refer to an appropriate section within the manual for recommended nutritional management: nutrient need, method (oral, tube, parenteral), and/or disease (cancer, diabetes, renal, etc.).

NUTRIENT ADEQUACY

Efficacy of nutrition therapy is evaluated by a favorable change in assessment parameters. More than one measure should be evaluated specific to the situation. For example, height increments in a young child are indicative of increasing protein stores, whereas weight changes are more reflective of fluid or fat gain. Reassessment is completed at intervals. Parameters that reflect fast change (e.g., weight and nitrogen balance) are measured most frequently (weekly, daily). Parameters that reflect slow change (e.g., height, triceps skinfold, serum albumin, skin tests) are measured less frequently (monthly).

TABLES

TABLE 1-1. Conditions Predisposing to Malnutrition

Weight
- 10% below ideal body weight
- Recent weight change of 10% or more

Hospitalizations
- More than once in last six months for surgery, infection, sepsis or other trauma (e.g., burn)
- Longer than two weeks

Ability to eat
- Unable to eat for three or more days and not expected to eat for an equal length of time
- Long-term use (ten days or more) of intravenous fluid and electrolytes without adequate protein, calorie, vitamin, mineral, or trace element supplementation
- Long-term use of clear liquid feeding

Gastrointestinal complications
- Frequent episodes of nausea, vomiting, and/or diarrhea
- Impaired gastrointestinal tract function (e.g., ulcerative colitis, regional enteritis, sprue)

Chronic diseases
- Arthritis, alcoholism, diabetes, uncorrected thyroid function, chronic obstructive pulmonary disease, cancer

Treatments
- Receiving chemo- and/or radiation therapy or other drugs that interfere with nutrient intake, absorption, utilization, synthesis, or storage

Prior eating habits
- Long-term use of chemically defined or highly refined fabricated foods or fad, weight loss, or other limiting nutrient(s) diets

Other
- Exposure to environmental contaminants (e.g., dust with lead or manganese)
- Over 70 years of age

TABLE 1-2. Physical Signs Indicative or Suggestive of Malnutrition (12, 18)

Body Area	Normal Appearance	Signs Associated with Malnutrition
Hair	Shiny; firm; not easily plucked	Lack of natural shine; hair dull and dry; thin and sparse; hair fine, silky and straight; color changes (flag sign); can be easily plucked
Face	Skin color uniform; smooth, pink, healthy appearance; not swollen	Skin color loss (depigmentation); skin dark over cheeks and under eyes (malar and supra-orbital pigmentation); lumpiness or flakiness of skin of nose and mouth; swollen face; enlarged parotid glands; scaling of skin around nostrils (nasolabial seborrhea)
Eyes	Bright, clear, shiny; no sores at corners of eyelids; membranes a healthy pink and are moist. No prominent blood vessels or mound of tissue or sclera	Eye membranes are pale (pale conjunctivae); redness of membranes (conjunctival injection); Bitot's spots; redness and fissuring of eyelid corners (angular palpebritis); dryness of eye membranes (conjunctival xerosis); cornea has dull appearance (corneal xerosis); cornea is soft (keratomalacia); scar on cornea; ring of fine blood vessels around corner (circumcorneal injection)
Lips	Smooth, not chapped or swollen	Redness and swelling of mouth or lips (cheilosis); especially at corners of mouth (angular fissures and scars)
Tongue	Deep red in appearance; not swollen or smooth	Swelling; scarlet and raw tongue; magenta (purplish color) of tongue; smooth tongue; swollen sores; hyperemic and hypertrophic papillae; and atrophic papillae
Teeth	No cavities; no pain; bright	May be missing or erupting abnormally; gray or black spots (fluorosis); cavities (caries)
Gums	Healthy; red; do not bleed; not swollen	"Spongy" and bleed easily; recession of gums
Glands	Face not swollen	Thyroid enlargement (front of neck); parotid enlargement (cheeks become swollen)
Skin	No signs of rashes, swellings, dark or light spots	Dryness of skin (xerosis); sandpaper feel of skin (follicular hyperkeratosis); flakiness of skin; skin swollen and dark; red swollen pigmentation of exposed areas (pellagrous dermatosis); excessive lightness or darkness of skin (dyspigmentation); black and blue marks due to skin bleeding (petechiae); lack of fat under skin
Nails	Firm, pink	Nails are spoon-shape (koilonychia); brittle, ridged nails
Muscular and skeletal systems	Good muscle tone; some fat under skin; can walk or run without pain	Muscles have "wasted" appearance; baby's skull bones are thin and soft (craniotabes); round swelling of front and side of head (frontal and parietal bossing); swelling of ends of bones (epiphyseal enlargement); small bumps on both sides of chest wall (on ribs)—beading of ribs; baby's soft spot on head does not harden at proper time (persistently open anterior fontanelle); knock-knees or bow-legs; bleeding into muscle (musculoskeletal hemorrhages); person cannot get up or walk properly

TABLE 1-2. Physical Signs Indicative or Suggestive of Malnutrition (12, 18) [*Concluded*]

Body Area	Normal Appearance	Signs Associated with Malnutrition
Internal Systems:		
Cardiovascular	Normal heart rate and rhythm; no murmurs or abnormal rhythms; normal blood pressure for age.	Rapid heart rate (above 100 tachycardia); enlarged heart; abnormal rhythm; elevated blood pressure
Gastrointestinal	No palpable organs or masses (in children, however, liver edge may be palpable)	Liver enlargement; enlargement of spleen (usually indicates other associated diseases)
Nervous	Psychological stability; normal reflexes	Mental irritability and confusion; burning and tingling of hands and feet (paresthesia); loss of position and vibratory sense; weakness and tenderness of muscles (may result in inability to walk); decrease and loss of ankle and knee reflexes

Reprinted with permission from American Public Health Association, Inc.

TABLE 1-3. Known Essential Vitamins, Minerals, and Trace Elements: Functions, Deficiency Signs, Toxicity Potential, Biochemical Measures of Status, and Common Food Sources (16, 19)

Element	Functions	Deficiency Signs	Toxicity Potential[1]	Biochemical Measures of Status	Common Food Sources[2]
FAT-SOLUBLE VITAMINS					
A (retinol)	Involved in maintenance of mucous membranes	Impaired dark adaptation Damaged ocular tissues; night blindness; Bitot's spots	Toxic; greater than 7,500 retinol equivalents per day not prudent	Plasma retinol	Dark green and dark yellow vegetables; fruits; tomatoes; egg yolk; butter; fortified margarine
D (ergocalciferol and cholecalciferol)	Regulates calcium and phosphorous metabolism Intestinal absorption of calcium or phosphorous Mineralization of bone matrix	Rickets Osteomalacia	Toxic; intakes should closely approximate RDAs	Serum alkaline phosphatase	Fatty fish, fish liver oils; egg yolk; liver; fortified milk Action of sunlight (ultraviolet irradiation)
E	Undefined	Fragility of red blood cells Muscle loss Deposition of ceroid pigment in musculature of small intestine	Undocumented	Plasma tocopherols	Vegetable oils; wheat germ; cereal and other whole grain products; egg yolk; greens; nuts; dried peas and beans
K (phylloquinone, menaquinones)	Catalysts in synthesis prothrombin and other blood-clotting factors (catalyst)	Defective blood coagulation[3]	Toxic, therapeutic preparation, menadione, may be toxic because of its configurations	Prothrombin	Green leafy vegetables; fruits; cereals; dairy products; meat
WATER-SOLUBLE VITAMINS					
C (ascorbic acid and dehydroascorbic acid)	Enhances iron absorption Possible role in hydroxylation of proline in collagen formation	Scurvy Decreased wound healing	Nontoxic[4]	Ascorbate in plasma, leukocyte, whole blood, red blood cells, urine	Citrus fruits; tomatoes; potatoes; leafy vegetables; cantaloupe; berries; fortified drinks

TABLE 1-3. Known Essential Vitamins, Minerals, and Trace Elements: Functions, Deficiency Signs, Toxicity Potential, Biochemical Measures of Status, and Common Food Sources (16, 19) [*Continued*]

Element	Functions	Deficiency Signs	Toxicity Potential[1]	Biochemical Measures of Status	Common Food Sources[2]
	Amino acid metabolism, may synthesize epinephrin and anti-inflammatory steroids, folic acid metabolism, microsomal drug metabolism, and leucocyte functions				
Thiamin	Co-enzyme in metabolism of α-keta acids and 2-keto sugars; co-factor in carbohydrate metabolism	Beriberi; mental confusion; anorexia; muscle weakness and wasting; ataxia; peripheral paralysis; ophthalmopegia; edema; trachycardia; enlarged heart; cardiac failure	Undocumented	Erythrocyte transketolase activity Urinary excretion of thiamin or its metabolites	Meat, especially pork; poultry; organ meats; oysters; milk; whole grain and enriched cereal products; potatoes; vegetable greens; melons; wheat germ; soybeans; brewer's yeast
Riboflavin	Co-factor in biological oxidations	Cheilosis; angular stomatitis; scrotal skin changes; seborrheic dermatitis	Undocumented	Urinary excretion of riboflavin; erythrocyte glutathione reductase (EGR)	Milk; organ meats; meats; poultry; eggs
Niacin (nicotinic acid and nicotinamide)	Component of co-enzymes NAD; NADP necessary for glycolysis, fat synthesis, tissue respiration	Diarrhea; pellagra; dermatitis; inflammation of mucous mem brane; dementia; death	Nontoxic but may produce vascular dilation or "flushing"	Urinary metabolites of niacin	Organ meats; meats; poultry; fish; peanut butter; whole grain and enriched cereal products; mushrooms
B_6 (pyridoxine, pyridoxal pyridoxamine)	Co-enzymes in amino acid metabolism	Epileptiform convulsions; loss of weight; abdominal distress; vomiting; hyperirritability; depression; confusion	Nontoxic[5]	Urinary excretion of B_6 or its metabolite, 4-pyridoxic acid	Meat, especially pork; organ meats; fish; milk; whole grain products; dried peas and beans

[*Continued*]

TABLE 1-3. Known Essential Vitamins, Minerals, and Trace Elements: Functions, Deficiency Signs, Toxicity Potential, Biochemical Measures of Status, and Common Food Sources (16, 19) [*Continued*]

Element	Functions	Deficiency Signs	Toxicity Potential[1]	Biochemical Measures of Status	Common Food Sources[2]
Folacin	Co-enzyme in synthesis of nucleic acid and metabolism of some amino acids	Megaloblastic anemia Unpaired cell division and alterations of protein synthesis	Undocumented	Serum folacin	Liver; kidney; leafy green vegetables
B_{12} (cobalamin)	Co-enzyme in TCA cycle nucleic acid metabolism and synthesis of polyglutamyl forms of folacin	Megaloblastic anemia Pernicious anemia	Undocumented	Urinary methylmalonate; serum B_{12}	Liver; kidney; meat
Biotin	Component of carboxylating enzymes in metabolism of fat and carbohydrate	Anorexia; vomiting; nausea; glossitis; pallor; mental depression; dry, scaly dermatitis	Nontoxic	Serum and urinary levels of biotin	Liver; kidney; egg yolk
Pantothenic acid	Component of co-enzyme A (co-factor for acyl group activations) Important for release of energy from carbohydrate in gluconeogenesis, in synthesis and degradation of fatty acids, in synthesis of sterols and steroid hormones	Tissue failure, including infertility, abortion, abnormalities of skin and hair	Nontoxic	Urinary pantothenic acid	Organ meats; meat; milk; eggs; whole grain products; peanuts, legumes
MINERALS					
Calcium	Skeleton formation Involved in excitability of peripheral nerves and muscle; blood coagulation; myocardial function	Poor skeletal growth and bone density May be associated with development of osteoporosis	Undocumented[6]	Plasma and urinary calcium	Milk, milk products

TABLE 1-3. Known Essential Vitamins, Minerals, and Trace Elements: Functions, Deficiency Signs, Toxicity Potential, Biochemical Measures of Status, and Common Food Sources (16, 19) [*Continued*]

Element	Functions	Deficiency Signs	Toxicity Potential[1]	Biochemical Measures of Status	Common Food Sources[2]
Phosphorus	Component of supportive structures of body Important in many chemical reactions within body: lipid, protein, carbohydrate, energy-transfer enzymes Many B-complex vitamins only effective when combined with phosphate	Weakness; anorexia; malaise; pain in bones[7]	Undocumented	Serum phosphate	Organ meats; meat; poultry; fish; milk; most foods
Magnesium	Predominant cation in living cells Component of many enzyme systems Important in maintaining electrical potential in nerves and muscle membranes	Neuromuscular dysfunction (tremor convulsions)[8]	Undocumented	Serum magnesium	Most foods, especially vegetables
TRACE ELEMENTS					
Iron	Constituent of hemoglobin, myoglobin, number of enzymes	Anemia	Toxic	Hemoglobin; free erythrocyte protoporphyrin (FEP); serum iron-binding capacity; transferrin saturation (TS); serum iron	Organ meats; meat; poultry; fish; oysters; egg yolk

[*Continued*]

TABLE 1-3. Known Essential Vitamins, Minerals, and Trace Elements: Functions, Deficiency Signs, Toxicity Potential, Biochemical Measures of Status, and Common Food Sources (16, 19) [*Continued*]

Element	Functions	Deficiency Signs	Toxicity Potential[1]	Biochemical Measures of Status	Common Food Sources[2]
Zinc	Constituent of enzymes involved in most major metabolic pathways	Decreased cellular growth and repair; loss of appetite; failure to grow; skin changes; impaired regeneration of wound tissues; decreased taste acuity; hypogonadism; dwarfism	Toxic	Serum zinc; urinary zinc	Meat; egg; seafood
Iodine	Integral part of thyroid hormones, thyroxin, and triiodothyronine	Thyroid enlargement	Toxic	Urinary iodine	Iodized salt; seafood
Copper	Component of enzyme systems	Bone disease; anemia; neutropenia; many skeletal defects, demyelination; degeneration of nervous system and defects in pigmentation and structure of hair[9]	Nontoxic	Serum copper	Liver; meat; fish; poultry; oysters; mushrooms; coffee; nuts; dried peas and beans
Manganese	Essential in several enzyme systems in protein and energy metabolism; formation of mucopolysaccharides	Undocumented	Undocumented by ingestion; injected or inhaled adverse effects on central nervous system	Serum manganese	Nuts; unrefined grains; vegetables; fruits
Fluoride(ine)	Increase caries-resistant teeth	Mottling of teeth Fluorosis	Toxic	Serum fluoride	Fluoridated water; seafood
Chromium	May be co-factor of insulin and in maintenance of glucose metabolism	Disturbances of glucose metabolism[9]	Undocumented	Urinary chromium	Brewer's yeast; meat; cheese; whole grains

TABLE 1-3. Known Essential Vitamins, Minerals, and Trace Elements: Functions, Deficiency Signs, Toxicity Potential, Biochemical Measures of Status, and Common Food Sources (16, 19) [*Concluded*]

Element	Functions	Deficiency Signs	Toxicity Potential[1]	Biochemical Measures of Status	Common Food Sources[2]
Selenium	Enzyme of glutathione peroxidase	Undocumented	Undocumented		Seafoods; kidney, liver; meat
Molybdenum	Essential to function of enzymes involved in production of uric acid and oxidation of aldehydes and sulfites	Undocumented	Toxic[10]	Serum molybdenum	Meat; grains; legumes

[1] Refer to Table A.2-2.
[2] Food tables have incomplete data on many nutrients and the nutrients' biological availability is not totally known.
[3] Uncommon and may require elimination of both dietary vitamin K and inhibition of intestinal microflora growth by antibiotics.
[4] Adverse effects of large doses of ascorbic acid have been reported; ascorbic acid-induced uricosuria, absorption of excessive amounts of iron, impaired activity of leukocytes.
[5] B_6 dependency has been induced in "healthy" adults given 200 mg pyridoxine for 33 days.
[6] Refer to Chapter 35.
[7] Prolonged and excessive intakes of nonabsorbable antacids.
[8] Complications of kwashiorkor.
[9] Associated protein–calorie malnutrition.
[10] Not recommended more than 0.5 mg/day. A goutlike syndrome with increased urinary copper; increased serum molybdenum, uric acid, and xanthine oxidase may result.

TABLE 1-4. Nutrition Assessment Worksheet (13, 15, 20, 22, 23)

Physical Appearance (signs indicative of malnutrition)

Diet History Summary

Nitrogen Balance	Positive	Negative

Nitrogen balance = Nitrogen in − nitrogen out

$$\text{Nitrogen balance} = \frac{\text{Protein intake (g)}}{6.25} - \left(\begin{matrix}\text{urinary} = \text{urea}\\ \text{nitrogen} + 4\end{matrix}\right)$$

Measures of Protein Deficit	Value	Deficit[1] Severe (<60%)	Moderate (60–90%)	Adequate (>90%)
Somatic				
Weight	kg			
Height	cm			
Head circumference (infant)[2]	cm			
Triceps skinfold[3]	mm			
Midarm circumference	cm			
Midarm muscle circumference[4]	cm			
Creatinine—height index[5]	%			
Urinary creatinine	mg/24 hr			
Visceral[6]				
Albumin	g/100 ml			
Total lymphocyte count	mm³			
Total iron-binding capacity	μg/100 ml			
Transferrin	mg/100 ml			

Other Measures Nutrient Specific[7]	Value	% Deficit

TABLE 1-4. Nutrition Assessment Worksheet (13, 15, 20, 22, 23) [*Concluded*]

Cell-Mediated Immunity	Positive	Negative
Candida		
Mumps		
PPD		
Streptokinase/streptodornase		

Nutritional Status	Adequate	At Risk	Inadequate
Type of malnutrition			
marasmus–kwashiorkor		Degree	
kwashiorkor (visceral)		severe	
marasmus (somatic)		moderate	
other			

Diseases Present and Treatments Planned (affect nutrient requirements)

Nutrition Support Plan

Goal

Type	Amount of nutrients
oral	calories
oral with supplements	protein
tube feeding	fat
parenteral	carbohydrate
fluid, electrolyte replacement	other

[1] Deficits are

$$\% \text{ Standard} = \frac{\text{Actual value}}{\text{Standard}} \times 100$$

$$\% \text{ Change} = \frac{\text{Usual} - \text{actual}}{\text{Usual}} \times 100$$

[2] Refer to Figures 49-1 and 49-3.

[3] Measure of fat status and nonprotein reserves.

[4] Measure of protein status. Midarm muscle circumference equals midarm circumference minus 3.14 × tricep skinfold.

[5] Creatinine height index equals actual urinary creatinine divided by ideal urinary creatinine × 100. (13)

[6] Refer to Table 1-7.

[7] Refer to reference 21 or another book of laboratory tests and/or Table 1-3.

TABLE 1-5. Standards for Tricep Skinfold, Midarm Circumference, and Midarm Muscle Circumference (18)

	Standard	90% Standard	90–60% Standard	60% Standard
Tricep skinfold (mm), adults				
Male	12.5	11.3	11.3–7.5	7.5
Female	16.5	14.9	14.9–9.9	9.9
Midarm circumference (cm), adults				
Male	29.3	26.3	26.3–17.6	17.6
Female	28.5	25.7	25.7–17.1	17.1
Midarm muscle circumference (cm), adults				
Male	25.3	22.8	22.8–15.2	15.2
Female	23.2	20.9	20.9–13.9	13.9

TABLE 1-6. Standards for Ideal Urinary Creatinine Values (mg), Adults (22)

Male Height[1] (cm)	Ideal Creatinine (mg)	Female Height[2] (cm)	Ideal Creatinine (mg)
157.5	1288	147.3	830
160.0	1325	149.9	851
162.6	1359	152.4	875
165.1	1386	154.9	900
167.6	1426	157.5	925
170.2	1467	160.0	949
172.7	1513	162.6	977
175.3	1555	165.1	1006
177.8	1596	167.6	1044
180.3	1642	170.2	1076
182.9	1691	172.7	1109
185.4	1739	175.3	1141
188.0	1785	177.8	1174
190.5	1831	180.3	1206
193.0	1891	182.9	1240

[1] Creatinine coefficient (males) = 23 mg/kg of ideal body weight.
[2] Creatinine coefficient (females) = 18 mg/kg of ideal body weight.

TABLE 1-7. Selected Normal Values for Visceral Proteins, Adults (21)

Biochemical Measure	Value
Albumin, serum	3.5–4.9 g/100 ml
Total lymphocyte count	1,500–3,000/mm^3
Total iron-binding capacity	250–450 μg/100 ml
Transferrin	200–400 mg/100 ml
Creatinine	1.0–1.8 g/24 hr

TABLE 1-8. Recommended Calorie and Protein Intakes for Healthy Adults (19)[1]

	Age	Weight (kg)	Height (cm)	kcal (range)	Protein (g)
Females	19–22	55	163	1700–2500	44
	23–50	55	163	1600–2400	44
	51–75	55	163	1400–2200	44
	76+	55	163	1200–2000	44
Males	19–22	70	177	2500–3300	56
	23–50	70	178	2300–3100	56
	51–75	70	178	2000–2800	56
	76+	70	178	1650–2450	56

[1] Refer to Chapter 2 for energy and protein needs during stress.

REFERENCES CITED

1. BISTRIAN, B. R.; BLACKBURN, G. L.; and HALLOWELL, E. 1974. Protein status of general surgical patients. *JAMA* 230:858.
2. BUTTERWORTH, C. E., and BLACKBURN, G. L. 1975. Hospital malnutrition. *Nutr. Today* 10:8.
3. BISTRIAN, B. R.; BLACKBURN, G. L.; VITALE, J.; COCHRAN, D.; and NAYLOR, J. 1976. Prevalence of malnutrition in general medical patients. *JAMA* 235:1567.
4. WILLCUTTS, H. D. 1977. Nutrition assessment of 1000 surgical patients in an affluent suburban community hospital. *JPEN* 1:25.
5. WEINSIER, R. L.; HUNKER, E. M.; KRUMDIECK, C. L.; and BUTTERWORTH, C. E. 1979. Hospital malnutrition: A prospective evaluation of general medical patients during the course of hospitalization. *Am. J. Clin. Nutr.* 32:418.
6. FAINTUCH, J.; FAINTUCH, J. J.; MACHADO, M. C. C.; and RAJA, A. A. 1979. Anthropometric assessment of nutritional depletion after surgical injury. *JPEN* 3:369.
7. PARSONS, H. D.; FRANCOEUR, T. E.; HOWLAND, P.; SPENGLER, R. D.; and PENCHARZ, P. B. 1980. The nutritional status of hospitalized children. *Am. J. Clin. Nutr.* 33:1140.
8. MERRITT, R. J., and SUSKIND, R. M. 1979. Nutritional survey of hospitalized pediatric patients. *Am. J. Clin. Nutr.* 32:1320.
9. SELTZER, M. H.; BASTIDAS, J. A.; COOPER, D. M.; ENGLER, P.; SLOCUM, B.; and FLETCHER, S. 1979. Instant nutritional assessment. *JPEN* 3:157.
10. MULLEN, J. L.; BUSBY, G. P.; WALDMAN, M. T.; GERTNER, M. H.; HOBBS, C. L.; and ROSATO, E. F. 1979. Prediction of operative morbidity and mortality by preoperative nutrition assessment. *Surgical Forum,* pp. 80–82. 65th Annual Clinical Congress, Chicago.
11. YARBROUGH, C.; HABICHT, J. P.; KLEIN, E.; MARTORELL, L.; LECHTIG, A.; and GUZMAN, G. 1978. Response of indicators of nutritional status to nutritional interventions in populations and individuals. In *Evaluations of child health services,* eds. S. J. Bosch, and J. Arias. DHEW Pub. No. (NIH) 78-1066. Washington, D.C.
12. CHRISTAKIS, G., ed. 1973. *Nutritional assessment in health programs.* Washington, D.C.: American Public Health Association.
13. BLACKBURN, G. L.; BISTRIAN, B. R.; MAINI, B. S.; SCHLAMM, H. T.; and SMITH, M. F. 1977. Nutritional and metabolic assessment of the hospitalized patient. *JPEN* 1:11.
14. KAMINSKI, M. V., and JEEJEEBHOY, K. N. 1979. Unit 1. Nutrition assessment—Diagnosis of malnutrition and selection of therapy. *J. Surg. Pract.* 64:45.
15. KAMINSKI, M. V., and RUGGIERO, R. P. 1979. Nutrition assessment: A guide to initiation and efficacy of enteral hyperalimentation. *Int. Surg.* 64:33.
16. SAUBERLICH, H. E.; SKALA, J. H.; and DOWDY, R. P. 1976. *Laboratory tests for the assessment of nutritional status.* Cleveland, Ohio: CRC Press.
17. International Classification of Diseases. *ICDA,* 8th rev. ed. DHEW Pub. No. 1693. Washington, D.C.
18. JELLIFFE, D. B. 1966. *The assessment of the nutritional status of the community.* WHO Monograph No. 53. Geneva: World Health Organization.
19. Food and Nutrition Board. 1980. *Recommended dietary allowances.* 9th rev. ed. Washington, D.C.: National Academy of Sciences.
20. MACKENZIE, T.; BLACKBURN, G. L.; and FLATT, J. P. 1974. Clinical assessment of nutritional status using nitrogen balance. *Fed. Proc.* 33:683.
21. BATSAKIS, J. G. 1979. *University Hospital, University of Michigan pathology laboratories handbook, 1979–80.* Stow, Ohio: Lexi-Comp.
22. SELTZER, C. C.; GOLDMAN, R. F.; and MAYER, J. 1965. The triceps skinfold as a predictive measure of body density and body fat in obese adolescent girls. *Pediatrics* 36:212.
23. DAMON, A., and GOLDMAN, R. F. 1964. Predicting fat from body measurements: Densitometric validation of ten anthropometric equations. *Human Biol.* 36:32.

2 High Calorie, High Protein

INDICATIONS FOR USE

The high-calorie, high-protein diet is indicated for individuals with conditions that result in a catabolic state and for individuals with protein–calorie malnutrition. Conditions resulting in a catabolic state include major burns, infection, cancer, fractures, surgery, and other major trauma. (1–4) The high-calorie, high-protein diet should be used until wound healing is completed, infection controlled, nitrogen balance maintained, and threat of malnutrition passed.

Modifications of the high-calorie, high-protein diet are indicated for pregnancy (Chapter 46), nephrotic syndrome (Chapter 27), and hypoglycemia (Chapter 34).

DESCRIPTION

The goals of increasing energy and protein intakes are to (1–3)

- Minimize nitrogen depletion from body stores and muscle mass.
- Provide adequate intake of calories so that protein will not be used for energy.
- Replenish the nitrogen stores during convalescence.
- Provide for an adequate intake of vitamins, minerals, and trace elements.

Nutritional requirements are affected by the extent of injury or disease state, the therapy used, and the nutritional status of the individual prior to the catabolic state. Nutrient requirements are assessed by monitoring of anthropometric, clinical, biochemical, and dietary parameters (Chapter 1).

Guidelines for determining energy and protein requirements for some catabolic conditions are as follows:

Major burns. Individual body size and magnitude of the burn injury are used to estimate energy and protein requirements. (3) The energy requirement of a burned individual can be estimated by using the formula kcal requirement = [25 kcal × weight (kg)] + [40 kcal × percent total body surface burned]. (3) The suggested protein intake is 2–3 g protein/kg of body weight. (2)

Infection. Energy requirements during infection are increased due to the increased basal metabolic rate that occurs with increased body temperature. The basal energy expenditure is increased approximately 12% for each degree centigrade (8% for each degree Fahrenheit) above normal body temperature. (3)

Negative nitrogen balance occurs during infection and may be due to decreased intake or altered metabolism. (6–8) Therapy with high-protein diets with adequate calories has been shown to produce a highly positive nitrogen balance and rapid weight gains in individuals who have had depletion of tissue proteins. (6, 7)

Cancer. Maintenance of nutritional status is important for the individual with cancer undergoing surgery, radiation, or chemotherapy. For specific recommendations, refer to Chapter 7.

Surgery. Catabolism frequently leading to weight loss is a usual consequence of surgical diseases and operations. (9) Performing major surgery in patients who are not prepared nutritionally is likely to lead to increased morbidity and mortality due to increased vulnerability to concurrent illnesses, infection, and other complications. When the gastrointestinal tract is used for feeding, the diet should contain at least 80–120 g of protein and 2000–3000 kcal from nonprotein sources.

GUIDELINES FOR NUTRITIONAL MANAGEMENT

The diet must be planned to meet the nutritional needs, willingness to eat, and the ability of each individual to eat. Modifications in consistency, meal size, and meal frequency may be necessary. Oral supplements, tube feedings, and parenteral nutrition, or a combination of these, may be necessary to provide adequate nutrient intake.

Whenever possible, meals are freely selected by the hospitalized patient and monitored and supplemented to provide a high-calorie, high-protein intake. Oral supplements are often provided between meals (Chapter 3). Sources of high-biological-value protein such as milk and milk products, eggs, meat, and poultry are emphasized in meeting the protein requirement.

Food intake is monitored when necessary to determine the patient's actual nutrient intake. Nutrient monitoring may be requested by the physician, nurse, or dietitian and involve monitoring and recording of the individual's calorie, protein, carbohydrate, and fat consumption. Other nutrients, for example, sodium or potassium, may be monitored.

NUTRIENT ADEQUACY

"The special nutritional needs arising from metabolic disorders, chronic diseases, injuries, prematurity, and many other medical conditions require therapeutic treatment not covered by the Recommended Dietary Allowances for healthy persons." (10) Nutritional adequacy of the diet can only be determined by ongoing assessment of nutrient intake and nutritional status.

REFERENCES CITED

1. Bistrian, B. R. 1977. Nutritional assessment and therapy of protein–calorie malnutrition in the hospital. *J. Am. Dietet. A.* 71:393.
2. Artz, C. P.; Soroff, H. S.; Pearson, E.; and Hummel, R. P. 1956. Some recent developments in oral feedings for optimal nutrition in burns. *Am. J. Clin. Nutr.* 4:642.
3. Curreri, P. W.; Richmond, D.; Marvin, J.; and Baxter, C. R. 1974. Dietary requirements of patients with major burns. *J. Am. Dietet. A.* 65:415.
4. Blackburn, G. L., and Bistrian, B. R. 1976. Nutritional care of the injured and/or septic patient. *Surg. Clin. N. Am.* 56:1195.
5. Harper, H. A.; Rodwell, V. W.; and Mayes, P. A. 1977. *Review of physiological chemistry,* p. 544. 16th ed. Los Altos, Calif.: Lange Medical Publications.
6. Co Tui, Kuo, N. H., and Schmidt, L. 1954. The protein status in pulmonary tuberculosis. *Am. J. Clin. Nutr.* 2:252.
7. Harrell, G. T.; Wolff, W. A.; Venning, W. L.; and Reinhart, J. B. 1946. The prevention and control of disturbances of protein metabolism in Rocky Mountain spotted fever. *Southern Med. J.* 39:551.
8. Wilson, D.; Bressani, R.; and Scrimshaw, N. S. 1961. Infection and nutritional status. I. The effect of chicken pox on nitrogen metabolism in children. *Am. J. Clin. Nutr.* 9:154.
9. MacFadyen, B. V., Jr.; Copeland, E. M., III; and Dudrick, S. J. 1977. Surgery. In *Nutritional support of medical practice,* eds. H. A. Schneider, C. E. Anderson, and D. B. Coursin, pp. 485–499. New York: Harper & Row.
10. Food and Nutrition Board. 1980. *Recommended dietary allowances.* 9th rev. ed., p. 9. Washington, D.C.: National Academy of Sciences.

Oral Supplements

INDICATIONS FOR USE

Oral supplements are indicated for individuals tolerating oral feedings who are unable to meet nutrient needs with a general diet (three meals and an evening nourishment).

DESCRIPTION

Oral supplements are foods and beverages designed to meet specific nutrient needs. Recipes for these are given in Table 3-1. Table 3-2 lists the nutrient composition of the standard oral supplements. When nutrient needs and patient acceptance cannot be met by use of standard oral supplements, others may be designed. Recipes are formulated using special dietary products, Table 3-3, and regular foods.

GUIDELINES FOR NUTRITIONAL MANAGEMENT

The dietitian, after assessing the individual's condition, food preferences, nutrient requirements, and the diet prescription, will choose or design an appropriate oral supplement.

Supplements are usually served between regular meal times.

NUTRIENT ADEQUACY

Oral supplements are nutritionally incomplete. When taken without other foods containing adequate calories and other nutrients, they will not provide individuals with nutrients adequate to improve nutritional status. They are meant to supplement, not replace, other forms of nutrient intake.

TABLES

TABLE 3-1. Oral Supplement Recipes (per 240 ml or 1 cup)

Supplement	Ingredients	Weight (g)	Household Measure[1]
Low-calcium drink	Egg white powder	13	2 tablespoons
	Orange juice conc.	43	3 tablespoons
	Sherbet	124	⅔ cup
	Water	140	½ cup
Low-protein drink	Sherbet	62	⅓ cup
	7-Up	201	¾ cup
	Lipomul	16	1 tablespoon
Eggnog	Eggnog mix	33	¼ cup
	Whole milk	230	1 cup
Vanilla milkshake	Vanilla ice cream	68	½ cup
	Whole milk	125	½ cup
	Skim milk powder	9	1 tablespoon
	Vanilla	1	⅛ teaspoon
Chocolate milkshake	Chocolate ice cream	67	½ cup
	Whole milk	122	½ cup
	Skim milk powder	10	1 tablespoon and 1 teaspoon
	Chocolate syrup	13	1 tablespoon
MCT drink	Sherbet	142	¾ cup
	Skim milk	150	⅔ cup
	MCT oil	17	1 tablespoon
Straw-ana drink	Ensure Plus	143	½ cup
	Baby bananas with tapioca	76	½ jar *or* 3½ tablespoons
	Vanilla ice cream	38	¼ cup
	Strawberry syrup	23	1½ tablespoons
High-protein MCT drink	Sherbet	135	⅔ cup
	Skim milk	142	⅔ cup
	Skim milk powder	24	3 tablespoons
	MCT oil	16	1 tablespoon
Swiss Miss drink	Whole milk	94	¼ cup and 2 tablespoons
	Vanilla ice cream	129	1 cup
	Swiss Miss	22	1 packet *or* ⅓ cup
	Eggnog milk	23	3 tablespoons
Zollinger cocktail	Whole milk	182	¾ cup
	Eggnog mix	79	⅔ cup
	Honey	9	2 teaspoons
	Lipomul	13	1 tablespoon
Creamy milkshake	Heavy whipping cream	140	½ cup and 2 tablespoons
	Vanilla ice cream	67	½ cup
	Egg white powder	14	2 tablespoons
	Sugar	14	1 tablespoon
Peanut butter drink	Heavy whipping cream	118	½ cup
	Smooth peanut butter	40	3 tablespoons
	Chocolate syrup	40	3 tablespoons
	Vanilla ice cream	67	½ cup

[1] Household measures approximately equal to gram weight.

TABLE 3-2. Nutrient Composition[1] of Oral Supplements (per 240 ml) Compared with Whole Milk and Skim Milk

Supplement[2]	kcal	kcal/ml	Protein (g)	Fat (g)	Carbohydrate (g)	Sodium (mg)
Whole milk	170	0.7	8	10	12	119
Skim milk	80	0.3	8	—	12	126
Low-calcium drink	234	1.0	10	2	44	176
Low-protein drink	257	1.1	0.5	11	39	49
Eggnog	268	1.1	14	8	35	202
Vanilla milkshake	289	1.2	12	13	31	200
Chocolate milkshake	321	1.3	11	13	40	176
MCT drink	332	1.4	5	16	42	118
Straw-ana drink	371	1.5	8	11	60	170
High-protein MCT drink	396	1.7	13	16	50	216
Swiss Miss drink	478	2.0	14	18	65	289
Zollinger cocktail	520	2.2	22	16	72	309
Creamy milkshake	678	2.8	16	54	32	261
Peanut butter drink	829	3.5	15	65	46	330
Other[3]	Varies					

[1] All figures are rounded to nearest whole number or .0.
[2] Supplements are listed in order of caloric density. See recipes in Table 3-2.
[3] Others may be developed to meet nutrient and taste requirements of individuals.

Sodium (mEq)	Potassium (mg)	Potassium (mEq)	Calcium (mg)	Calcium (mEq)	Nitrogen (g)	Supplement[2]
5.2	370	9.5	290	14.5	1.3	Whole milk
5.5	401	10.3	298	14.9	1.3	Skim milk
7.7	448	11.5	75	3.8	1.6	Low-calcium drink
2.1	58	1.5	32	1.6	0.1	Low-protein drink
8.8	543	13.9	432	21.6	2.2	Eggnog
8.7	573	14.7	416	20.8	1.9	Vanilla milkshake
7.6	595	15.3	411	20.6	1.8	Chocolate milkshake
5.1	325	8.3	215	10.8	0.8	MCT drink
7.4	370	9.5	140	7.0	1.3	Straw-ana drink
9.4	658	16.9	448	22.4	2.1	High-protein MCT drink
12.6	565	14.5	448	22.4	2.2	Swiss Miss drink
13.4	745	19.1	599	30.0	3.5	Zollinger cocktail
11.3	359	9.2	175	8.8	2.6	Creamy milkshake
14.3	539	13.8	177	8.9	2.4	Peanut butter drink
						Other[3]

TABLE 3-3. Nutrient Composition and Description of Some Dietary Products Used to Formulate Oral Supplements or Tube Feedings (per 100 g)[1]

Product (Manufacturer)	kcal	Protein (g)	Fat (g)	Carbo-hydrate (g)	Sodium (mg)	Potas-sium (mg)	Calciur (mg)
Protein sources							
Egg white powder	376	82	—	4	1238	1116	89
Skim milk powder	362	36	1	52	535	1794	1257
Lonalac (Mead Johnson)	512	27	28	38	20	960	880
Eggnog mix (Delmark)	404	20	2	75	287	627	514
Fat sources							
Lipomul, oral (Upjohn)	600	—	67	—	42	2	9
MCT oil (Mead Johnson)	830	—	100	—	—	—	—
Carbohydrate sources							
Polycose (powder) (Ross)	380	—	—	94	115	39	60
Controlyte (Doyle)	504	—	24	72	10	4	4
Swiss Miss (Beatrice Foods)	388	10	7	78	388	317	359

[1] Any common foodstuffs may be incorporated into oral supplements or tube feedings; dependent on the specifi nutrient requirements or restrictions, adaptability to feeding method, and patient's taste preferences.

Description	Preparation Methods	Product (Manufacturer)
		Protein sources
Lactose and fat-free protein supplement	Mix with milk or other foods	Egg white powder
Dehydrated skim milk	Mix with milk or other foods	Skim milk powder
High-protein beverage mix, low in sodium	Mix with water or other foods	Lonalac (Mead Johnson)
Institutional product consisting mainly of eggs and milk products	Mix with milk or other foods	Eggnog mix (Delmark)
		Fat sources
Corn oil	Mix with foods and beverages or ingest alone	Lipomul, oral (Upjohn)
Semisynthetic lipid consisting of medium-chain triglycerides (C_8 and C_{10})	Blend with foods and beverages or ingest alone	MCT oil (Mead Johnson)
		Carbohydrate sources
Glucose polymers that provide calories without sweet taste	Add to most semisolid foods and beverages	Polycose (powder) (Ross)
High-calorie, no protein, low-electrolyte supplement	Add to most semisolid foods and beverages	Controlyte (Doyle)
Chocolate-flavored milk based	Mix with beverages or semisolid foods	Swiss Miss (Beatrice Foods)

Tube Feedings

INDICATIONS FOR USE

Tube feedings are indicated for individuals with a functioning gastrointestinal tract who cannot or will not eat. Such individuals include those with neurologic disorders affecting ability to swallow, those with head or neck tumors causing obstruction or pain upon eating, and those not eating because of general weakness or psychological factors. (1)

Tube feedings may be safely administered in a hospital setting or, after appropriate education, in a home setting. (2) They may be required for a short period of time or indefinitely.

Vomiting is a contraindication to feeding by tube.

DESCRIPTION

A wide variety of tube-feeding formulas are available to meet different nutritional needs. To determine which tube feeding is appropriate, the patient's condition, including function of the gastrointestinal tract and metabolic needs, must be considered. (3) An appropriate tube feeding is one that is nutritionally adequate, provides nutrients in forms that will be utilized by the individual without causing side effects such as cramping or diarrhea, and is reasonable in terms of cost and preparation. (4)

Factors to consider in choosing a tube feeding are the following:

Osmolality.[1] Osmolality is the concentration of solute per unit of solvent and is measured in terms of milliosmoles per kilogram of water (mOsm/kg). The osmolality is a measure of the ability of a solution to hold water or draw it through a semipermeable membrane. (6) A formula of high osmolality, administered quickly, will draw fluid into the intestines and may result in cramps, nausea, vomiting, or diarrhea. (5) Osmolality may be a critical factor for individuals who have had gastric surgery or have a jejunostomy feeding tube. (7) Osmolality may not be a problem for other patients if the formula is administered slowly or by constant drip. (7) Generally, the lower the osmolality of the formula, the more rapidly it can be infused. (8)

A well-balanced diet of natural foodstuffs has an osmolality of approximately 600 mOsm/kg of water compared with serum, which is approximately 300 mOsm/kg of water. (9) The osmolality of tube feedings is increased by the presence of free amino acids, monosaccharides, disaccharides, and electrolytes. Fats, whole proteins, and starches are less osmotically active. (5)

Carbohydrate. Carbohydrate may come from many sources including fruits, cereals, vegetables, corn syrup, glucose, sucrose, lactose, glucose oligosaccharides, and dextrins. (10) Cornstarch, maltodextrin, and oligosaccharides have been used to provide carbohydrate while minimizing formula osmolality and sweetness. (10)

A relative lactose intolerance has been identified in some hospitalized patients. (11) The lactose content of many formulas has been reduced, and lactose-free formulas are available.

[1] *Osmolarity* (mOm) is the concentration of solute per total volume of solution and is measured in terms of milliosmoles per liter of solution. The osmolarity of liquid diets is approximately 80% of their osmolality. (5)

Dietary fiber is present in formulas containing fruits, vegetables, or cereals. Dietary fiber can be increased by adding banana flakes, applesauce, or pureed fruit and may be beneficial for individuals with diarrhea or constipation. Low-fiber, low-residue formulas are available.

Protein. Protein may be supplied in formulas as whole protein, hydrolyzed protein, or as free amino acids. Formulas that provide protein in the form of free amino acids, dipeptides, or tripeptides are rarely indicated (Chapter 5). A formula low in protein may be indicated for individuals with hepatic or renal impairment. A high-protein formula may be indicated for individuals who are malnourished, septic, or pre- or postsurgical or have experienced other trauma (Chapter 2). Individuals receiving high-protein formulas, particularly those who are unconscious or cannot communicate thirst, should be monitored for adequate water intake and fluid and electrolyte balance. (6, 12)

Fat. Fat adds calories to formulas without increasing the osmolality. Fat is generally provided in the form of vegetable oils. If fat malabsorption is present, a formula low in fat or one that contains medium-chain triglycerides (MCT) in place of long-chain fatty acids is indicated. (7)

Vitamins, minerals, trace elements. Vitamins, minerals, and trace elements are generally provided in commercial formulas in amounts to meet the recommended dietary allowances. For individuals with malabsorption or for those under stress, these amounts may be inadequate. These nutrients should be monitored and supplemented when necessary. (7)

Modified commercial formulas or house-blenderized formulas may be necessary when electrolyte or mineral intake must be controlled. The portions of sodium, potassium, and/or phosphorus may need to be altered for individuals with renal, hepatic, or cardiac failure.

Cost and preparation time. House-blenderized formulas prepared from regular foods permit flexibility in meeting nutrient needs, are inexpensive, and may be more acceptable to the patient psychologically as the formula may be perceived as regular food. Commercial preparations require minimal preparation time, are convenient for storage and administration, are presterilized, and have consistent composition. (4) Choice between house-blenderized or commercial feeding will depend upon home or hospital setting, storage and refrigeration space available, cost and time constraints, and the nutrient requirements of the individual.

GUIDELINES FOR NUTRITIONAL MANAGEMENT

Nutrition management includes choice of an appropriate tube feeding, use of a safe and effective method of administration, and monitoring of nutritional status.

Tube-feeding formula. Tube feedings are commercial preparations or house-blenderized food mixtures. Tube feedings are selected based on nutrient content, cost, and availability. When standard commercial or house-blenderized formulas do not satisfy an individual's nutrient needs or restrictions, other house-blenderized formulas may be designed to meet specified requirements. Skim milk, whole milk, or milk substitutes may be used initially for the malnourished patient. Not all tube feedings commercially available are stocked in every hospital. Generally three or four choices are available that meet different requirements. For example, the ones starred in Table 4-1 are stocked at University Hospital. Refer to Table 4-2 for the vitamin, mineral, and trace element content of 1000 ml of tube feedings and to Tables 4-3, 4-4, and 4-5 for recipes of three hospital-prepared blenderized tube feedings. Other formulas or ingredients appropriate for tube feedings are listed in Chapters 3 and 5 and in Chapter 48, Tables 48-1 and 48-2.

Concentration of feeding. Initially a dilute concentration of $\frac{1}{4}$ to $\frac{1}{2}$ kcal/ml should be given. The concentration of the feeding can be increased to 1 to $1\frac{1}{2}$ kcal/ml over a three- to four-day period. This gradual increase in concentration allows the gastrointestinal tract to adapt to the osmolality of the formula (1, 10) and to regain other functions (e.g., enzyme activity) when the gastrointestinal tract has not been utilized for a long period of time.

Administration of feeding. Both commercial and house-blenderized formulas should be well shaken immediately prior to administration.

A recent study suggests that, when a refrigerated tube feeding is used, it should be allowed to come to room temperature or should be given at a slow rate (240 ml/30 min) to allow for warming prior to reaching the stomach. (13) A primate study indicated that the temperature of the feeding had only a slight effect on gastric motility and had no effect on transit time. (14) Tube feedings are excellent mediums for bacterial growth and heating of the formulas may increase this growth rate. Therefore, warming tube feeding is not recommended.

The feeding should be administered slowly to help prevent gastric retention and esophageal regurgitation. The initial volume is approximately 200 ml administered over 45 minutes every 4 to 6 hours. (1) The volume and frequency are increased as tolerated but not at the same time. If the feeding is to be given continuously, a Barron pump may be used to regulate flow rate and decrease the potential for gastric retention and vomiting. (1) When administering the tube feeding, the individual's chest should be kept at a 30° angle or higher, minimizing the possibility of aspiration. (7)

Storage of formula. House-blenderized formulas and opened commercial feedings are to be refrigerated and should be discarded if not used within 24 hours.

Tube selection and placement. Tube feedings may be administered through nasopharyngeal, esophagostomy, gastrostomy, or jejunostomy tubes. Nasopharyngeal tubes are generally indicated when tube feedings are used for brief periods of time. Gastrostomy and jejunostomy tubes are preferred for long-term feeding. (3, 10)

For a nasopharyngeal tube feeding, a pliable tube with the smallest gauge that will allow the feeding to flow freely should be used to minimize discomfort. (15) The Dobbhoff nasojejunal feeding tube (a no. 8 French polyurethane tube) is generally well tolerated because of its size and softness. (8) The tube requires a low-viscosity formula. Placement in the duodenum or jejunum needs to be confirmed by X ray 12 to 24 hours after placement. (8) Initial feeding should be started after confirmation of placement is received.

Care of feeding tube. The feeding tube should be flushed with a small amount of water (approximately 60 ml) immediately before and after the feeding is given. (16) This ensures that the tube is open and clear before administration of the formula and that the tube has been rinsed following the feeding to minimize the potential for bacterial growth and/or blockage of the tube.

Monitoring of patient's condition. The tube-fed patient's fluid and electrolyte balance, weight changes, and intake and output must be monitored and recorded to identify problems. Malnourished patients should have liver function monitored to prevent nitrogen overload. Various problems may occur with the tube-fed patient; the majority of these problems should not be viewed as natural side effects but as problems that can be corrected by changing the type of feeding or the administration technique. Table 4-6 identifies common problems in tube-fed patients and possible solutions.

NUTRIENT ADEQUACY

Nutritional adequacy of tube feedings must be assessed on an individual basis. Variables affecting the nutritional adequacy of the feeding are nutrient content of the formula, volume and concentration of the feeding, presence of other forms of nutrient intake, the individual's physical condition including catabolic or anabolic state, and use of medications or therapy that affect nutritional status.

TABLES

TABLE 4-1. Nutrient Composition and Food Sources of Tube Feedings (per 1000 ml)[1]

Product (Manufacturer)	kcal	Protein (g)	Fat (g)	Carbohydrate (g)	Sodium (mg)	Sodium (mEq)	Potassium (mg)	Potassium (mEq)	Chloride (mg)	Chloride (mEq)	Nitrogen (g)
*Whole milk (3.3% fat)	622	34	34	48	500	21.7	1550	39.7			5
*Skim milk	357	35	2	49	530	23.0	1693	43.4			5
Instant Breakfast[2] (Carnation)	1072	59	32	136[a]	921[a]	40.0[a]	2810[a]	72.1[a]			10
*Compleat B (Doyle)	1000	40	40	120	1188	51.7	1313	33.7	813	22.9	6
Compleat modified (Doyle)	1066	43	37	141	666	29.0	1399	35.9	466	13.3	7
*Ensure (Ross)	1060	37	37	144	741	32.2	1270	32.6	1058	29.8	6
*Ensure Plus (Ross)	1500	55	53	200	1050	45.7	1890	48.5	1596	45.0	9
Formula II (Cutter)	1000	38	40	123	600	26.1	1760	45.1	1900	53.5	6
*Isocal (Mead Johnson)	1060	34	45	131	530	23.0	1323	33.9	1060	29.9	5
Magnacal (Organon)	2000	70	80	250	1000	43.5	1250	32.1	950	26.8	11
Meritene Liquid (Doyle)	1000	61	34	117	932	40.5	1696	43.5	1696	47.8	10
Osmolite (Ross)	1060	37	38	145	551	24.0	890	22.8	806	22.7	6
*Portagen (Mead Johnson)	1000	35	48	115	468	20.3	1248	32.0	858	24.2	6
Precision HN (Doyle)	1050	44	1	216	980	42.6	910	23.3	1190	33.5	7

Lactose (g)	Osmolality (mOsm/kg)	Food Sources			Product (Manufacturer)
		Protein	Fat	Carbohydrate	
48	288	Casein	Butterfat	Lactose	* Whole milk (3.3% fat)
49	270	Casein	Butterfat	Lactose	* Skim milk
95[b]		Casein; soy protein; sodium caseinate	Butterfat	Lactose; sucrose; corn syrup solids	Instant Breakfast[2] (Carnation)
24[b]	390	Beef; nonfat dry milk	Corn oil	Hydrolyzed cereal solids; vegetables; malto dextrin; fruits; orange juice; nonfat dry milk	* Compleat B (Doyle)
0	300	Beef; calcium caseinate	Corn oil	Hydrolized cereal solids; vegetables; fruits—peach, orange	Compleat modified (Doyle)
0	450	Sodium caseinate; calcium caseinate; soy protein isolate	Corn oil	Corn syrup solids; sucrose	* Ensure (Ross)
0	600	Sodium caseinate; calcium caseinate; soy protein isolate	Corn oil	Corn syrup solids; sucrose	* Ensure Plus (Ross)
38	470	Nonfat dry milk; beef	Corn oil; egg yolk	Lactose; sucrose; vegetables; orange juice; wheat flour	Formula II (Cutter)
0	350	Sodium caseinate; calcium caseinate; soy protein isolate	Soy oil; MCT oil	Corn syrup solids	* Isocal (Mead Johnson)
0	520	Calcium caseinate; sodium caseinate	Soy oil	Malto dextrin; corn syrup solids; sucrose	Magnacal (Organon)
57[a]	550–610[a]	Caseinate; sodium caseinate	Corn oil	Lactose; corn syrup solids; sucrose	Meritene Liquid (Doyle)
0	300	Sodium caseinate; calcium caseinate; soy protein isolate	MCT oil; corn oil; soy oil	Corn syrup solids	Osmolite (Ross)
	357	Sodium caseinate	MCT oil; corn oil	Malto dextrin; sucrose	* Portagen (Mead Johnson)
0	557	Egg white solids	MCT oil; soy oil	Malto dextrin; sucrose	Precision HN (Doyle)

[*Continued*]

TABLE 4-1. Nutrient Composition and Food Sources of Tube Feedings (per 1000 ml)[1] [*Concluded*]

Product (Manufacturer)	kcal	Protein (g)	Fat (g)	Carbo-hydrate (g)	Sodium (mg)	Sodium (mEq)	Potas-sium (mg)	Potas-sium (mEq)	Chlor-ide (mg)	Chlor-ide (mEq)	Nitro-gen (g)
Precision Isotonic (Doyle)	1000	30	31	151	804	35.0	1005	28.3	1072	30.2	5
Precision LR (Doyle)	1110	24	1	225	636	27.7	795	20.4	1007	28.4	4
Renu (Organon)	1012	33	40	130	500	21.7	1250	32.1	950	26.8	5
Sustacal Liquid (Mead Johnson)	1000	60	23	138	926	40.3	2057	52.7	1555	43.8	10
Vitaneed (Organon)	1020	35	40	130	550	23.9	1250	32.1	750	21.1	6
*High protein (hospital)	1037	95	10	145	1163	50.6	4225	108.3			15
*High protein–low sodium (hospital)	1002	76	24	116	689	30.0	3044	78.1			12
*Maintenance (hospital)	977	49	44	101	409	17.8	1995	51.2			8

[1] Blank spaces under nutrients indicate inadequate information available.
[2] Made with whole milk (3.3% fat).
[a] Values for vanilla flavor; additional flavors vary.
[b] Taken from Shils et al., Liquid formulas and tube feedings, 1979.
* Available at Department of Dietetics, University Hospital.

Lactose (g)	Osmolality (mOsm/kg)	Food Sources			Product (Manufacturer)
		Protein	Fat	Carbohydrate	
0	300	Egg white solids; sodium caseinate	Partially hydrogenated soy oil	Glucose oligosaccharides; sucrose	Precision Isotonic (Doyle)
0	525	Egg white solids	MCT oil; partially hydrogenated soy oil	Malto dextrin; sucrose	Precision LR (Doyle)
0	330	Sodium caseinate; calcium caseinate; soy protein isolate	Soy oil; mono- and diglycerides	Sucrose; dextrin; citrate	Renu (Organon)
16.7	625	Skim milk; sodium caseinate; calcium caseinate; soy protein isolate	Partially hydrogenated soy oil	Sucrose; skim milk; corn syrup solids	Sustacal Liquid (Mead Johnson)
0	400	Beef; calcium caseinate	Soy oil	Corn syrup solids; malto dextrin; vegetables; fruit	Vitaneed (Organon)
92	868 ± 50	Strained meat; nonfat dry milk; eggnog mix	Strained meat; eggnog mix	Strained applesauce; strained vegetables; nonfat dry milk; dry yeast; orange juice	*High protein (hospital)
65	737 ± 50	Strained meat; nonfat dry milk; Lonalac; eggnog mix	Strained meat; eggnog mix	Strained applesauce; strained vegetables; orange juice concentrate; eggnog mix	*High protein–low sodium (hospital)
22	915 ± 50	Strained meat; whole milk	Whole milk; corn oil	Strained applesauce; strained vegetables; orange juice; baby rice cereal; sugar	*Maintenance (hospital)

TABLE 4-2. Vitamin and Mineral Composition of Tube Feedings (per 1000 ml) Compared with Recommended Dietary Allowances[1]

	Fat-Soluble Vitamins			Water-Soluble Vitamins									
Product (Manufacturer)	Vitamin A (μg RE)	Vitamin D (μg)	Vitamin E (mg α TE)	Vitamin K (μg)	Vitamin C (mg)	Thiamin (mg)	Riboflavin (mg)	Niacin (mg NE)	Vitamin B_6 (mg)	Folacin (μg)	Vitamin B_{12} (μg)	Biotin (μg)	Pantothenic Acid (mg
Male (age 23–50)[2]	1000	5	10	70–140[a]	60	1.4	1.6	18	2.2	400	3.0	100–200[a]	4–7[a]
Female (age 23–50)[3]	800	5	8	70–140[a]	60	1.0	1.2	13	2.0	400	3.0	100–200[a]	4–7[a]
Milk (3.3% fat)	386	11[b]			10	0.4	1.7	1	0.4	51	3.6		3
Skim milk	625	11[b]			10	0.4	1.4	1	0.4	51	3.9		3
Instant Breakfast (Carnation)	1500	10	43[c]		111	1.5	1.9	20	1.9	427	4.4		11
Compleat B (Doyle)	938	6	29		56	1.4	1.6	13	1.9	250	3.8	190	6
Compleat Modified (Doyle)	3330	11	20	67	60	1.5	1.7	13	2.0	277	4.0	200	6.6
Ensure (Ross)	796	5	48	1000	161	1.6	1.8	21	2.1	210	6.3	160	5
Ensure Plus (Ross)	796	5	72	1590	159	2.7	2.8	32	3.2	210	9.5	300	9
Formula II (Cutter)	751	6	32		39	0.8	0.9	10	1.4	200	3.0		5
Isocal (Mead Johnson)	796	5	60	131	159	2.0	2.3	26	2.6	212	8.0	170	13
Magnacal (Organon)	1502	10	45		60	1.5	1.7	20	2.0	400	6.0	300	10
Meritene Liquid (Doyle)	1273	8	38		76	1.9	2.2	17	2.5	339	5.0	254	8
Osmolite (Ross)	796	5	48	1000	170	1.6	1.8	21	2.1	210	6.3	170	5
Portagen (Mead Johnson)	339	20	47	156	78	1.6	1.9	21	2.0	156	6.0	78	10
Precision HN (Doyle)	76	4	16	35	32	0.8	0.9	7	1.1	140	2.1	110	4
Precision Isotonic (Doyle)	1006	7	20	67	60	1.5	1.7	13	2.0	268	4.0	200	7
Precision Low Residue (Doyle)	796	5	24	53	48	1.2	1.4	11	1.6	212	3.2	160	5
Renu (Organon)	901	6	30		60	1.3	1.4	15	1.5	400	4.0	250	8
Sustacal (Mead Johnson)	1394	9	42	232	56	1.4	1.7	19	1.9	369	5.6	278	10
Vitaneed (Organon)	1051	6	38		60	1.3	1.5	18	1.0	400	5.0	250	8
High-protein (hospital)	6360	1[d]			126	1.7	4.2	12	0.5[d]	280[d]	10.0[d]		7[d]
High-protein–low-sodium (hospital)	6463	1[d]			120[d]	1.2	3.3	11	0.7[d]	235[d]	6.3[d]		4[d]
Maintenance (hospital)	4961				196	0.7	2.6	14	0.8	299	5.3[d]		3[d]

[1] Blank spaces under nutrients indicate inadequate information available.
[2] 1980 RDA for 178 cm, 70 kg adult male.
[3] 1980 RDA for 163 cm, 55 kg adult female (non-pregnant, non-lactating).
[a] Estimated safe and adequate daily dietary intakes from 1980 RDAs.
[b] Values from Bowes and Church, *Food values of portions commonly used,* 12th ed., 1975.
[c] Values are for powder composition only; milk values not available.
[d] Actual values may be slightly higher due to lack of information on vitamin and mineral content of some ingredients.

Minerals			Trace Elements									
Calcium (mg)	Phosphorus (mg)	Magnesium (mg)	Iron (mg)	Zinc (mg)	Iodine (μg)	Copper (mg)	Manganese (mg)	Fluoride (mg)	Chromium (mg)	Selenium (mg)	Molybdenum (mg)	Product (Manufacturer)
800	800	350	10	15	150	2.3[a]	2.5–5[a]	1.5–4[a]	0.05–0.2[a]	0.05–0.2[a]	0.15–0.5[a]	Male (age 23–50)[2]
800	800	350	18	15	150	2.3[a]	2.5–5[a]	1.5–4[a]	0.05–0.2[a]	0.05–0.2[a]	0.15–0.5[a]	Female (age 23–50)[3]
1214	947	133	1	4								Milk (3.3% fat)
1255	1030	112	—	4								Skim milk
1319	1071	428	18	15	29[c]	1.9[c]						Instant Breakfast (Carnation)
625	1250	250	11	9	94	1.3	2.5					Compleat B (Doyle)
700	900	266	12	10	100	1.3	2.7					Compleat Modified (Doyle)
530	530	210	10	16	79	1.1	2.1					Ensure (Ross)
636	636	318	14	24	106	1.6	2.1					Ensure Plus (Ross)
720	560	100	13	8	75	1.0	0.2					Formula II (Cutter)
636	530	212	10	11	81	1.1	2.5					Isocal (Mead Johnson)
1000	1000	400	18	15	150	2.0						Magnacal (Organon)
1272	1272	339	15	13	127	1.7	3.3					Meritene Liquid (Doyle) 550
550	550	210	10	16	81	1.1	2.2					Osmolite (Ross)
936	707	208	19	9	73	1.6	3.0					Portagen (Mead Johnson)
350	350	140	6	5	53	0.7	1.4					Precision HN (Doyle)
670	670	268	12	10	101	1.3	2.7					Precision Isotonic (Doyle)
530	530	212	10	8	80	1.1	2.1					Precision Low Residue (Doyle)
500	500	200	10	10	75	2.0						Renu (Organon)
1000	917	375	17	14	139	1.9	2.8					Sustacal (Mead Johnson)
575	525	250	12	10	150	1.5						Vitaneed (Organon)
2492	2145	229[d]	7[d]	17[d]		1.0[d]						High-protein (hospital)
1795	1630	166[d]	7	7[d]		1.0[d]						High-protein–low-sodium (hospital)
775	839	134	13	7		1.5[d]						Maintenance (hospital)

TABLE 4-3. Recipe: Hospital-Blenderized High-Protein Tube Feeding (per 1000 ml) (approximately 1037 kcal or 1 kcal/ml)

Ingredients	Weight (g)	Household Measure[1]	Protein (g)	Fat (g)	Carbo-hydrate (g)	Sodium (mg)	Potas-sium (mg)	Chlor-ide (mg)[2]
Strained baby meat[3]	150	11 tablespoons	21	9	1	101	294	
Strained baby vegetable[4]	50	3½ tablespoons	1	—	3	10	89	
Strained baby applesauce	50	3½ tablespoons	—	—	5	1	36	
Orange juice concentrate	50	1⅓ tablespoons	1	0	19	1	329	
Nonfat dry milk[5]	180	1¾ cups	65	—	94	963	3229	
Delmark eggnog mix	30	4 tablespoons	6	1	22	84	201	
Dry yeast	3	1 tablespoon	1	—	1	3	47	
Water to 1000 ml								
Total			95	10	145	1163	4225	

[1] Approximate measure for home use that most nearly equals the gram weight.
[2] Values of chloride content of food incomplete.
[3] Alternate use of strained baby liver, beef, and chicken.
[4] Alternate use of strained baby green beans and carrots.
[5] Instant high-density type (⅞ cup powder + 3¾ cup water = 1 quart).

TABLE 4-4. Recipe: Hospital-Blenderized High-Protein, Low-Sodium Tube Feeding (per 1000 ml) (approximately 1002 kcal or 1 kcal/ml)

Ingredients	Weight (g)	Household Measure[1]	Protein (g)	Fat (g)	Carbo-hydrate (g)	Sodium (mg)	Potas-sium (mg)	Clor-ide (mg)[2]
Strained baby meat[3]	150	11 tablespoons	21	9	1	101	294	
U.S. strained baby vegetable[4]	50	3½ tablespoons	1	—	3	10	89	
Strained baby applesauce	50	3½ tablespoons	—	—	5	1	36	
Nonfat dry milk[5]	90	¾ cup and 2 tablespoons	33	1	47	482	1615	
Orange juice concentrate	50	1 tablespoon and 1 teaspoon	1	—	19	1	329	
Delmark eggnog mix	30	4 tablespoons	6	1	22	84	201	
Lonalac	50	6½ tablespoons	14	13	19	10	480	
Water to 1000 ml								
Total			76	24	116	689	3044	

[1] Approximate measure for home use that most nearly equals the gram weight.
[2] Values of chloride content of food incomplete.
[3] Alternate use of strained baby liver, beef, and chicken.
[4] Alternate use of strained baby green beans and carrots.
[5] Instant high-density type (⅞ cup powder + 3¾ cup water = 1 quart).

TABLE 4-5. Recipe: Hospital-Blenderized Maintenance Tube Feeding (per 1000 ml) (approximately 976 kcal or 1 kcal/ml)

Ingredients	Weight (g)	Household Measure[1]	Protein (g)	Fat (g)	Carbohydrate (g)	Sodium (mg)	Potassium (mg)	Chloride (mg)[2]
Strained baby meat[3]	200	$\frac{7}{8}$ cup	27	12	1	135	392	
Strained baby vegetable[4]	128	9 tablespoons	1	—	8	25	226	
Strained baby applesauce	128	9 tablespoons	—	—	14	2	91	
Whole milk (3.3%)	488	2 cups	19	16	23	242	752	
Orange juice, diluted	249	1 cup	2	—	29	2	502	
Baby rice cereal	8	3 tablespoons and 1 teaspoon	—	1	6	3	31	
Corn oil	15	1 tablespoon	0	15	0	0	0	
Sugar	20	1 tablespoon	0	0	20	—	1	
Water to 1000 ml								
Total			49	44	101	409	1995	

[1] Approximate measure for home use that most nearly equals the gram weight.
[2] Values of chloride content of food incomplete.
[3] Alternate use of strained baby liver, beef, and chicken.
[4] Alternate use of strained baby green beans and carrots.

TABLE 4-6. Problems Associated with the Tube-Fed Patient and Suggested Treatment (1, 6, 7, 11, 12, 17)

Complications	Possible Reasons	Suggested Treatment
Gastrointestinal disturbances Diarrhea Nausea Vomiting Cramping Delayed gastric emptying Constipation	Osmotic overload	Change concentration of formula and/or change source of nutrients
	Volume overload	Decrease flow rate Decrease total volume of formula
	Fat malabsorption	Decrease fat content of feeding and/or use MCT oil
	Lactose intolerance	Use lactose-free feeding
Dehydration	Too little additional water administered	Increase water given
	Too high protein concentration	Decrease protein concentration
Overhydration	Too much fluid administered	Decrease volume of feeding and/or water given
	Renal or pulmonary involvement	Decrease sodium content of feeding
Aspiration	Too rapid administration of feeding	Decrease flow rate Decrease volume of feeding
	Position of patient during feeding	Arrange position of patient with head and chest at 30° angle from supine position
	Position of end of tube	
Electrolyte imbalance	Receiving peripheral and/or central alimentation plus tube feeding	Monitor electrolytes administered
	Renal involvement	Modify tube feeding
Insufficient weight gain	Insufficient calories	Increase concentration and/or volume of feeding given
	Malabsorption	Modify nutrient composition of formula
	Catabolic state	

TABLE 4-6. Problems Associated with the Tube-Fed Patient and Suggested Treatment (1, 6, 7, 11, 12, 17) [*Concluded*]

Complications	Possible Reasons	Suggested Treatment
Rapid weight gain	Excess calories	Decrease concentration and/or volume of feeding given
	Fluid electrolyte imbalance	Evaluate fluid electrolyte status
Increased blood urea nitrogen (BUN) with liver or renal disease	Excess protein (nitrogen) intake	Decrease or change protein content of formula

REFERENCES CITED

1. SCHNEIDER, H. A.; ANDERSON, C. E.; and COURSIN, D. B., eds. 1977. *Nutritional support of medical practice,* pp. 487–488. New York: Harper & Row.
2. SIMPSON, S.; BESKITT, P.; NEWMARK, S. R.; BLACK, J.; and DURHAM, D. 1980. Home tube feeding can be used for long-term nutritional support. Paper presented at 4th Clinical Congress of ASPEN, Chicago, January 1980.
3. SHILS, M. E. 1977. Enteral nutrition by tube. *Cancer Res.* 37:2432.
4. ROBINSON, C. H., and LAWLER, M. R. 1977. *Normal and therapeutic nutrition,* p. 482. 15th ed. New York: Macmillan.
5. Massachusetts General Hospital Dietary Department. 1976. *Diet manual,* pp. 10–11. Boston: Little, Brown.
6. KUBO, W.; GRANT, M.; WALIKE, B.; BERGSTROM, N.; WONG, H.; HANSON, R.; and PADILLA, G. 1976. Fluid and electrolyte problems of tube-fed patients. *Am. J. Nurs.* 76:912.
7. SHILS, M. E.; BLOCH, A. S.; and CHERNOFF, R. 1979. *Liquid formulas for oral and tube feeding.* 2nd ed. New York: Memorial Sloan-Kettering Cancer Center.
8. WESLEY, J. R.; SARAN, P. A.; KHALIDI, N.; MUNN, C. J.; and FAUBION, W. C. 1980. *Parenteral and enteral nutrition manual.* Ann Arbor, Mich.: University Hospital, University of Michigan.
9. GORMICAN, A., and LIDDY, E. 1973. Nasogastric tube feedings. *Postgrad. Med.* 53:71.
10. CHERNOFF, R., and BLOCH, A. S. 1977. Liquid feedings: Considerations and alternatives. *J. Am. Dietet. A.* 70:389.
11. WALIKE, B. C., and WALIKE, J. W. 1977. Relative lactose intolerance: A clinical study of tube-fed patients. *JAMA* 238:948.
12. WALIKE, B. C.; PADILLA, G.; BERGSTROM, N.; HANSON, R. L.; KUBO, W.; GRANT, M.; and WONG, H. L. 1975. Patient problems related to tube feeding. In *Communicating nursing research,* ed., M. V. Batey. Vol. 7. Boulder, Colo.: WICHE.
13. KAGAWA-BUSBY, K. S.; HEITKEMPER, M. M.; HANSEN, B. C.; HANSON, R. L.; and VANDERBURG, V. V. The effects of diet temperature on tolerance of enteral feedings. Accepted for publication in *Nursing Research.*
14. WILLIAMS, K. R., and WALIKE, B. C. 1975. Effect of the temperature of tube feeding on gastric motility in monkeys. *Nurs. Res.* 24:4.
15. KAMINSKY, M. V., JR. 1973. *Tube feeding: Tips and techniques.* Norwich, N.Y.: Eaton Laboratories.
16. DOBBIE, R. P., and HOFFMEISTER, J. A. 1976. Continuous pump-tube enteric hyperalimentation. *Surg. Gyn. Obstet.* 143:273.
17. WALIKE, B. C.; WALIKE, J. W.; HANSON, R. L.; GRANT, M.; KUBO, W.; BERGSTROM, N.; WONG, H. L.; PADILLA, G.; and WILLIAMS, K. 1975. Nasogastric tube feeding: Clinical complications and current progress of research. *Health Team* 2:33.

5 Elemental (Defined Formula)

INDICATIONS FOR USE

The elemental diet may be indicated for individuals who

- Have decreased digestive capability and are unable to adequately digest and/or absorb regular food. Whole protein foods or formulas should be used for a trial period and elemental diets initiated only if these whole protein foods are unsuccessful.
- Require minimal intestinal residue. Research has demonstrated that for healthy subjects a low-residue diet (Chapter 20) of common foods is as effective as the commercial low-residue formulas tested at reducing fecal output. The common food diet produces a harder stool than the elemental diets. (1)
- Require clear liquids as the sole source of nutrients for an extended period of time.

Such individuals may include those with short bowel syndrome, fistulas of the small intestine, and Crohn's disease. (2, 3)

CONTRAINDICATIONS FOR USE

Elemental diets *are not* indicated for individuals who are able to digest and absorb regular foods or whole protein formulas. (2, 4)

Elemental diets *are not* designed to be used as high-protein supplements for individuals who are able to tolerate regular foods or whole protein formulas.

DESCRIPTION

Elemental diets are liquid formulas with nutrients in easily absorbable forms. These nutrients require minimal amounts of biliary, pancreatic, and intestinal secretions for digestion and are almost completely absorbed in the proximal intestine, leaving little residue for excretion. (2, 5)

Protein is usually provided in the form of purified L-amino acids, dipeptides, tripeptides, and/or protein hydrolysates. The rate of amino acid uptake from solutions containing individual dipeptides, individual tripeptides, or partially hydrolyzed proteins has been shown to be greater than the rate from solutions composed solely of free amino acids. (6) Carbohydrate is in the form of glucose oligosaccharides, corn syrup solids, or sucrose. Glucose oligosaccharides can be hydrolyzed by enzymes in the intestinal mucosa and, therefore, do not require pancreatic amylase. Fat is generally provided from vegetable oil but may include medium-chain triglycerides. Vitamins, minerals, trace elements, and electrolytes are included in the formulations to provide nutritionally complete feedings. Tables 5-1 and 5-2 list nutrient composition and food sources of commercially available elemental diets. Not all are stocked in every hospital; for example, the ones starred in Table 5-1 are stocked at University Hospital.

GUIDELINES FOR NUTRITIONAL MANAGEMENT

Elemental diets may be taken orally but are unpalatable; oral ingestion rarely reaches optimal caloric intake. If taken orally, the individual is advised to sip the feeding slowly and in small quantities to prevent hyperosmolar diarrhea, nausea, and abdominal distention. (2) The formula can be mixed with various fruit juices, served over ice, put in broths, or made into gelatins, slushes, or popsicles to slightly improve palatability.

Elemental formulas are most appropriately given via nasopharyngeal, esophagostomy, gastrostomy, or jejunostomy tubes. When given via tube, the feeding should be administered by constant drip. Instead of the usual Levin feeding tube, a French infant feeding tube may be used. Additional water is not needed unless evaporative or dynamic losses are excessive. Elemental tube feedings should be started at half strength ($\frac{1}{2}$ kcal/ml) solution infused at 25–50 ml/hr. Increases in concentration or rate of flow should be gradual (2) and not at the same time. Possible complications include abdominal cramps, distention, nausea, and mild watery diarrhea. (2) These problems are managed by slowing the rate of administration, reducing the concentration of the feeding, or changing to another type of formula. Refer to Table 4-6 for monitoring problems associated with tube-fed patients and suggested treatments.

NUTRIENT ADEQUACY

Nutritional adequacy of elemental diets must be assessed on an individual basis. Variables affecting the nutritional adequacy of the feeding are nutrient content of the formula, volume and concentration of the feeding, presence of other forms of nutrient intake, the individual's physical condition including catabolic or anabolic state, and use of medications or therapy that affect nutritional status.

TABLES

TABLE 5-1. Nutrient Composition and Food Sources of Elemental Diets (per 1000 ml)

Product (Manufacturer)	kcal	Protein (g)	Fat (g)	Carbohydrate (g)	Sodium (mg)	Sodium (mEq)	Potassium (mg)	Potassium (mEq)	Chloride (mg)	Chloride (mEq)	Nitrogen (g)
Flexical (Mead Johnson)	1000	23	34	152	350	15.2	1250	32.1	1000	28.1	4
Vipep (Cutter)	1000	25	25	175	750	32.6	850	21.8	1700	48.0	4
Vital (Ross)	1000	42	10	185	383	16.7	1167	29.9	666	18.5	4
*Vivonex (Norwich-Eaton)	1000	20	1	230	860	37.4	1172	30.1	1839	51.8	3
*Vivonex-HN (Norwich-Eaton)	1000	43	1	211	771	33.5	702	18.0	1858	52.3	7

[a] Unflavored Flexical.
[b] Flavored Flexical.
* Available at Department of Dietetics, University Hospital.

TABLE 5-2. Vitamin and Mineral Composition of Elemental Diets (per 1000 ml) Compared with Recommended Dietary Allowances[1]

Product (Manufacturer)	Fat-Soluble Vitamins: Vitamin A (μg RE)	Vitamin D (μg)	Vitamin E (mg αTE)	Vitamin K (μg)	Water-Soluble Vitamins: Vitamin C (mg)	Thiamin (mg)	Riboflavin (mg)	Niacin (mg NE)	Vitamin B_6 (mg)	Folacin (μg)	Vitamin B_{12} (μg)	Biotin (μg)	Pantotheni Acid (mg)
Male (age 23–50)[3]	1000	5	10	70–140[a]	60	1.4	1.6	18	2.2	400	3.0	100–200[a]	4–7[a]
Female (age 23–50)[4]	800	5	8	70–140[a]	60	1.0	1.2	13	2.0	400	3.0	100–200[a]	4–7[a]
Flexical (Mead Johnson)	751	5	33	125	150	1.9	2.2	25	2.5	200	7.5	150	12
Vipep (Cutter)	751	5	23	75	45	0.8	0.8	10	1.0	200	3.0	150	5
Vital (Ross)	1000	7	30	133	60	1.0	1.1	13	1.3	266	4.0	200	6.7
Vivonex (Norwich-Eaton)	834	6	25	37	33	0.8	0.9	11	1.1	200	3.3	170	5.6
Vivonex HN (Norwich-Eaton)	501	3	15	22	20	0.5	0.6	7	0.7	130	2.0	100	3.3

[1] Blank spaces in table indicate incomplete nutrient analysis available.
[2] Fluoride level depends on fluoride content of water.
[3] 1980 RDA for 178 cm, 70 kg adult male.
[4] 1980 RDA for 163 cm, 55 kg adult female (nonpregnant, nonlactating).
[a] Estimated safe and adequate daily dietary intakes from 1980 recommended dietary allowances.

Lactose (g)	Osmolality (mOsm/kg)	Food Sources: Protein	Food Sources: Fat	Food Sources: Carbohydrate	Product (Manufacturer)
0	550[a]/723[b]	Hydrolyzed casein; pure crystalline amino acids	Soy oil; MCT oil	Corn syrup solids; modified tapioca starch	Flexical (Mead Johnson)
0	520	Hydrolyzed fish protein; free amino acids	MCT oil; corn oil	Corn syrup solids; sucrose; cornstarch; potassium gluconate; tapioca starch	Vipep (Cutter)
0	450	Hydrolyzed soy, whey, and meat proteins; pure crystalline amino acids	Sunflower oil	Glucose oligo- and polysaccharides; sucrose; cornstarch	Vital (Ross)
0	550	Pure crystalline amino acids	Safflower oil	Glucose oligosaccharides	*Vivonex (Norwich-Eaton)
0	810	Pure crystalline amino acids	Safflower oil	Glucose oligosaccharides	*Vivonex-HN (Norwich-Eaton)

Minerals			Trace Elements										
Calcium (mg)	Phosphorus (mg)	Magnesium (mg)	Iron (mg)	Zinc (mg)	Iodine (μg)	Copper (mg)	Manganese (mg)	Fluoride[2] (mg)	Chromium (mg)	Selenium (mg)	Molybdenum (mg)	Product (Manufacturer)
800	800	350	10	15	150	2–3[a]	2.5–5[a]	1.5–4.0[a]	0.05–0.2[a]	0.05–0.2[a]	0.15–0.5[a]	Male (age 23–50)[3]
800	800	300	18	15	150	2–3[a]	2.5–5[a]	1.5–4.0[a]	0.05–0.2[a]	0.05–0.2[a]	0.15–0.5[a]	Female (age 23–50)[4]
600	500	200	9	10	75	1	2.5					Flexical (Mead Johnson)
600	500	200	9	8	75	1	1.3					Vipep (Cutter)
666	666	266	12	10	100	1.3	1.3					Vital (Ross)
570	570	222	10	8	83	1.1	1.6					Vivonex (Norwich-Eaton)
330	330	133	6	5	50	0.7	0.9					Vivonex HN (Norwich-Eaton)

REFERENCES CITED

1. Bondy, R. A.; Beyer, P. L.; and Rhodes, J. B. 1979. Comparison of two commercial low residue diets and a low residue diet of common foods. *JPEN* 3:226.
2. Freeman, J. B.; Egan, M. C.; and Millis, B. J. 1976. The elemental diet. *Surg. Gyn. Obstet.* 142:925.
3. Chernoff, R., and Bloch, A. S. 1977. Liquid feedings: Considerations and alternatives. *J. Am. Dietet. A.* 70:389.
4. Shils, M. E. 1977. Enteral nutrition by tube. *Cancer Res.* 37:2432.
5. Kaminski, M. V., Jr. 1976. Enteral hyperalimentation. *Surg. Gyn. Obstet.* 143:12.
6. Matthews, D. M., and Adibi, S. A. 1976. Peptide absorption. *Gastroenterology* 71:151.
7. Shils, M. E.; Bloch, A. S.; and Chernoff, R. 1979. *Liquid formulas for oral and tube feeding.* 2nd ed. New York: Memorial Sloan-Kettering Cancer Center.

6 Parenteral

INDICATIONS FOR USE

Parenteral nutrition is the administration of nutrients via a peripheral or central vein. (1, 2) Parenteral nutrition is indicated for individuals at risk for malnutrition and for those who are unable to obtain sufficient nutrients by enteral means alone. (2) Parenteral nutrition should not be confused with the intravenous administration of fluid, carbohydrate, and electrolytes utilized to maintain hydration, maintain electrolyte balance, and provide glucose.

Parenteral nutrition may be required as the primary nutrition therapy or as supplemental or supportive nutrition therapy. (1–6)

Parenteral nutrition may be indicated as the primary nutrition therapy in the following conditions:

- *Inability to retain, digest, or absorb food* as may occur with peritonitis, bowel obstruction, prolonged ileus, peritoneal sepsis, severe vomiting or diarrhea, enterocutaneous fistula, pernicious vomiting of pregnancy, regional enteritis, ulcerative colitis, malabsorption syndrome, stricture or carcinoma of the stomach, severe peptic ulcer with gastric outlet obstruction, transmural and mucosal colitis, diverticulitis, gastroenteritis, short bowel syndrome.

Parenteral nutrition may be used as supportive therapy for individuals who are eating and/or being tube fed but are unable to consume enough calories and other nutrients to meet their nutritional needs. The following conditions may require parenteral nutrition as supportive nutrition therapy:

- *Preoperatively* with individuals who are emaciated, nutritionally depleted, or have lost more than 10% of their body weight.
- *Postoperatively* in individuals who will be unable to eat normally for five days or longer.
- *Traumatic conditions* such as burns or multiple fractures with other complications such as sepsis where the requirement for nutrients is very high.
- *Cancer,* especially as adjunct to surgery, radiation, or chemotherapy.
- *Protein or protein–calorie malnutrition* or when edema-free weight has fallen 10% below ideal body weight.
- *Refusal or inability to eat* with such conditions as coma, anorexia nervosa, or neurological conditions such as pseudobulbar palsy that interfere with eating.

DESCRIPTION

Parenteral solutions are prepared by the pharmacy. The nutritional content of the solution varies according to the needs of the individual and is based on specific orders written by the physician. For the nutritional content and indications for use of standard solutions utilized at University Hospital, refer to Table 6-1. Solutions other than standard are ordered at the physician's discretion. The following factors are considered in providing appropriate parenteral nutrition solutions.

Energy. The energy requirement for a normal, healthy adult at normal weight with restricted activity is about 30 kcal per kilogram of body weight per day. (3) Stress conditions such as fever, multiple surgeries, tumors, burns, trauma, or sepsis or a required weight gain may increase energy requirements 50 to 100% (Chapter 2). Patient response to therapy may be measured by small increments in body weight, height (infant, child), and/or a less negative or positive nitrogen balance.

Carbohydrate. Glucose (dextrose) is the carbohydrate source most commonly used. (1, 3, 6) Concentrations range from 5% to 70%; however, 20% to 50% is most common. Hydrous glucose provides 3.4 kcal/g. (6)

Protein. The protein source in the parenteral nutrition solution is in the form of crystalline amino acids and protein hydrolysates. (1, 3, 6) The total amount of nitrogen given must be enough to meet the daily requirements, and all eight essential amino acids must be present in sufficient amounts and in the proper balance. (1) For individuals requiring parenteral nutrition, protein ranges of 0.8–2.5 g protein per kilogram of body weight have been recommended for adults and 3–4 g protein per kilogram of body weight have been recommended for children. (1, 3, 4) The amount required will depend on the adequacy of energy intake, the presence of stress conditions, and the presence of protein wastage as occurs in burns or enteropathy. (3, 4) Protein cannot be stored without adequate caloric intake and some physical movement.

Solutions with nonprotein kilocalorie-to-gram nitrogen ratios of approximately 150:1 to 220:1 are necessary and sufficient for most adult patients for promoting positive nitrogen balance, protein synthesis, and weight gain as well as for minimizing gluconeogenesis. Children generally require a higher ratio, 230–300:1, to remain in positive nitrogen balance. (6)

Modifications of protein content may be necessary for individuals with renal or hepatic insufficiency or for those who have had severe protein deprivation. (1, 4, 6)

Fat. Fat is administered as a fat emulsion through a separate intravenous line or piggyback into a line containing other nutrients. Administration of a fat emulsion is indicated to provide sufficient calories when adequate carbohydrate calories cannot be infused and to avoid or reverse essential fatty acid deficiency. (6, 7) Table 6-2 lists the composition of two commercial fat emulsions.

Vitamins. A multivitamin concentrate is added to the parenteral solution daily. To avoid toxicity of vitamins A and D, a multivitamin complex containing fat-soluble vitamins (Table 6-3) is used only every other day. A multivitamin complex containing only water-soluble vitamins (Table 6-4) is used on the alternate days.

Vitamin B_{12} (cyanocobalamin) and vitamin K^1 cannot be added to parenteral nutrition solutions; they may be deactivated. A dosage of 100 μg of vitamin B_{12} should be given intramuscularly each month. Vitamin K is given intramuscularly or in a peripheral IV as required by prothrombin time, the usual dose is 10 mg/wk. Folic acid is incompatible with riboflavin and should be given intramuscularly, 5 mg/wk. (6)

Electrolytes. Electrolyte requirements are individualized for each patient. Table 6-5 lists approximate ranges of electrolytes usually present in a parenteral nutrition solution.

Trace minerals. Patients receiving parenteral nutrition for a period longer than one month may become depleted in trace minerals. A trace element solution containing zinc, copper, chromium, and magnesium, following the guidelines of the American Medical Association (Table 6-6), is recommended. Cobalt is provided in vitamin B_{12} and does not have to be added to the solution. Iodine is obtained from the Betadine solution used to clean the catheter insertion site. Iron dextran may be added prophylactically to parenteral nutrition solutions. (8) However, at University Hospital it is not routinely added to adult solutions but is to infant solutions (1.0 mg/day). (6) Other trace minerals including selenium, vanadium, molybdenum, nickel, tin, silicon, and arsenic are believed to be essential nutrients, but at present there is insufficient information to recommend their use in parenteral nutrition therapy. (9)

Many institutions have either nutrition or metabolic support services or parenteral–enteral nutrition teams who may be consulted about specific recommendations for solutions and for monitoring efficacy of therapy. At University Hospital, refer to the *Parenteral and Enteral Nutrition Manual* and/or consult the Parenteral–Enteral Nutrition team. (6)

GUIDELINES FOR NUTRITIONAL MANAGEMENT

Although parenteral nutrition solutions have been developed for use in peripheral veins, the hypertonicity of most of the solutions requires rapid dilution by high blood flow to prevent phlebitis or thrombosis. (1, 3, 6) This is accomplished by use of a central vein such as the subclavian for infusion of the solution through a catheter. Insertion of the catheter is a surgical procedure and must be performed with strict attention to aseptic technique. (1, 6)

Complications of parenteral nutrition include (6)

- *Technical complications* related to the catheter: pneumothorax, puncture of the subclavian artery, air embolism, thromboembolism.
- *Metabolic complications* relating to glucose, acid–base, and electrolyte imbalances: hyperglycemia, hypoglycemia, hyperkalemia, hypokalemia, hypercalcemia, hypermagnesemia, hyperphosphatemia, hypocalcemia, hypomagnesemia, hypophosphatemia.
- *Septic complications* suggested by a temperature elevation, sudden glucose intolerance, hypotension, oliguria, or a general deterioration in clinical condition. Absolute indications for catheter removal include septic shock, bacteremia, or fungemia confirmed by laboratory; focal infection at catheter insertion site; embolic phenomena; and persistent fever with no other source found.

The potential for complications is minimized by strict attention to sterile technique in catheter insertion and care of the insertion site, regular monitoring of fluid and electrolyte balance, and ongoing assessment of nutritional status.

As soon as the individual's gastrointestinal tract can function and its use is not contraindicated, the gastrointestinal tract should be used. If the individual is also able and willing to eat, oral nutrition support is the choice; otherwise, an appropriate tube feeding is used. If the gastrointestinal tract has not been utilized for a long period of time, transient malabsorption of nutrients (e.g., lactose, fat) may appear. Adjustments can be made in the composition of the tube feeding or oral intake to decrease this effect. The parenteral nutrition solution should be tapered as enteral nutrient intake is established to support maintenance or improvement of nutritional status.

NUTRIENT ADEQUACY

Nutrient adequacy of parenteral nutrition must be assessed on an individual basis. Variables affecting nutrient adequacy include the nutrient content of the solution, the volume of solution administered, the presence of other forms of nutrient intake, the individual's physical condition including catabolic or anabolic state, and use of medications or therapy that affect nutritional status.

TABLES

TABLE 6-1. Indications for Use and Composition of Standard Parenteral Nutrition Solutions

Solution	Mixed Amino Acid Formulation	Mixed Amino Acid Formulation and Added Sodium	Mixed Amino Acid Formulation and Added Sodium Low Potassium	Mixed Amino Acid Cardiac Formulation	Essential Amino[1] Acid Renal Formulation	Mixed Amino Acid[2] Peripheral Formulation
Indications for use		Standard indications		Cardiac disease	Renal disease	When peripheral alimentation is preferred
Volume	1050 ml	1050 ml	1050 ml	1050 ml	750 ml	1050 ml
Total caloric value	1010 kcal	1010 kcal	1010 kcal	1351 kcal	1249 kcal	455 kcal
Nitrogen content (g)	5.5	5.5	5.5	5.5	1.4	4
Nonprotein kcal: g nitrogen	155:1	155:1	155:1	216:1	820:1	Refer to footnote 2
Approximate osmolarity	1750 mOm	1750 mOm	1750 mOm	2250 mOm	1900 mOm	880 mOm
Amino acid	35 g (3.5%)	35 g (3.5%)	35 g (3.5%)	35 g (3.5%)	13.5 g (2.5%)	25 g (2.5%)
Dextrose	250 g (25%)	250 g (25%)	250 g (25%)	350 g (35%)	350 g (47%)	100 g (12.5%)
Calcium	4.5 mEq	4.5 mEq	4.5 mEq	4.5 mEq	—	4.5 mEq
Magnesium	5.0 mEq	5.0 mEq	5.0 mEq	8.0 mEq	—	5.0 mEq
Potassium	40.0 mEq	40.0 mEq	23.0 mEq	40.0 mEq	—	23.0 mEq
Sodium	35.0 mEq	55.0 mEq	51.0 mEq	—	1.5 mEq	47.0 mEq
Acetate	73.5 mEq	73.5 mEq	73.5 mEq	44.0 mEq	—	73.5 mEq
Chloride	35.0 mEq	55.0 mEq	35.0 mEq	20.0 mEq	—	35.0 mEq
Gluconate	—	—	—	4.5 mEq	—	—
Phosphorus	12 mM	12 mM	12 mM	12 mM	—	9 mM
Vitamin complex[3]	5 ml	5 ml	5 ml	5 ml	5 ml	5 ml

[1] Electrolytes may be added.

[2] This solution must be administered with 500 ml of fat emulsion to achieve appropriate osmolarity for a peripheral vein. The nonprotein kcal:g nitrogen ratio is then 222:1.

[3] Vitamin complex containing water-soluble and fat-soluble vitamins is provided every other day. Vitamin complex containing only water-soluble vitamins is provided on the alternate days.

TABLE 6-2. Composition of Two Fat Emulsions, Liposyn and Intralipid

Nutrient	Liposyn[1] (Abbott)	Intralipid (Cutter)
	(10% fat emulsions)	
Oil	Safflower, 10%	Soybean, 10%
Glycerine	2.5%	2.5%
Egg yolk phospholipids	1.2%	1.2%
Major fatty acid components:		
Linoleic acid	77.0%	54.0%
Oleic acid	13.0%	26.0%
Palmitic acid	7.0%	9.0%
Stearic acid	2.5%	—
Linolenic acid	—	8.0%
Osmolality	300 mOsm/l	280 mOsm/l
kcal/ml	1.1	1.1

[1] Available at University Hospital.

TABLE 6-3. Composition of Multivitamin Complex Containing Water-Soluble and Fat-Soluble Vitamins (6)

Vitamins	Amount Per 5 ml MVI Concentrate
Ascorbic acid (C)	500 mg
Thiamine HCl (B_1)	50 mg
Riboflavin (B_2)	10 mg
Pyridoxine HCl (B_6)	15 mg
Niacinamide	100 mg
Dexpanthenol (pantothenic acid)	25 mg
Vitamin A	10,000 IU
Vitamin D (ergocalciferol)	1,000 IU
Vitamin E	5 IU

TABLE 6-4. Composition of Multivitamin Complex Containing Only Water-Soluble Vitamins (6)

Vitamins	Amount Per 5 ml Solu-B with Ascorbic Acid
Thiamine HCl (B_1)	10 mg
Riboflavin (B_2)	10 mg
Niacinamide	250 mg
Ascorbic acid (C)	500 mg
Pyridoxine HCl (B_6)	5 mg
Sodium pantothenate	50 mg

TABLE 6-5. Ranges of Electrolytes in Parenteral Nutrition Solution (6)

Electrolytes	Per 24 Hours	Per Liter	Per Liter
Potassium	90–240 mEq	20–50 mEq	80 m Eq
Sodium	60–150 mEq	24–50 mEq	wide range
Magnesium	8–24 mEq	2–8 mEq	12 mEq
Calcium	9–11 mEq	10 mEq/L once daily	10 mEq
Phosphate	40–50 mM	10–20 mM	20 mEq
Chloride	80–120 mEq	20–40 mEq	wide range
Acetate	80–120 mEq	20–40 mEq	wide range

TABLE 6-6. Suggested Daily Intravenous Intakes of Essential Trace Elements (1)

Trace Elements	Pediatric Patients μg/kg[1]	Stable Adult	Adult in Acute Catabolic State	Stable Adult with Intestinal Losses[2]
Zinc	300[a] 100[b]	2.5–4.0 mg	Additional 2 mg	Add 12.2 mg/L small bowel fluid lost; 17.1 mg/kg of stool or ileostomy output
Copper	20	0.5–1.5 mg	—	—
Chromium	0.14–0.2	10–15 μg	—	20 μg
Manga-nese	2–10	0.15–0.8 mg	—	—

Expert Panel, AMA Department of Foods and Nutrition: 1979. Guidelines for essential trace element preparations for parenteral use. *JAMA* 241:2051. Copyright 1979, American Medical Association.

[1] Limited data are available for infants weighing less than 1500 g. Their requirements may be more than the recommendations because of their low body reserves and increased requirements for growth.

[2] Frequent monitoring of blood levels in these patients is essential to provide proper dosage.

[a] Premature infants (weighing less than 1500 g) up to 3 kg of body weight. Thereafter, the recommendations for full-term infants apply.

[b] Full-term infants and children up to 5 yr old. Thereafter, the recommendations for adults up to a maximum dosage of 4 mg/day.

REFERENCES CITED

1. Meng, H. C. 1977. Parenteral nutrition: Principles, nutrient requirements, techniques, and clinical applications. In *Nutritional support of medical practice,* eds., H. A. Schneider, C. E. Anderson, and D. B. Coursin, pp. 152–183. New York: Harper & Row.
2. Abbott, W. M. 1976. Indications for parenteral nutrition. In *Total parenteral nutrition,* ed., J. E. Fisher, pp. 3–14. Boston: Little, Brown.
3. Shils, M. E. 1972. Guidelines for total parenteral nutrition. *JAMA* 220:1721.
4. Weinsier, R. L.; Butterworth, C. E.; and Sahm, D. W. 1977. *Handbook of clinical nutrition,* pp. 65–68. Birmingham: University of Alabama, Department of Nutrition Sciences.
5. Kaminski, M. V.; Burke, W. A.; and Blackburn, G. L. 1977. *Intravenous hyperalimentation in modern hospital practice.* Tuckahoe, New York: USV Pharmaceutical Corporation.
6. Wesley, J. R.; Saran, P. A.; Khalidi, N.; Munn, C. J.; and Faubion, W. C., eds. 1980. *Parenteral and enteral nutrition manual.* Ann Arbor: University Hospital, University of Michigan.
7. Meng, H. C., and Wilmore, D. W., eds. 1976. *Fat emulsions in parenteral nutrition.* Chicago: American Medical Association.
8. Kwong, K. W., and Tsallas, G. 1980. Dilute iron dextran formulation for addition to parenteral nutrient solutions. *Am. J. Hosp. Pharm.* 37:206.
9. Expert Panel for Nutrition Advisory Group, AMA Department of Foods and Nutrition. 1979. Guidelines for essential trace element preparations for parenteral use. *JAMA* 241:2051.
10. Chernoff, R. 1979. The team concept: The dietitian's responsibility. *JPEN* 3:89.

chain fatty acid intake and using medium-chain triglycerides and providing water-soluble forms of fat-soluble vitamins (Chapter 29). Intestinal resection may also result in hyperoxaluria and renal oxalate stone formation. Modifications in fat and oxalate intake are indicated (Chapter 36).

Massive intestinal resection, leaving three feet or less of small bowel, presents problems of severe malabsorption of nutrients, water, and electrolytes. Principles of nutrition therapy then include appropriate use of total parenteral nutrition, elemental diets, and diets modified in fat and other nutrients. The absorptive capacity of the intestines of patients with intestinal resections improves with time. Nutritional management is then reevaluated and modified as necessary. Nutrition assessment is essential to ensure adequate provision of all nutrients, including minerals and trace elements. (7)

Radiation. Radiation therapy will affect nutritional status depending upon the location of the tumor and the dose of radiation.

Radiation to the head and neck region results in complications that interfere with nutrient intake. These may include the following:

1. *Dysgeusia.* Dysgeusia is the condition of mouth blindness or altered taste. It is believed to be caused by radiation damage to the microvilli of the taste cells or their surfaces. (10) The damage may result in increased taste recognition threshholds for sweetness and decreased taste recognition threshholds for bitterness. (11)
2. *Xerostomia.* Xerostomia is dry mouth. Radiation to the salivary glands results in decreased saliva production. Xerostomia may occur within one to two weeks after therapy has been initiated. (12) When therapy is completed, saliva production may gradually return to normal. A permanent loss of saliva production occurs in some individuals. (12) Artificial saliva may be used and is available from the dentist or pharmacist.
3. *Excessive mucus.* The quality of saliva may change to a viscid acid mixture containing abnormally high amounts of organic material. (10) Changes in saliva may occur early and be permanent or may after many months gradually return to normal.
4. *Soreness of oral cavity; difficulty swallowing.* A sore throat or mouth and difficulty swallowing may develop due to increased sensitivity and inflammation of the mucous membrane. Superficial ulceration to the oral epithelium may also develop. (10) This soreness may be seen in the second or third week of therapy and may increase in severity. The soreness gradually subsides after therapy is terminated.
5. *Dental caries.* Decreased saliva production alters the composition of the oral bacteria flora, increasing the risk of dental caries. (10) The teeth seem brittle and pieces of the enamel may break away from the tooth. Damage to the teeth or "radiation caries" may not appear until several years after radiation. When developing teeth are subjected to radiation, tooth growth may be stunted. (12)
6. *Osteoradionecrosis.* Osteoradionecrosis is a pathological process that may affect the mandible or maxilla following heavy radiation. Infection, necrosis, pain, and sometimes permanent deformity are present. Radiation damages the vascular bed of the bone with subsequent disturbance of the inflammatory response. This damage is usually permanent. Danger to the patient occurs when infection is

able to enter the bone as occurs with the mandible and maxilla where infection enters through dental caries in the teeth. Extraction of teeth in the area of bone to be irradiated may be indicated. (12)

The stomach generally tolerates irradiation, although anorexia and nausea may occur. (10) Radiation to the intestines often results in nausea, vomiting, and diarrhea. (4, 10) Malabsorption of glucose, fats, and electrolytes results to a variable degree. (10) Colitis can occur with high doses of irradiation to the colon or rectum. (10) Radiation to the pelvic region induces intestinal changes that may result in cramping, diarrhea, and nausea. (4)

Chemotherapy. Most chemotherapeutic agents used in the treatment of cancer inhibit one or more steps in cell metabolism, especially those involving the synthesis of purines, pyrimidines, DNA, and RNA. (7) Several different classes of drugs are used. These include the following:

1. *Alkylating agents.* Alkylating agents such as nitrogen mustard and Cytoxan[R] cause cross-linking of the DNA strands by inserting an alkylchemical group, thus interfering with cell replication. (13) Cells in all phases of the cell cycle are affected.
2. *Antimetabolites.* Antimetabolites such as methotrexate are active during DNA synthesis and are effective against rapidly dividing cells. (13, 14)
3. *Antitumor antibiotics.* Antitumor antibiotics such as Adriamycin[R] appear to directly complex with DNA and disrupt its function. (13) Such corticosteroids (e.g., prednisone) are given along with chemotherapeutic agents to enhance effectiveness. Prednisone will stimulate the appetite to a degree, but it may also cause impaired glucose tolerance, hypertension, peptic ulcers, and fluid retention. (13) Side effects of androgens (e.g., fluoxymesterone) and estrogens (e.g., diethylstilbestrol) include nausea, vomiting, fluid retention, and hypercalcemia.

Chemotherapy is usually administered cyclically in high doses with a combination of drugs. These regimens are designed to destroy cells in different phases of the cell cycle, overcome the frequent development of resistance of cells to the action of a single drug, and allow time between doses for recovery of normal cells. (7, 15)

The toxic action of chemotherapeutic agents is not restricted to tumor cells. Normal cells, particularly those that are constantly renewing such as blood, epidermal, and gastrointestinal mucosal cells, are affected. (16) Side effects of the therapy affecting nutritional status will depend on the drugs used, drug dosage, duration of treatment, rates of metabolism, and the individual's condition. (7) Common side effects affecting nutrient intake and nutritional status include (refer to Table 7-1) the following:

1. *Stomatitis.* Stomatitis in the form of oral ulceration, cheilosis, glossitis, and pharyngitis reflect toxicity to cells of the oral mucosa. (4)
2. *Nausea and vomiting.* Nausea and vomiting are the most common and immediate effects of chemotherapy.
3. *Diarrhea or constipation.* Diarrhea results from drug effects on the intestinal mucosa. (7) Constipation and adynamic ileus have been observed with vincristine. (4)

4. *Central nervous system effects.* Some drugs result in lassitude, apathy, confusion, and impaired oral intake. (17)

5. *Anorexia.* Anorexia occurs frequently and may be a result of nausea or altered taste sensation or hepatic injury. (17)

Because of the side effects associated with administration of the chemotherapy, encouraging oral intake for maintenance of nutritional status is most effective in the periods between drug treatment. There is evidence that use of total parenteral nutrition as an adjunct to cancer chemotherapy may, in some cases, decrease the incidence of side effects and increase the patient's tolerance to the drug. (18, 19)

GUIDELINES FOR NUTRITIONAL MANAGEMENT

Nutritional support is designed to provide nutrients in adequate amounts in forms that can be utilized by the individual. Parenteral feedings, tube feedings, and use of foods modified in composition or consistency may be necessary. Body weight, immunocompetence, serum albumin, serum transferrin, anthropometric measurements, and dietary intake records must be monitored to assess current treatment and to identify appropriate nutritional support. Continuous reassessment is necessary. (20, 21)

Energy and protein. A maintenance or anabolic calorie and protein level is required to minimize the effect of the increased metabolic rate and to promote wound healing. The energy requirement for maintenance can be estimated at 35 kcal/kg/day and for anabolism at 45 kcal/kg/day. The protein requirement is estimated at 1 g nitrogen/150 nonprotein kcal. (22) Children require adequate calories and protein to allow for normal growth and development and should be assessed on an individual basis.

Dietary modifications suggested for specific side effects of cancer therapy. (Refer to Table 7-2 for food items recommended to increase calorie and protein intakes of individuals with cancer.)

Anorexia

Provide small, frequent meals.

Breakfast may be more acceptable than meals later in the day. Provide nutritious foods at breakfast.

Avoid noncaloric items.

Small amounts of wine or other alcoholic beverages served with meals or just before may improve appetite.

Foods brought in from home may be better accepted than foods prepared in the institution.

Dental caries

Avoid excess sucrose-containing sticky foods such as regular candy and caramels.

Consult a dentist for recommendations for dental care.

Dysgeusia

Use flavorings and seasonings added to food to mask the "bad" taste as long as these flavorings and seasonings do not hurt the mouth. Mint, vanilla extract, oregano, bay leaf, barbecue sauce, and smoked meats are often well tolerated.

Gargle or rinse the mouth before eating with baking soda and water mixture (1 tablespoon baking soda per 1 quart water).

Substitute chicken, fish, cheese, egg, or turkey when beef is not well accepted.

Use eye appeal and aroma to enhance appetite.

Excessive mucus

Rinse mouth frequently with baking soda–water mixture (1 tablespoon baking soda per 1 quart water).

Eliminate sticky foods such as peanut butter, cheese spread, and thick hot cereals.

Citrus fruit juices, diet carbonated beverages, diet lemon drops, and lemon juice in tea may help to decrease excess mucus.

Soybean milk substitutes and skim milk may be acceptable when whole milk and milk products are not tolerated.

Nausea and vomiting

Restrict oral intake if necessary. Peripheral or central parenteral nutrition may be utilized to provide adequate nutrition when vomiting is severe or prolonged.

Provide small, frequent meals.

Avoid foods with odors that induce nausea. Cold foods may be more acceptable due to less odor.

Provide liquids for hydration.

Antiemetic should be used one hour prior to eating.

Soreness of the oral cavity; difficulty chewing or swallowing

Eat small, frequent meals, five to eight times per day.

Allow plenty of time to eat each meal.

Modify the texture of foods. A soft, mechanical soft, or pureed diet may be indicated (see Chapters 13–15).

Blenderize foods or cook foods in a pressure cooker. When blenderizing foods follow these basic guidelines:

Choose a variety of foods from the basic four food groups.

When regular meats, fruits, and vegetables are used, add liquid such as broth, juices, and oils to obtain a thin consistency.

Avoid using foods with nuts, seeds, or fibers. These may be difficult to blend.

Pureed baby meats, vegetables, and fruits may be used.

Special dietary products (refer to Table 3-3) may be added to increase nutrient content.

Use milder foods prepared without spices, such as boiled chicken, mashed potatoes, plain rice, cottage cheese, and cooked cereal.

Citrus fruits often irritate the oral cavity; substitute with apple, grape, or cranberry juice or peach, pear, or apricot nectar. Fruit-flavored drinks generally do not irritate and, if fortified, provide a good source of ascorbic acid.

Use foods of moderate temperature—not too hot or too cold.

Oral supplements may be used to provide concentrated sources of nutrients (Chapter 3). Liquid supplements are often well accepted when provided as between-meal feedings.

NUTRIENT ADEQUACY

"The special nutritional needs arising from metabolic disorders, chronic diseases, injuries, prematurity, and many other medical conditions require therapeutic treatment not covered by RDA for healthy persons." (23) Nutritional adequacy of the diet can only be determined by ongoing assessment of nutrient intake and nutritional status.

TABLES

TABLE 7-1. Chemotherapeutic Agents: Potential Side Effects That Affect Nutrient Intake or Nutritional Status (10, 13, 17, 24, 25)

Chemotherapeutic Agents			Potential Side Effects									
Generic Name	Trade Name or Abbreviation	Classification	Nausea and Vomiting	Stomatitis or Mouth Ulcerations	Diarrhea	Constipation	Taste Alteration	Hepatic Impairment	Fever and Chills	Abdominal Pain	CNS Involvement	Renal Impairment
L-Asparaginase	Elspar	Natural enzyme,	x					x	x		x	x
5-Azacytidine		Antimetabolite	x	x	x			x	x			
Bleomycin	Blenoxane	Antitumor antibiotic	x	x					x			
Busulfan	Myleran	Alkylating agent	x	x	x							
Carmustine	BCNU	Alkylating agent	x					x[1]				
Chlorambucil	Leukeran	Alkylating agent	x[2]					x				
Cis-Diammine-dichloroplatinum	Platinol, with Cis-Platinum	Heavy metal, alkylating agent	x				x				x	x
Cyclophosphamide	Cytoxan	Alkylating agent	x	x								x
Cytosine Arabinoside	Cytosar, Ara-C	Antimetabolite	x	x	x			x[1]		x		
Dacarbazine	DTIC	Alkylating agent	x					x				x
Dactinomycin	Cosmegen, Actinomycin D	Antitumor antibiotic	x	x	x					x		
Daunorubicin	Daunomycin, Cerubidine	Antitumor antibiotic	x	x	x				x			x
Doxorubicin	Adriamycin	Antitumor antibiotic	x	x	x			x				
5-Fluorouracil	Fluorouracil, 5-FU	Antimetabolite	x	x	x					x		
Hydroxyurea	Hydrea	Miscellaneous	x	x	x							x
Lomustine	CCNU	Alkylating agent	x	x				x[1]			x	x
Mechlorethamine	Mustargen	Alkylating agent	x	x								
Melphalan	Alkeran	Alkylating agent										
6–Mercaptopurine	6 MP, Purinethol	Antimetabolite	x	x	x			x				
Methotrexate	MTX	Antimetabolite	x	x	x			x[1]		x		x
Mithramycin	Mithracin	Antitumor antibiotic	x	x	x			x	x		x	x
Mitomycin C	Mutamycin	Antitumor antibiotic	x	x					x			x
Procarbazine	Matulane	Miscellaneous (methyl-hydrazine derivative)	x								x	
Semustine	Methyl-CCNU	Alkylating agent	x	x								
Streptozotocin	Zanosar	Alkylating agent	x		x			x[1]				x
6-Thioguanine	6-TG	Antimetabolite	x[3]	x[3]	x[3]							
Vinblastine	Velban	Vinca alkaloid	x	x	x	x				x		
Vincristine	Oncovin	Vinca alkaloid	x	x	x	x				x	x	

[1] Reversible.
[2] Mild.
[3] High doses.

TABLE 7-2. Food Items Recommended for Increasing Calorie and Protein Intake of the Individual with Cancer

Food Group	Recommendations
Milk and calcium equivalents	Custards; milkshakes; ice cream; yogurt; cheeses; cheese cake; double-strength milk (1 quart fluid milk mixed with 1 cup skim milk powder); cottage cheese; flavored milk; pudding; eggnogs; cream soups; milk powder; skim milk powder added to casseroles and mixed dishes
Meat and protein equivalents	Diced meat; casseroles; smooth peanut butter; cheese; eggs and egg dishes; cut, diced, or pureed meats mixed with soups, sauces, and gravies; fish, poultry, and vegetable protein meat substitutes; tuna, meat, or cheese in cream sauce
Fruit and vegetable	Fruit juice added to mashed or canned fruit; mashed or pureed fruit added to milk beverages, cereals, pudding, ice cream; jello made with fruit juice in place of water; tender, cooked vegetables such as mashed white or sweet potatoes, squash, spinach, carrots, beets; vegetables in soups and sauces; vegetables in cream or cheese sauces such as escalloped potatoes and cream-style corn
Grain	Hot cereals prepared with milk instead of water; ready-to-eat cereals softened in milk; high-protein noodles; noodles or rice in casseroles and soups; breaded or floured meats; bread or rice pudding
Other	
Beverage	Milk beverages; shakes made with fruit juice and sherbet when milk is not tolerated
Fat	Margarine or oil added to vegetables, hot cereals, and casseroles; cream used in place of milk or added to fruits and desserts; sour cream; salad dressings; mayonnaise mixed with tuna, egg, chicken, or fruit salad
Sweet	Desserts made with dry milk powder, peanut butter, or eggs

REFERENCES CITED

1. SHILS, M. E. 1979. Principles of nutritional therapy. *Cancer* 43:2093.
2. DEWYS, W. D. 1977. Anorexia in cancer patients. *Cancer Res.* 37:2354.
3. SCHMALE, A. H. 1979. Psychological aspects of anorexia. *Cancer* 43:2087.
4. LAWRENCE, W., JR. 1979. Effects of cancer on nutrition. *Cancer* 43:2020.
5. BRENNAN, M. F. 1977. Uncomplicated starvation versus cancer cachexia. *Cancer Res.* 37:2359.
6. BRENNAN, M. F. 1978. Host vs tumor metabolism. *Cancer Bull.* 30:72.
7. SHILS, M. E. 1980. Nutrition and neoplasia. In *Modern nutrition in health and disease,* eds., R. S. Goodhart and M. E. Shils, pp. 1153–1192. 6th ed. Philadelphia: Lea & Febiger.
8. LAWSON, D. 1980. Nutritional effects of TPN in the cancer patient—lean tissue or fat? Nutrition and Cancer postgraduate course presented at 4th Clinical Congress of ASPEN, Chicago, January 1980.
9. SHILS, M. E., and GILAT, T. 1966. The effect of esophagectomy on absorption in man: Clinical and metabolic observations. *Gastroenterology* 50:347.
10. DONALDSON, S. S., and LENON, R. A. 1979. Alterations of nutritional status: Impact of chemotherapy and radiation therapy. *Cancer* 43:2036.
11. DEWYS, W. D. 1979. Anorexia as a general effect of cancer. *Cancer* 43:2013.
12. SHAFER, W. G.; HINE, M. K.; and LEVY, B. M., eds. 1974. *A textbook of oral pathology,* pp. 515–519. 3rd ed. Philadelphia: W. B. Saunders.
13. SATHER, M. R.; WEBER, C. E., JR.; PRESTON, J. D.; LYMAN, G. H.; and SLEIGHT, S. M. 1978. *Cancer chemotherapeutic agents. Handbook of clinical data.* Boston: G. K. Hall.
14. MAYER, J., ed. 1971. Nutrition and cancer. *Postgrad. Med.* 50:57.
15. DEVITA, V. T., JR.; YOUNG, R. C.; and CANELLOS, G. P. 1975. Combination versus single agent chemotherapy: A review of the basis for selection of drug treatment of cancer. *Cancer* 35:98.
16. SILVER, R. T.; YOUNG, R. C.; and HOLLAND, J. F. 1977. Some new aspects of modern cancer chemotherapy. *Am. J. Med.* 63:772.
17. OHNUMA, T., and HOLLAND, J. F. 1977. Nutritional consequences of cancer chemotherapy and immunotherapy. *Cancer Res.* 37:2395.
18. COPELAND, E. M.; MACFADYEN, B. V.; LANZOTTI, V. J.; and DUDRICK, S. J. 1975. Intravenous hyperalimentation as an adjunct to cancer chemotherapy. *Am. J. Surg.* 129:167.
19. SOUCHON, E. A.; COPELAND, E. M.; WATSON, P.; and DUDRICK, S. J. 1975. Intravenous hyperalimentation as an adjunct to cancer chemotherapy with 5-Fluorouracil. *J. Surg. Res.* 18:451.
20. DWYER, J. T. 1979. Dietetic assessment of ambulatory cancer patients. *Cancer* 43:2077.
21. HARVEY, K. B.; BOTHE, A., JR.; and BLACKBURN, G. L. 1979. Nutritional assessment and patient outcome during oncological therapy. *Cancer* 43:2065.
22. COPELAND, E. M., III; DALY, J. M.; and DUDRICK, S. J. 1979. Nutritional concepts in the treatment of head and neck malignancies. *Head & Neck Surg.* 1:350.
23. Food and Nutrition Board. 1980. *Recommended dietary allowances.* 9th rev. ed. Washington, D.C.: National Academy of Sciences.
24. CARTER, S. K., and SOPER, W. T. 1974. Integration of chemotherapy into combined modality treatment of solid tumors. 1. The overall strategy. *Cancer Treatment Rev.* 1:1.
25. DEL REGATO, J. A., and SPJUT, H. J.: *Cancer diagnosis, treatment, and prognosis.* 5th ed. St. Louis, Mo.: C. V. Mosby.

OTHER REFERENCES

AKER, S. N. 1979. Oral feedings in the cancer patient. *Cancer* 43:2103.

FLEMING, S. M.; WEAVER, A. W.; and BROWN, J. M. 1977. The patient with cancer affecting the head and neck: Problems in nutrition. *J. Am. Dietet. A.* 70:391.

Hegedus, S., and Pelham, M. 1975. Dietetics in a cancer hospital. *J. Am. Dietet. A.* 67:235.

REFERENCES FOR THE LAY PUBLIC

Aker, S., and Lenssen, P. 1979. *A guide to good nutrition: During and after chemotherapy and radiation.* 2nd ed. Seattle, Wash.: Research Dietary Service, Fred Hutchinson Cancer Research Center.

American Cancer Society. 1974. *Nutrition: For patients receiving chemotherapy and radiation therapy.* New York: American Cancer Society.

National Cancer Institute. 1979. *Diet and nutrition: A resource for parents with children.* NIH pub. number 80-2038. Bethesda, Md.: National Cancer Institute.

———. 1980. *Eating habits: Recipes and tips for better nutrition during treatment.* NIH pub. number 80-2079. Bethesda, Md.: National Cancer Institute.

Tiernan, C. 1980. *Meal planning for children with cancer.* Ann Arbor, Mi.: Department of Dietetics, U. Hospital, U. of Michigan.

Zwahten, B. 1976. *Basic nutrition for patients receiving radiation therapy to the head and neck.* Ann Arbor, Mi.: Department of Dietetics, University Hospital, University of Michigan.

PART II
Basic

8

General for Adults

INDICATIONS FOR USE

The general diet, a self-selected menu, is designed for individuals who do not require extensive dietary modifications. This diet may be used when limited modifications in texture, nutrients, fluid, or calories are needed. Food choices must be monitored to assure appropriateness.

DESCRIPTION

The general diet is planned to offer the hospitalized patient a selection of foods that provides nutrients to repair, rebuild, or maintain body tissues. A modification of the "Guide to Good Eating" is the basis of the general diet. (1) Individuals can select foods to meet the U.S. dietary goals (Appendix 2) and/or the guidelines recommended by the American Heart Association (Chapter 10) for the general population at risk for premature atherosclerotic disease. (2, 3)

GUIDELINES FOR NUTRITIONAL MANAGEMENT

To maintain optimal nutrition, an individual should include a wide variety of foods from the basic four food groups. Adequate fluids (Appendix 4) should be consumed. Other foods, including fats, desserts and sweets, condiments, and alcohol, supplement, do not replace, foods from the basic food groups. Table 8-1 lists food groups and the minimum daily servings recommended for an adult.

NUTRIENT ADEQUACY

Actual nutrient intake depends upon the individual's appetite, preferences, and ability to eat. Provided that the individual consumes a wide variety of foods in adequate amounts, the diet will meet the recommended dietary allowances, 1980. It may be difficult for the premenopausal woman to meet the RDAs for iron (Chapter 38). When individuals are under stressful conditions, the recommended dietary allowances may not be adequate to meet nutrient needs.

TABLES

TABLE 8-1. Basic Food Groups and Minimum Daily Amounts for Adults

Food Group	Minimum Daily Servings
Milk and calcium equivalents	2 servings
1 cup milk or yogurt	
Calcium equivalents	
1½ ounces cheese[1]	
1¾ cups ice cream	
2 cups cottage cheese[1]	
Meat and protein equivalents	2 servings
2 ounces cooked lean meat, fish, or poultry	
Protein equivalents	
2 eggs	
2 ounces cheese[1]	
½ cup cottage cheese[1]	
1 cup cooked dried beans, peas	
4 tablespoons peanut butter	
Fruit and vegetable	4 servings
1 cup raw or medium-sized whole fruit	
½ cup cooked or juice	
A dark green or dark yellow at least every other day and a citrus fruit or its juice daily	
Grain	4 servings
1 slice bread	
½ cup cooked cereal, rice, or noodles	
1 ounce ready-to-eat cereal	
Whole grain, fortified, or enriched grain products	

[1] Count cheese as either milk or meat, not both simultaneously.

REFERENCES CITED

1. National Dairy Council. 1977. *Guide to good eating: A recommended daily pattern. Rosemont, Ill.: National Dairy Council.*
2. U.S. Senate: Select Committee on Nutrition and Human Needs. 1977. *Dietary goals for the United States.* 2nd ed. Washington, D.C.: GPO.
3. Turpeinen, O. 1979. Effect of cholesterol-lowering diet on mortality from coronary heart disease and other causes. *Circulation* 59: 1.

OTHER REFERENCES

Michigan Department of Public Health, Office of Nutrition Services. 1980. *Basic nutrition facts.* MDPH Pub. No. H-808. Lansing, Michigan.: Bureau of Personal Health Services, Michigan Department of Public Health.

Nutrition Foundation. 1977. *Index of nutrition education materials.* Washington, D.C.: Nutrition Foundation.

Page, L., and Phipard, E. F. 1956. *Essentials of an adequate diet.* USDA Agriculture Information Bulletin No. 160. Washington, D.C.: GPO.

RECOMMENDED REFERENCES FOR THE LAY PUBLIC

Cumming, C., and Newman, V. 1979. *Eater's guide: Nutrition basics for busy people.* San Diego, Calif.: Wellspring Publications.

Deutsch, R. M. 1973: *The family guide to better food and better health.* New York: Bantam Books.

McGill, M., and Pye, O. 1978. *The no-nonsense guide to food and nutrition.* New York: Butterick Publishing.

Rhode Island Department of Health, Office of Nutrition Services. 1980. *The way we eat.* Providence: State of Rhode Island and Providence Plantations, Department of Health, Office of Health Promotion.

U.S. Department of Agriculture. 1976. *Food is more than just something to eat.* Home and Garden Bulletin No. 216. Washington, D.C.: GPO.

9 Vegetarian

INDICATIONS FOR USE

Vegetarian diets are used by individuals who abstain from various foods of animal origin for religious, personal, or economic reasons.

DESCRIPTION

The three main categories of vegetarian diets are (1–3)

- *Lacto-ovo-vegetarian,* consisting of milk, milk products, eggs, and foods of plant origin.
- *Lacto-vegetarian,* consisting of milk, milk products, and foods of plant origin.
- *Total or strict vegetarian (vegan),* consisting only of foods of plant origin.

The quality and quantity of dietary proteins are of primary importance in vegetarian diets. Dietary proteins supply several amino acids that cannot be synthesized by the human body. These essential amino acids are listed in Table 9-1.

Dietary proteins also supply nitrogen and nonessential amino acids. A combination of essential and nonessential amino acids are the building blocks for synthesis of tissue proteins and nitrogen-containing compounds. (5) More than 20 essential and nonessential amino acids must be present simultaneously in sufficient quantities for protein synthesis to occur. If an adequate amount of one or more of the essential amino acids is not present, protein synthesis will be diminished. The remaining amino acids, even if present in excess, will not be used for protein synthesis but will be degraded and used for energy or stored as fat.

The quality or nutritive value of a food protein is determined by its amino acid composition and, less importantly, by its digestibility. (5) The essential amino acid composition of different food proteins varies widely. Animal protein has a characteristic amino acid pattern that closely resembles that of human protein. Animal proteins supply essential amino acids in amounts that produce optimum protein synthesis and are considered high-quality proteins. The essential amino acid patterns of individual plant proteins are not as complete as are those of animal proteins. They are called incomplete or lower-quality proteins because they may contain limited quantities of one or more of the essential amino acids.

Vegetarian diets are deficient when dietary amino acids are supplied from a single protein source. However, normally, diets contain a mixture of food proteins. By combining foods from several plant protein sources in the same meal, it is possible to obtain a pattern of amino acids that is equivalent to that obtained from animal protein. (3) For example, legumes are adequate in lysine but contain little methionine. Cereal grains such as wheat, rice, and corn are adequate in methionine but low in lysine. When legumes and grains are eaten at the same meal, they provide a mixture of amino acids that yields a higher-quality protein than either food would alone. (1, 3)

An adequate quantity of protein is supplied in the vegetarian diet by including adequate quantities of high-protein foods such as milk products, milk substitutes, eggs, legumes, nuts, and seeds.

For the total or strict vegetarian, attention must be given to providing sufficient energy, iron, calcium, riboflavin, vitamin D, and vitamin B_{12}. Energy requirements may be difficult to meet as the total or strict vegetarian diet is often high in bulk. If energy requirements are not met, amino acids will be used for energy rather than for protein synthesis. (1, 2) Iron requirements are more difficult to meet as iron absorption from nonheme iron sources is relatively poor (Chapter 38). Calcium, riboflavin, and vitamin D intake may be inadequate if neither dairy products nor fortified milk substitutes are included in the diet. Vitamin B_{12} is found only in foods of animal origin. The total or strict vegetarian must include either vitamin B_{12}-fortified foods in the diet or a vitamin B_{12} supplement. (2)

GUIDELINES FOR NUTRITIONAL MANAGEMENT

To maintain optimal nutrition, an individual should consume a wide variety of foods from the food groups listed in Table 9-2. It is particularly important for the vegetarian to consume a variety of vegetable protein sources to achieve the desired amino acid complementarity. Table 9-3 lists recommended minimum daily servings for each food group and their approximate protein content (in grams).

The following food combinations will supply a mixture of essential amino acids that mutually complement one another. When eaten at the same meal, they will provide the amino acid pattern of high-quality protein. (1–3, 6)

grains *plus* legumes
grains *plus* egg
grains *plus* milk products
legumes *plus* milk products
soy *plus* sesame

Other foods, including fats, beverages, sugar, and various condiments, supplement, do not replace, foods from the four vegetarian food groups. Use of these other foods should be determined by the individual's energy requirements.

NUTRIENT ADEQUACY

Lacto-ovo- and lacto-vegetarian diets are nutritionally adequate when a variety of foods as unprocessed as is practical is consumed in adequate amounts. (3, 7–9)

A total vegetarian diet is deficient in vitamin B_{12} and may be deficient in energy, iron, calcium, riboflavin, and vitamin D. It is recommended that a minimum of 2 cups a day of fortified soybean milk be included in this diet to obtain an adequate intake of these nutrients. (2) When fortified soybean milk is not used, vitamin B_{12} supplementation is indicated along with an increased consumption of green leafy vegetables. It is essential that lactating women following a total vegetarian diet supplement their diet with vitamin B_{12}. (10) Children following a total vegetarian diet can be deficient in vitamin D unless vitamin D-fortified soybean milk is included in the diet. (11)

TABLES

TABLE 9-1. Essential Amino Acids for Humans (4)

Isoleucine	Histidine (essential for infants)[1]	Phenylalanine
Leucine		Threonine
Lysine		Tryptophan
Methionine		Valine

[1] There is some documentation that dietary histidine may be required for adults and that dietary arginine may be limiting under special circumstances. (5)

Table 9-2. Vegetarian Food Groups and Serving Sizes

Food Group	Serving Size
Milk and calcium equivalents	
Milk[1]	1 cup
Yogurt	1 cup
Cheese, natural[1]	1½ ounces
Ice cream	1¾ cups
Cottage cheese[1]	2 cups
Soy milk, calcium fortified	1 cup
Broccoli, collards[2]	1 cup
Turnip greens[2]	1¼ cups
Kale, mustard greens[2]	1½ cups
Beet greens[2]	2 cups
Meat alternatives and protein equivalents[3]	
Eggs, small	2
Cheese, natural[1]	1½ ounces
Cottage cheese[1]	½ cup
Milk[1]	1⅓ cups
Soybeans cooked	½ cup
Tofu (soybean curd)	4 ounces
Meat analog[4]	various
Textured vegetable protein (TVP)[4]	various
Peanut butter	2½ tablespoons
Peanuts	⅓ cup
Split peas, common dried bean varieties, lentils (cooked)	⅔ cup
Blackeye, cowpeas	¾ cup
Almonds, cashews	½ cup
Walnuts, filberts	⅔ cup
Pecans	1 cup
Sesame seeds	⅓ cup
Sunflower seeds	½ cup
Fruit and vegetable[5]	
Cooked or juice	½ cup
Raw	1 cup or piece or portion only served
Grain[6]	
Bread	1 slice
Cereal, ready-to-eat	1 cup
Cereal, cooked	½ cup
Pasta, grits, rice	½ cup

[1] Count milk and cheese as either milk or meat alternate, not both simultaneously.
[2] If these vegetable items are used to supply calcium requirements, extra protein should be obtained from the meat alternate food group.
[3] Protein equivalent is ½ cup soybeans or 9.9 g protein.
[4] Read the nutrition label to determine serving size of these products.
[5] Include a citrus fruit daily and a dark green leafy or deep yellow vegetable three to four times per week.
[6] Use whole grain, fortified, or enriched grain products.

TABLE 9-3. Recommended Minimum Daily Servings and Protein Contribution of Vegetarian Food Groups (3, 6)

Food Group	Minimum Daily Servings		
	Child	Teenager	Adult
Milk and calcium equivalents	3–4	4–5	2
(protein, g)	(24–32)	(32–40)	(16)
Meat alternates	2	3	2–3
(protein, g)	(20)	(30)	(20–30)
Fruit and vegetable	4	4	4
(protein, g)	(8)	(8)	(8)
Grain	4	4	4
(protein, g)	(8)	(8)	(8)
Total protein, g	*60–68*	*78–86*	*52–62*

Courtesy, National Dairy Council, *Vegetarian nutrition.*

REFERENCES CITED

1. Committee on Nutrition, American Academy of Pediatrics. 1977. Nutritional aspects of vegetarianism, health foods, and fad diets. *Pediatrics* 59:460.
2. Register, U. D., and Sonnenberg, L. M. 1973. The vegetarian diet. *J. Am. Dietet. A.* 62:253.
3. Vyhmeister, I. B.; Register, U. D.; and Sonnenberg, L. M. 1977. Safe vegetarian diets for children. *Pediatr. Clin. N. Am.* 24:203.
4. Committee on Amino Acids, Food and Nutrition Board, National Research Council. 1974. *Improvement of protein nutriture.* Washington, D.C.: National Academy of Sciences.
5. Food and Nutrition Board. 1980. *Recommended dietary allowances.* 9th rev. ed. Washington, D.C.: National Academy of Sciences.
6. National Dairy Council. 1979. *Vegetarian nutrition.* Rosemont, Ill.: National Dairy Council.
7. Hardinge, M. G., and Stare, F. J. 1954. Nutritional studies of vegetarians. I. Nutritional, physical, and laboratory studies. *J. Clin. Nutr.* 2:73.
8. Hardinge, M. G.; Crooks, H.; and Stare, F. J. 1966. Nutritional studies of vegetarians. Proteins and essential amino acids. *J. Am. Dietet. A.* 48:25.
9. Committee on Nutritional Misinformation, National Academy of Sciences. 1975. Can a vegetarian be well nourished? *JAMA* 233:898.
10. Higginbottom, M. C.; Sweetman, L.; and Nyhan, W. L. 1978. A syndrome of methylmalonic aciduria, homocystinuria, megaloblastic anemia and neurologic abnormalities in a vitamin B_{12} deficient breast-fed infant of a strict vegetarian. *N. Eng. J. Med.* 299:317.
11. Dwyer, J. T.; Dietz, W. H.; Hass, G.; and Suskind, R. 1979. Risk of nutritional rickets among vegetarian children. *Amer. J. Dis. Child.* 133:134.

OTHER REFERENCES

Smith, E. B. 1975. A guide to good eating the vegetarian way. *J. Nutr. Ed.* 7:109.

Zolber, K. 1975. Producing meals without meat. *Hospitals* 49:81.

RECOMMENDED REFERENCES FOR THE LAY PUBLIC

Lappe, F. M. 1976. *Diet for a small planet.* New York: Ballantine.

Moore, S. T., and Byers, M. P. 1978. *A vegetarian diet.* Santa Barbara, Calif.: Woodbridge Press.

National Dairy Council. 1979. *Vegetarian nutrition.* Rosemont, Ill.: National Dairy Council.

Robertson, L.; Flinders, C.; and Godfrey, B. 1976. *Laurel's kitchen: A handbook for vegetarian cookery and nutrition.* Petaluma, Calif.: Nilgiri Press.

Smith, E. B. 1979. *Vegetarian meal-planning guide.* Winnipeg, Canada: Hyperion Press.

10

Prudent

INDICATIONS FOR USE

The prudent diet is recommended for the general population at risk for premature atherosclerotic diseases. (1) Along with dietary modifications, other risk factors including hypertension, smoking, and diabetes should be eliminated or controlled. (2)

The prudent diet is not indicated for individuals who have lipoprotein abnormalities or for individuals who are overweight. Individuals with hyperlipoproteinemias follow a diet modified specifically for the lipoprotein abnormality (Chapter 32). Individuals who are overweight without lipoprotein abnormalities should follow a weight reduction diet with prudent guidelines (Chapter 24).

DESCRIPTION

The goal of the prudent diet is to help prevent hypercholesterolemia, a primary risk factor for coronary heart disease. (2) Decreasing cholesterol in the diet can decrease serum cholesterol levels. (3–5) Diets reduced in saturated fat and cholesterol and increased in polyunsaturated fat have been shown to decrease serum cholesterol. (6, 7) Epidemiological studies identify that populations who consume diets high in saturated fat have an increased incidence of coronary heart disease. (8)

The prudent diet recommendations differ from an average American diet and are summarized in Table 10-1. The prudent diet is not controlled in energy, carbohydrate, or protein. However, it is controlled in total fat, percentage of polyunsaturated and saturated fat, and cholesterol.

GUIDELINES FOR NUTRITIONAL MANAGEMENT

The diet is planned using the prudent food exchange groups (Table 10-2). These food exchange groups were established to facilitate meal planning. Foods with similar total fat, saturated fat, polyunsaturated fat, cholesterol, and calorie content are grouped together. Table 10-3 lists the nutrient composition of the food exchange groups.

Diets are planned with a fat intake equal to or less than 35% of total calories. Intake of meat, eggs, milk, cheese, vegetable fats, and animal fats must be controlled to meet this requirement. To achieve the recommended polyunsaturated-to-saturated fat ratio of 1 : 1, use equal amounts of fats or oils with high concentrations of saturated fat and those with high concentrations of polyunsaturated fats. High concentrations of saturated fats are found in animal fats, coconut oil, palm oil, and hydrogenated vegetable oils. Oils high in polyunsaturated fat are safflower, sunflower, corn, and soybean. Cholesterol intake should be equal to or less than 300 mg/day. Cholesterol is found only in foods of animal origin. Egg yolks, organ meats, and other meats are major sources and must be limited.

The procedure for calculating a prudent diet is as follows:

Steps	*Example*
1. Obtain diet history.	
2. Determine calories needed to maintain ideal body weight (Chapter 23).	2700 kcal (reference human)
3. Calculate number of calories to come from fat (35% of total calories).	2700 kcal × .35 = 945 kcal from fat
4. Calculate total grams of fat allowed.	945 kcal ÷ 9 kcal/g fat = 105 g fat
5. Calculate total fat allowance to achieve P:S ratio of at least 1:1 and a cholesterol level of less than or equal to 300 mg/day. Use nutrient values for food groups listed in Table 10-3.	(see table below)
6. The remainder of the calorie requirement is obtained from a variety of nonfat foods from the Fruit–vegetable, Grain, and Other food groups.	

Food Group	No. Exchanges	Fat (g)	Saturated Fat (g)	Polyunsaturated Fat (g)	Cholesterol (mg)	kcal
Meat	7	21	8.4	0.7	210	420
Fat	14	70	11.2	26.6	—	630
Egg ($\frac{1}{7}$)	1	1	0.3	0.1	40	15
2% Milk	2	10	5.8	0.4	40	250
Total		102	25.7	27.8	290	1315

NUTRIENT ADEQUACY

This diet can be planned to meet the recommended dietary allowances, 1980, provided that the individual consumes a variety of foods in adequate amounts. It may be difficult for the premenopausal woman to meet the recommended dietary allowances for iron (Chapter 38).

TABLES

TABLE 10-1. Prudent Diet Recommendations Compared with an Average American Diet (1, 9, 10)

Diet Components	kcal from Fat as % of Total Calories	P:S	Cholesterol (mg/day)
Prudent diet recommendations	≤35	1:1	≤300
Average American diet	40	1:2	600

TABLE 10-2. Prudent Food Exchange System

Food Group/Foods Allowed	Serving Size	Foods to Avoid
Meat		
Poultry	1 ounce	Poultry skin, goose, duck
Fish, shellfish	1 ounce	Shrimp except as egg substitute
Lean beef, lamb, pork, veal, wild game	1 ounce	Fatty, well-marbled meats; bacon, frankfurters, luncheon meats, sausage, hamburger, canned meats; organ meats except as egg substitute
Tuna, salmon, cottage cheese	¼ cup	Cheese spreads, cheese foods
Peanut butter	2 tablespoons	
Polyunsaturated Fat		
Liquid safflower, sunflower, corn, or soybean oil	1 teaspoon	Coconut, cottonseed, olive, palm, and peanut oil and products made with these
Margarine made with an allowed oil listed as the first ingredient	1 teaspoon	Dietetic margarines, butter
Mayonnaise	1 teaspoon	Dietetic mayonnaise
Commercial or homemade salad dressing with an allowed oil listed as the first ingredient	2 teaspoons	Dietetic salad dressings
Nondairy creamers made from a polyunsaturated fat	Varies with brand	Sweet or sour cream, imitation sour cream, whipped topping; cream cheese; most cream substitutes
Almonds	9	Cashews, macadamia nuts; peanuts and pistachios
Pecan or walnut halves	6	
		Cream sauces, thickened gravies, and French-fried foods unless homemade using allowed fats and skimmed meat drippings
		Olives, avocados

[*Continued*]

TABLE 10-2. Prudent Food Exchange System [*Concluded*]

Food Group / Foods Allowed	Serving Size	Foods to Avoid
Egg yolks (serving sizes are for servings per week)		
Egg	1	Amounts in excess of those planned in the diet
Heart	4 ounces	
Kidney	1½ ounces	
Liver	2 ounces	
Shrimp	5 ounces	
Sweet bread (thymus gland)	1½ ounces	
2% Milk		
2% Milk	8 ounces	Whole milk, whole milk drinks; evaporated or condensed
Low-fat yogurt	8 ounces	Whole milk; eggnog; malted beverage mixes
Cheese		
Natural cheese	1 ounce	Processed cheese; cream cheese
Skim milk		
Skim milk, buttermilk, yogurt made from skim milk	Unlimited	Whole milk, whole milk products
Fruit and vegetable		
Fresh, frozen, canned	Unlimited	Coconut; buttered, creamed, or fried vegetables
Grain		
Enriched or whole grain bread and cereal products	Unlimited	Biscuits, muffins, sweet rolls, pancakes, French toast, waffles, and cornbread unless made from allowed ingredients
Miscellaneous		
Angel food cake; fruit ices; jello and gelatins; skim milk junket or pudding; popsicles; meringues; beverages; condiments; seasonings; sweets; soups or broths that do not contain fat	Unlimited	Desserts made with chocolate, whole milk, egg yolk, butter, lard, and margarines or shortenings made with hydrogenated fats, including commercial cakes, cookies, pies, cake and cookie mixes (except angel food cake mix), chocolates

TABLE 10-3. Nutrient Composition of Prudent Food Exchange System

Food Group	Total Fat (g)	Saturated Fat (g)	Polyunsaturated Fat (g)	Cholesterol (mg)	kcal
Meat	3	1.2	0.1	30	60
Polyunsaturated fat	5	0.8	1.9	—	45
Egg yolk ($\frac{1}{7}$)	1	0.3	0.1	40	15
2% Milk	5	2.9	0.2	20	125
Cheese	8	5.4	0.2	30	100

REFERENCES CITED

1. Report of Inter-Society Commission for Heart Disease Resources. 1972. Primary prevention of the atherosclerotic diseases. *Circulation* 42:18.
2. GLUECK, C. J.; MATTSON, F.; and BIERMAN, E. L. 1978. Diet and coronary heart disease: Another view. *N. Eng. J. Med.* 298:1471.
3. MATTSON, F. H.; ERICKSON, B. A.; and KLIGMAN, A. M. 1972. Effect of dietary cholesterol on serum cholesterol in man. *Am. J. Clin. Nutr.* 25:589.
4. KEYS, A.; ANDERSON, J. T.; and GRANDE, F. 1965. Serum cholesterol response to changes in the diet. II. The effect of cholesterol in the diet. *Metabolism* 14:759.
5. CONNOR, W. E.; STONE, D. B.; and HODGES, R. E. 1964. The interrelated effects of dietary cholesterol and fat upon human serum lipid levels. *J. Clin. Invest.* 43:1691.
6. TURPEINEN, O. 1979. Effect of cholesterol-lowering diet on mortality from coronary heart disease and other causes. *Circulation* 59:1.
7. ANDERSON, J. T.; GRANDE, F.; and KEYS, A. 1973. Cholesterol-lowering diets. *J. Am. Dietet. A.* 62:133.
8. KEYS, A., ed. 1970. Coronary heart disease in seven countries. XVII. The diet. *Circulation* 41 (Suppl. I): 162.
9. KEYS, A. 1968. Official collective recommendation on diet in the Scandinavian countries. *Nutr. Rev.* 26:259.
10. U.S. Senate Select Committee on Nutrition and Human Needs. 1977. *Dietary goals for the United States.* 2nd ed. Washington, D.C.: GPO.

OTHER REFERENCES

NORUM, K. R. 1978. Some present concepts concerning diet and prevention of coronary heart disease. *Nutr. Rev.* 36:194.

REFERENCES FOR LAY PUBLIC

CONNOR, W. E.; CONNOR, S. L.; FRY, M. M.; and WARNER, S. L. 1976. *The alternative diet book.* Iowa City: University of Iowa Press.

JONES, J. 1975. *Diet for a happy heart.* San Francisco, Calif.: 101 Productions.

ROBERTSON, L.; FLINDERS, C.; and GODFREY, B. 1976. *Laurel's kitchen: A handbook for vegetarian cookery and nutrition.* Petaluma, Calif.: Nilgiri Press.

PART III
Modifications in Consistency

11

Clear Liquid

INDICATIONS FOR USE

The clear liquid diet may be indicated for short-term use following periods of acute vomiting or diarrhea, when minimal residue in the gastrointestinal tract is desired, and to test the ability of the individual to tolerate oral feedings.

Due to its high concentration of simple carbohydrates, the clear liquid diet may be contraindicated following gastric surgery (Chapter 33). The diet must be modified for the individual with diabetes mellitus (Chapter 25) or hypoglycemia (Chapter 34).

DESCRIPTION

The clear liquid diet provides clear fluids to relieve thirst, prevent dehydration, yield minimal bowel residue, and/or test the ability of the individual to tolerate oral feedings.

GUIDELINES FOR NUTRITIONAL MANAGEMENT

The clear liquid diet is composed of clear fluids and other food items as listed in Table 11-1. A sample menu follows:

SAMPLE MENU

Breakfast	*Lunch*	*Supper*
Grape juice	Apple juice	Cranberry juice
Chicken broth	Beef broth	Beef broth
High-calorie jello[1]	High-calorie jello[1]	High-calorie jello[1]
Carbonated beverage	Carbonated beverage	Carbonated beverage
Coffee or tea	Popsicle	Popsicle
Sugar	Coffee or tea	Coffee or tea
	Sugar	Sugar

[1] High-calorie jello is made by substituting fruit juice for water in preparation.

NUTRIENT ADEQUACY

The clear liquid diet is inadequate in all nutrients and should be used for only a brief period of time.

TABLES

TABLE 11-1. Foods Allowed and Foods to Avoid for a Clear Liquid Diet

Food Group	Foods Allowed	Foods to Avoid
Milk and calcium equivalents	None	All
Meat and protein equivalents	None	All
Fruit and vegetable	Grape, cranberry, apple juice; other strained fruit juices	All other
Grain	None	All
Other		
Beverage	Carbonated beverages; tea, coffee, cereal grain beverages (e.g., Postum); clear broth; clear fruit-flavored drinks	All other
Fat	None	All
Sweet	Clear candies; honey; sugar; popsicles; plain jello; syrup	All other

12

Full Liquid

INDICATIONS FOR USE

The full liquid diet may be indicated for individuals who are unable to chew, swallow, or tolerate solid foods. The full liquid diet has traditionally been used as a step in the progression from clear liquid to solid foods. This step is generally unnecessary. (1) Oral supplements may be used with the full liquid diet to increase nutrient intake (Chapter 3).

Due to its high concentration of simple carbohydrates, the full liquid diet may be contraindicated following gastric surgery (Chapter 33). The diet may be modified to accommodate other dietary restrictions.

DESCRIPTION

Individuals unable to tolerate solid foods can be provided with a nutritionally adequate diet using the full liquid diet.

GUIDELINES FOR NUTRITIONAL MANAGEMENT

The full liquid diet is composed primarily of foods that are liquid at room temperature as listed in Table 12-1. Soft foods that require little mastication may be added to the diet as individual tolerance improves. A sample menu follows:

Sample Menu

Breakfast	*Lunch*	*Supper*
Orange juice	Pineapple juice	Tomato juice
Farina	Cream of chicken soup	Cream of mushroom soup
Eggnog	Whipped potatoes	Whipped potatoes
Milk	Chicken gravy	Beef gravy
Margarine	Jello	Chocolate pudding
Coffee or tea	Custard	Milk
Sugar	Milk	Margarine
	Margarine	Coffee or tea
	Coffee or tea	Sugar
	Sugar	

NUTRIENT ADEQUACY

The full liquid diet can be planned to meet the recommended dietary allowances. However, due to the difficulty of consuming adequate amounts of liquid foods from the meat and grain food groups, a vitamin–mineral supplement is recommended when the diet is to be used for more than a few days.

TABLES

TABLE 12-1. Foods Allowed and Foods to Avoid for a Full Liquid Diet

Food Group	Foods Allowed	Foods to Avoid
Milk and calcium equivalents	Milk and milk beverages; eggnog; yogurt; ice cream; pudding; cream soup	All other
Meat and protein equivalents	Custard; pureed meats added to cream soups	All other
Fruit and vegetable	All juices; whipped potatoes	All other
Grain	Cooked refined cereals	All other
Other		
Beverage	All beverages	None
Fat	Margarine, butter; gravy; cream	All other
Sweet	Clear candies, honey, sugar; popsicles; plain jello; syrup; sherbet	All other

REFERENCES CITED

1. Moss, G. 1980. Clinical absorption and motility studies documenting full enteral nutrition immediately following colectomy. Unpublished data presented at 4th Clinical Congress, American Society for Parenteral and Enteral Nutrition, Chicago, January 30–February 2, 1980.

General Soft (Diet as Tolerated)

INDICATIONS FOR USE

The soft diet is considered to be a "diet as tolerated"; foods are included or excluded from the diet based on individual tolerance. The soft diet has traditionally been used as a step in the progression from liquid to solid foods. This step is generally unnecessary.

DESCRIPTION

The soft diet has been based on tradition and individual tolerances to food rather than on scientific evidence. The soft diet has been described as providing foods that are easily digested and soft in texture and avoiding highly seasoned, fried, and "gassy" foods. (1) Foods in the traditional soft diet vary with individual eating habits and the geographic region. (2)

The characteristics ascribed to the soft diet may or may not be applicable to the diet for the individual patient.

Easily digested and soft in texture. The basis for this restriction is generally for ease of mastication and digestion. (1) A more appropriate diet prescription may be a mechanical soft diet (Chapter 14).

Elimination of spicy or highly seasoned foods. There is controversy as to the effect of various spices on the gastrointestinal tract. (3, 4) Individuals should be encouraged to eat a regular diet, avoiding those foods or condiments that produce pain or symptoms such as heartburn, belching, or indigestion. (5)

Elimination of fried or rich foods. Studies indicate that symptoms related to fat ingestion are not the result of the fat but of personal prejudices about fat. (6, 7) Traditionally, dairy fats were thought to inhibit gastric secretion and were encouraged; other fats were avoided. This has not been confirmed by experimental observations. (2) Fats are included in the diet unless fat ingestion is related to specific symptoms.

Avoidance of "gassy" foods. Flatus arises from bacterial fermentation of indigestible carbohydrate in the colon. (8, 9) Foods that contain large amounts of indigestible carbohydrate may need to be avoided. Individual tolerance varies. Alterations in gastrointestinal bacteria also change luminal gas production. For example, antibiotic therapy that alters the bacterial populations of the gastrointestinal tract may induce gaseousness or relieve it. (8)

GUIDELINES FOR NUTRITIONAL MANAGEMENT

Dietary management is based on the individual's nutrient requirements and food preferences and tolerances. A wide variety of foods from the basic four food groups is encouraged and provided in forms that the individual is able to tolerate.

NUTRIENT ADEQUACY

Actual nutrient intake depends upon the individual's appetite, preferences, and ability to eat. Provided that the individual consumes a wide variety of foods in adequate amounts, the diet will meet the recommended dietary allowances, 1980. When individuals are under stressful conditions, the recommended dietary allowances may not be adequate to meet nutrient needs.

REFERENCES CITED

1. Krause, M. V., and Hunscher, M. 1972. *Food, nutrition, and diet therapy,* pp. 318–319. 5th ed. Philadelphia: W. B. Saunders.
2. Weinstein, L.; Olson, R. E.; Van Itallie, T. B.; Caso, E.; Johnson, D.; and Ingelfinger, F. J. 1961. Diet as related to gastrointestinal function. *JAMA* 176:935.
3. Schneider, M. A.; DeLuca, V., Jr.; and Gray, S. J. 1956. The effect of spice ingestion upon the stomach. *Am. J. Gastroenterol.* 26:722.
4. Demling, L., and Koch, H. 1974. Condiments. *Acta Hepato-Gastroenterol.* 716:377.
5. Dunkerley, R. C.; Dunn, G. D.; and Wilson, F. A. 1976. Gastrointestinal disorders: The role of diet in cause and management. *Postgrad. Med.* 59:182.
6. Manier, J. W. 1970. Diet in gastrointestinal diseases. *Med. Clinics N. Amer.* 54:1357.
7. Taggart, D., and Billington, B. P. 1969. Fatty foods and dyspepsia. *Lancet* 2:464.
8. Polish, E. O. 1974. Belching and flatulence. In *Gastrointestinal pathophysiology,* ed., F. P. Brooks, pp. 21–26. New York: Oxford University Press.
9. Davies, P. J. 1971. Influence of diet on flatus volume in human subjects. *Gut* 12:713.

14
Mechanical Soft

INDICATIONS FOR USE

The mechanical soft diet is indicated for individuals who have difficulty chewing or swallowing. Conditions that affect chewing or swallowing are absence of teeth, loose dentures, sore gums, cancer of the head or neck region (Chapter 7), esophageal repair, and certain neurologic disorders.

DESCRIPTION

The mechanical soft diet is designed to provide an adequate nutrient intake for individuals unable to eat a regular diet.

GUIDELINES FOR NUTRITIONAL MANAGEMENT

The mechanical soft diet is composed of foods that are easily masticated and swallowed. Foods may be modified as necessary by mechanical processing such as blenderizing, mashing, or chopping.

The major considerations in meal planning are the individual's ability to chew and swallow foods and the individual's food preferences and tolerances. A wide variety of foods from the basic four food groups is encouraged and provided in forms that the individual is able to tolerate.

The list of foods allowed and foods to avoid appears in Table 14-1 to provide suggestions for meal planning. It is not meant to be restrictive. The individual's condition should determine the restrictions of the diet.

NUTRIENT ADEQUACY

Actual nutrient intake depends upon the individual's appetite, preferences, and ability to eat. Provided that the individual consumes a wide variety of foods in adequate amounts, the diet will meet the recommended dietary allowances, 1980. When individuals are under stressful conditions, the recommended dietary allowances may not be adequate to meet nutrient needs.

TABLES

TABLE 14-1. Foods Allowed and Foods to Avoid for a Mechanical Soft Diet

Food Group	Foods Allowed	Foods to Avoid
Milk and calcium equivalents	Milk and milk beverages; eggnog; yogurt; ice cream; pudding; cream soups; cottage cheese; cheese	None
Meat and protein equivalents	Eggs; custard; tender meats or meats processed by pressure cooking, grinding, or chopping; peanut butter; creamed meats; casseroles	Tough meat
Fruit and vegetable	All juices; all pureed fruits and vegetables; applesauce; ripe banana; cooked or canned tender fruits and vegetables; mashed potatoes	Fruits or vegetables with membranes, tough skins, or tough fibers
Grain	Cooked cereals; dry cereals served with milk; cookies or crackers served with a beverage; cooked noodles, rice; bread, toast	Hard rolls
Other		
Beverage	All	None
Fat	Butter, margarine; cream salad dressings; cream sauces; gravies	Bacon; nuts
Sweet	Puddings; cakes; pies; sherbet; gelatin desserts	Caramels
Miscellaneous	Soups; seasonings	

15

Pureed

INDICATIONS FOR USE

A pureed diet is indicated for individuals who are unable to chew solid foods or have impaired ability to swallow. Included are individuals with fractured and/or wired jaws or with neurologic disorders that affect the eating function. (1, 2) Individuals receiving radiation to the head and neck may require a pureed diet with other modifications (Chapter 7).

DESCRIPTION

The foods included in the pureed diet require no mastication and are easily swallowed.

Individuals with fractured and/or wired jaws must be provided with foods that require minimal jaw movement. Foods that the individual can consume will depend on the extent of the fracture and wiring.

For individuals with neurologic disorders, the pureed diet may be used in retraining the individual to swallow and avoid aspiration. (1, 2)

GUIDELINES FOR NUTRITIONAL MANAGEMENT

The pureed diet consists of liquids and semiliquid foods. Individual food tolerance must be considered in the selection of foods.

Foods allowed and foods to avoid are presented in Table 15-1 to provide suggestions for meal planning. It is not meant to be restrictive. The individual's condition should determine the restrictions of the diet.

NUTRIENT ADEQUACY

Actual nutrient intake depends upon the individual's appetite, preferences, and ability to eat. Provided that the individual consumes a wide variety of foods in adequate amounts, the diet will meet the recommended dietary allowances, 1980. When individuals are under stressful conditions, the recommended dietary allowances may not be adequate to meet nutrient needs.

TABLES

TABLE 15-1. Foods Allowed and Foods to Avoid for a Pureed Diet

Food Group	Foods Allowed	Foods to Avoid
Milk and calcium equivalents	Milk and milk beverages; eggnog; yogurt; ice cream; pudding; cream soups	All other
Meat and protein equivalents	Soft poached and soft scrambled eggs; custard; pureed meat; cheese sauce	All other
Fruit and vegetable	All juices; all pureed fruits and vegetables	All other
Grain	Cooked cereals	All other
Other		
Beverage	All	None
Fat	Butter, margarine; gravy; cream; cream sauces	All other
Sweet	Sherbet; plain jello; popsicles; sugar; honey; syrup	All other
Miscellaneous	Soups; seasonings	All other

REFERENCES CITED

1. LARSEN, G. L. 1972. Rehabilitation for dysphagia paralytica. *J. Speech and Hearing Disorders* 37:187.
2. GRIFFIN, K. M. 1974. Swallowing training for dysphagic patients. *Arch. of Phys. Med. Rehab.* 55:467.

Postsupraglottic Laryngectomy

INDICATIONS FOR USE

This diet is indicated for individuals who have had a supraglottic laryngectomy. The diet is initiated seven to ten days postoperatively and is used for two to three days while the individual is taught new swallowing techniques. When an adequate swallowing technique has been achieved, the individual is advanced to a diet as tolerated. Nasogastric tube feedings are utilized prior to initiation of the diet.

DESCRIPTION

The supraglottic laryngectomy removes the portion of the larynx above the vocal cord. The ability to speak is retained; the ability to swallow is impaired. The function of the larynx, which prevents passage of food into the trachea, is lost.

New swallowing techniques must be learned by the individual to avoid aspiration. (1–3) The diet provides foods that are easiest to swallow without aspiration.

GUIDELINES FOR NUTRITIONAL MANAGEMENT

Initially a pureed diet is provided (Chapter 15), omitting liquids. As the individual improves the swallowing technique, liquids are added. Experience has shown that carbonated beverages are the best tolerated and that milk and milk products are the least well tolerated. The individual slowly progresses to a general diet of solid foods and liquids.

NUTRIENT ADEQUACY

Because intake is minimal in the early stages of transition, the diet is nutritionally inadequate. Individuals may be supplemented with tube feedings until they are adept at eating (Chapter 4).

REFERENCES CITED

1. Ogura, J. H., and Mallen, R. W. 1965. Partial laryngopharyngectomy for supraglottic and pharyngeal carcinoma. *Trans. Amer. Acad. Ophth. and Otolaryn.*, pp. 832–845.
2. Ogura, J. H.; Jurema, A. A.; and Watson, R. K. 1960. Partial laryngopharyngectomy and neck dissection for pyriform sinus cancer. Conservation surgery with immediate reconstruction. *Laryngoscope* 70:1399.
3. Ogura, J. H. 1958. Supraglottic subtotal laryngectomy and radical neck dissection for carinoma of the epiglottis. *Laryngoscope* 68:983.

Bland

INDICATIONS FOR USE

The bland diet may be indicated for individuals with gastric or duodenal ulcers, gastritis, irritable bowel, or ulcerative colitis. The diet may be liberalized as symptoms subside and as the medical condition improves.

DESCRIPTION

The bland diet is a general diet with the omission of foods that produce pain and those that are strong stimulators of gastric acid secretion and motility. (1–3)

Meals are on a regular schedule to act as a timing mechanism for antacid or other drug therapy. (1) A bedtime feeding is discouraged for the individual with ulcers due to the increase in gastric acid and possible nocturnal pain that may occur two to four hours after the meal. (1)

Use of the traditional bland diet—generally milk based and excluding spices, condiments, high-fiber foods, and highly seasoned foods—has not been shown to increase the rate of healing of gastric or duodenal ulcers. (4–6)

GUIDELINES FOR NUTRITIONAL MANAGEMENT

A general diet is provided with the omission of alcohol and caffeine-containing beverages (Table A. 8-4). (2, 3) Decaffeinated coffee has been shown to increase gastric acid secretion (7) and should be limited. If these beverages are included in the diet, they should be used in moderation and consumed with food at meals.

Other foods, condiments, or spices that produce symptoms in the individual should be avoided. Black pepper, chili pepper, cloves, mustard seed, and nutmeg have been demonstrated to be gastric irritants in some individuals. (8) Other spices may increase gastric secretion. (9, 10)

Three meals at regularly scheduled times are provided each day. Eating at bedtime is discouraged.

NUTRIENT ADEQUACY

Actual nutrient intake depends upon the individual's appetite, preferences, and ability to eat. Provided that the individual consumes a wide variety of foods in adequate amounts, the diet will meet the recommended dietary allowances, 1980. When individuals are under stressful conditions, the recommended dietary allowances may not be adequate to meet nutrient needs.

REFERENCES CITED

1. Borland, J. L. 1976. Rational management of peptic ulcer disease. *Hospital Practice* 11:33.
2. Dunkerley, R. C.; Dunn, G. D.; and Wilson, F. A. 1976. Gastrointestinal disorders. The role of diet in cause and management. *Postgrad. Med.* 59:182.
3. Isenberg, J. I. 1975. Therapy of peptic ulcer. *JAMA* 233:540.
4. Buchman, E.; Kaung, D. T.; Dolan, K.; and Knapp, R. N. 1969. Unrestricted diet in the treatment of duodenal ulcer. *Gastroenterology* 56:1016.
5. Doll, R.; Friedlander, P.; and Pygott, F. 1956. Dietetic treatment of peptic ulcer. *Lancet* 1:5.
6. The American Dietetic Association. 1971. Position paper on bland diet in the treatment of chronic duodenal ulcer disease. *J. Am. Dietet. A.* 59:244.
7. Cohen, S., and Booth, G. H., Jr. 1975. Gastric acid secretion and lower-esophageal-sphincter pressure in response to coffee and caffeine. *N. Eng. J. Med.* 293:897.
8. Schneider, M. A.; DeLuca, V., Jr.; and Gray, S. J. 1956. The effect of spice ingestion upon the stomach. *Am. J. Gastroenterol.* 26:722.
9. Demling, L., and Koch, H. 1974. Condiments. *Acta Hepato-Gastroenterol.* 716:377.
10. Sanchez-Palomera, E. 1951. The action of spices on the acid gastric secretion, on the appetite, and on the caloric intake. *Gastroenterology* 18:254.

OTHER REFERENCES

Caron, H. S., and Roth, H. P. 1972. Popular beliefs about the peptic ulcer diet. *J. Am. Dietet. A.* 60:306.

Gastroesophageal Reflux

INDICATIONS FOR USE

This diet is indicated for individuals with gastroesophageal reflux. (1–3) Symptoms of gastroesophageal reflux are regurgitation, esophagitis, heartburn, and dysphagia. (3–5) Gastroesophageal reflux results from dysfunction of the lower esophageal sphincter mechanism and may occur with hiatus hernia or scleroderma. (1, 3, 6)

Gastroesophageal reflux can generally be corrected by surgery. The diet is indicated prior to surgery and for those individuals for whom surgery is not indicated. (3)

DESCRIPTION

The lower esophageal sphincter functions as a barrier to the reflux of acid contents from the stomach into the esophagus. (4, 5) Normally there is a pressure zone at the lower esophageal sphincter of 10–20 mm Hg above the pressure in the stomach. (3) When this pressure falls, the gastric contents may flow from the stomach into the esophagus. This gastroesophageal reflux may progress to esophagitis, the inflammation of the esophageal mucosa. Dysphagia results from incoordination of esophageal peristalsis induced by the esophageal irritation. (3, 5)

Goals of nutrition therapy are the following:

Increase lower esophageal sphincter tone. Intake of protein, which raises lower esophageal sphincter pressure, is increased. (1, 2, 7, 8) Intake of items that lower esophageal sphincter pressure is decreased. (1–3, 8–14) The latter includes fat, chocolate, alcohol, peppermint and spearmint oils, and tobacco smoke.

Decrease esophageal irritation. Acidic or spicy foods that may directly irritate the esophageal mucosa are avoided. (1, 2, 8, 14)

Avoid dysphagia. Foods that may stick in the esophagus or produce the sensation of a "lump in the throat" are avoided. A mechanical soft or pureed diet may be indicated. (3)

Reduce the potential for gastroesophageal reflux. Large meals increase reflux by increasing intragastric pressure; small, frequent meals are provided. (1, 3) Reflux is increased in the prone position; sitting or standing after meals is encouraged, and eating is avoided for at least two hours before bedtime. Excess adiposity may increase abdominal pressure and increase reflux; overweight individuals are encouraged to lose weight (Chapter 24). (1)

GUIDELINES FOR NUTRITIONAL MANAGEMENT

The following criteria are used when planning a diet to decrease gastroesophageal reflux:

A source of protein is provided with each meal. A minimum of 80 g protein is provided each day.

Fat intake is limited to approximately 50 g per day.

The following items are avoided (1–3, 8–14):

alcohol
caffeine-containing beverages (Table A.8-4)
chocolate
citrus fruits and juices
smoking tobacco

tomato and tomato-based foods
other foods that the individual has identified as irritating

Foods are provided that are easily masticated and moist. (3)

Five to six small meals are provided each day. (1, 3)

The individual is instructed to maintain an upright sitting or standing posture during and after eating and to avoid food two hours before bedtime.

NUTRIENT ADEQUACY

Actual nutrient intake depends upon the individual's appetite, preferences, and ability to eat. Provided that the individual consumes a wide variety of foods in adequate amounts, the diet will meet the recommended dietary allowances, 1980. If a vitamin C-fortified fruit juice or food is not included in the daily diet, vitamin C intake may be inadequate and should be supplemented.

REFERENCES CITED

1. Castell, D. O., and Frank, B. B. 1979. How to treat heartburn with diet therapy. *Nutr. Today* 14:12.
2. Castell, D. O. 1975. Diet and the lower esophageal sphincter. *Am. J. Clin. Nutr.* 28:1296.
3. Communication with M. B. Orringer, M.D., Associate Professor of Surgery, Esophageal Clinic, University Hospital, University of Michigan, Ann Arbor, Mich., 1980.
4. Chodosh, P. L. 1977. Gastro-esophago-pharyngeal reflux. *Laryngoscope* 87:1418.
5. Edwards, D. A. W. 1973. Symposium on gastroesophageal reflux and its complications. Section 1. Definitions, the antireflux mechanism, and symptoms. *Gut* 14:233.
6. Castell, D. O. 1975. The lower esophageal sphincter. *Ann. Intern. Med.* 83:390.
7. Nebel, O. T., and Castell, D. O. 1972. Lower esophageal sphincter pressure changes after food ingestion. *Gastroenterology* 63:778.
8. Babka, J. C., and Castell, D. O. 1973. On the genesis of heartburn. The effects of specific foods on the lower esophageal sphincter. *Am. J. Dig. Dis.* 18:391.
9. Nebel, O. T., and Castell, D. O. 1973. Kinetics of fat inhibition of the lower esophageal sphincter. *J. Appl. Physiol.* 35:6.
10. Hogan, W. J.; Viegas de Andrade, S. R.; and Winship, D. H. 1972. Ethanol-induced acute esophageal motor dysfunction. *J. Appl. Physiol.* 32:755.
11. Dennish, G. W., and Castell, D. O. 1972. Caffeine and the lower esophageal sphincter. *Am. J. Dig. Dis.* 17:993.
12. Sigmund, C. J., and McNally, E. F. 1969. The action of a carminative on the lower esophageal sphincter. *Gastroenterology* 56:13.
13. Dennish, D. W., and Castell, D. O. 1971. Inhibitory effect of smoking on the lower esophageal sphincter. *N. Eng. J. Med.* 284:1136.
14. Price, S. F.; Smithson, K. W.; and Castell, D. O. 1978. Food sensitivity in reflux esophagitis. *Gastroenterology* 75:240.

PART IV
Fiber Modifications

19

Introduction

The terms residue, roughage, and bulk have been used to describe the indigestible components of foods. The term fiber is used in these sections.

Dietary fiber is defined as the sum of the polysaccharides and lignin not digested by the enzymes of the human gastrointestinal tract and includes hemicelluloses, pectin substances, gums, mucilages, and cellulose. (1–3) Because it is a mixture of complex components, no single procedure can be used as a satisfactory measurement of dietary fiber. The most popular methods in the past measured crude fiber, acid detergent fiber, and neutral detergent fiber and underestimated the total dietary fiber content of foods. (1, 3) Crude fiber, the value most generally found in food composition tables, is primarily a measure of the lignin and cellulose content of the food and may represent as little as one seventh of the total dietary fiber of the food. (2) Values for dietary fiber content of foods are incomplete. Table 19-1 provides a comparison of dietary fiber content of some foods per 100 g.

Foods rich in dietary fiber may contain a variety of fiber components. The physiological properties observed will be dependent on the specific fiber components present. (2) Proposed actions of dietary fiber components on the gastrointestinal tract include modifying gastric and intestinal transit time, increasing fecal weight and volume, decreasing intraluminal pressure, increasing fecal mineral excretion, increasing bile salt and cholesterol excretion, and altering nutrient absorption. (4–6)

The effect of cooking and food processing on the dietary fiber content of foods and on their physiological effect has not been adequately studied. The main effect of processing appears to be on particle size, making the plant cell wall more accessible to bacterial attack in the large bowel. (7)

TABLES

TABLE 19-1. Dietary Fiber Content of Some Foods (per 100 g)

Food Item	Dietary Fiber Per 100 g Edible Food (g)
Almonds	14.3
Peanuts	8.1
Peanut butter, smooth	7.6
Coconut, desiccated	23.5
Beans, baked, canned in tomato sauce	7.3
Lentils, cooked	3.7
Split peas, cooked	5.1
Apple, pared	2.0
Apricots, dried	24.0
Banana	3.4
Peach, fresh	1.4
Pear, pared	2.3
Pineapple, fresh	1.2
Broccoli tops, cooked	4.1
Carrots, raw	2.9
Celery, raw	1.8
Corn, sweet, canned	5.7
Lettuce	1.5
Onions, raw	1.3
Peas, fresh, cooked	5.2
Potatoes, boiled, pared	1.0
Spinach, cooked	6.3
Tomatoes, canned, drained	0.9
Bran	44.0
Oatmeal, cooked	0.8
Rice, cooked	0.8
Bread	
Whole meal	8.5
Brown	5.1
White	2.7
Cereals	
All Bran	26.7
Cornflakes	11.0
Puffed Wheat	15.4
Rice Krispies	4.5
Shredded Wheat	12.3
Special K	5.5

Values for dietary fiber from Paul, A. A., and Southgate, D. A. T. 1978. *McCance and Widdowson's the composition of foods.* 4th ed. London: Her Majesty's Stationery Office.

REFERENCES CITED

1. SOUTHGATE, D. A. T.; BAILEY, B.; COLLINSON, E.; and WALKER, A. F. 1976. A guide to calculating intakes of dietary fibre. *J. Hum. Nutr.* 30:303.
2. The Institute of Food Technologists' Expert Panel on Food Safety and Nutrition and the Committee on Public Information. 1979. Dietary fiber. *Food Tech.* 33:35.
3. VAN SOEST, P. J. 1978. Dietary fibers: Their definition and nutritional properties. *Am. J. Clin. Nutr.* 31:S12.
4. ANDERSON, J. W., and CHEN, W. L. 1979. Plant fiber. Carbohydrate and lipid metabolism. *Am. J. Clin. Nutr.* 32:346.
5. EASTWOOD, M. A., and KAY, R. M. 1979. An hypothesis for the action of dietary fiber along the gastrointestinal tract. *Am. J. Clin. Nutr.* 32:364.
6. KELSAY, J. L. 1978. A review of research on effects of fiber intake on man. *Am. J. Clin. Nutr.* 31:142.
7. Communication with D. A. T. Southgate, Head, Nutrition and Food Quality, Agricultural Research Council, Food Research Institute, Norwich, England, November 1979.

OTHER REFERENCES

SPILLER, G. A., and KAY, R. M. 1979. Recommendations and conclusions of the dietary fiber workshop of the XI International Congress of Nutrition, Rio de Janeiro, 1978. *Am. J. Clin. Nutr.* 32:2102.

Low Fiber, Low Residue

INDICATIONS FOR USE

The low-fiber, low-residue diet may be indicated during acute phases of diverticulitis, ulcerative colitis, or infectious enterocolitis. (1, 2)

The low-fiber, low-residue diet is contraindicated when a soft stool is desired and for the individual with intestinal obstruction or diverticulosis. (1, 3)

DESCRIPTION

The low-fiber, low-residue diet provides foods that produce a small fecal mass. Foods high in dietary fiber and foods that increase fecal output are avoided.

GUIDELINES FOR NUTRITIONAL MANAGEMENT

The low-fiber, low-residue diet omits fruits and vegetables high in dietary fiber, nuts, seeds, and whole grains. Milk is limited as it may increase fecal output. (2, 4) Prune juice is avoided as it contains the laxative principal diphenyllisatin. (2) Fruits and vegetables that contain less than or equal to 2.0 g of dietary fiber per 100 g edible food are allowed in the diet. (5)

Table 20-1 lists foods allowed and foods to avoid on a low-fiber, low-residue diet. As more information becomes available regarding dietary fiber content of foods and the effect of cooking and processing on the physiological effects of fiber, these food listings may be modified.

NUTRIENT ADEQUACY

Actual nutrient intake depends upon the individual's appetite, preferences and ability to eat. Provided that the individual consumes a wide variety of foods in adequate amounts, the diet will meet the recommended dietary allowances, 1980. When individuals are under stressful conditions, the recommended dietary allowances may not be adequate to meet nutrient needs.

TABLES

TABLE 20-1. Foods Allowed and Foods to Avoid for a Low-Fiber, Low-Residue Diet

Food Groups	Foods Allowed	Foods to Avoid
Milk and calcium equivalents	Cottage cheese; cheeses; limit milk to 2 cups per day including that used in cooking	Milk in excess of 2 cups per day
Meat and protein equivalents	Eggs; meat; poultry; fish	Any prepared with legumes, nuts, peanut butter, seeds
Fruit	All juices except prune; pared apple; avocado; cherries; white grapes; grapefruit, oranges, and tangerines with membrane removed; cantaloupe and honeydew melon; mulberries; peaches; pineapple	Prune juice All other
Vegetable	All juices; raw or cooked celery, cucumber (flesh only), lettuce, onions, green pepper (flesh only), pumpkin, radishes, tomatoes; cooked asparagus soft tips, cauliflower, potatoes	All other
Grain	Baked products made from refined flour	Products containing whole grains, whole grain flour, bran, nuts, or seeds
	Cooked, refined cereals; fine-cut oatmeal; ready-to-eat cereals made from refined corn, rice, or oats; noodles; white rice	Whole grain, bran, or high-fiber cereals Brown or wild rice
Other		
Beverage	All except milk, limited to 2 cups daily	None
Fat	All	None
Sweet	Candy; cake; jello; pie; sherbet	Any made with foods to avoid
Miscellaneous	Soups made with allowed ingredients	Coconut; olives; popcorn

REFERENCES CITED

1. Goldstein, F. 1972. Diet and colonic disease. *J. Am. Dietet. A.* 60:499.
2. Bogoch, A. 1973. *Gastroenterology,* p. 90. New York: McGraw-Hill.
3. Bondy, R. A.; Beyer, P. L.; and Rhodes, J. B. 1979. Comparison of two commercial low residue diets and a low residue diet of common foods. *JPEN* 3:226.
4. Carter, H. S.; Howe, P. E.; and Mason, H. H. 1923. *Nutrition and clinical dietetics,* p. 47. 3rd ed. Philadelphia: Lea & Febiger.
5. Paul, A. A., and Southgate, D. A. T. 1978. *McCance and Widdowson's the composition of foods.* 4th ed. London: Her Majesty's Stationery Office.

21 Modified Fiber

INDICATIONS FOR USE

The modified fiber diet may be indicated during and following radiation to the pelvic area. (1)

DESCRIPTION

Radiation to the pelvic area causes alterations in the gastrointestinal tract. The bacterial state is altered, motility is modified, and mucus production is decreased. Irritation, bleeding, and diarrhea may be present. Acute inflammation lasts for four to six weeks and effects may exist for one year following cessation of radiation. (1)

The fiber content of the diet is modified to produce a soft stool and to avoid foods that may irritate the gastrointestinal tract.

GUIDELINES FOR NUTRITIONAL MANAGEMENT

Nutrition management must be individualized depending on the individual's tolerance to foods and the presence of symptoms. A general diet is selected with the avoidance of fruits with skins or seeds, gas-forming vegetables, large amounts of raw vegetables, seeds, nuts, popcorn, and any foods identified as irritating by the patient.

NUTRIENT ADEQUACY

Actual nutrient intake depends upon the individual's appetite, preferences, and ability to eat. Provided that the individual consumes a wide variety of foods in adequate amounts, the diet will meet the recommended dietary allowances, 1980. When individuals are under stressful conditions, the recommended dietary allowances may not be adequate to meet nutrient needs.

REFERENCES CITED

1. Communication with G. W. Morley, M.D., Professor of Obstetrics and Gynecology, University Hospital, University of Michigan, Ann Arbor, Mich., June 1979.

22 High Fiber

INDICATIONS FOR USE

The high-fiber diet may be used for the prevention and treatment of constipation and diverticulosis. (1–3) Studies are being conducted to determine the role of a high-fiber diet in diabetes, obesity, fat metabolism, and gastrointestinal disturbances. (4)

The high-fiber diet is contraindicated pre- and postoperatively for surgery of the colon and during acute phases of diverticulitis and ulcerative colitis. (5, 6) The high-fiber diet may be contraindicated during and following radiation to the pelvic area (Chapter 21).

DESCRIPTION

The high-fiber diet includes a variety of foods high in dietary fiber. The increase in dietary fiber intake is designed to produce frequent, soft, bulky stools and increase fecal transit rate. (7, 8) These conditions may make the colon less likely to develop spasms that cause pressure, pain, and development and/or inflammation of diverticula. (3, 9)

The beneficial effects of dietary fiber are best obtained by consumption of a wide variety of foods rich in dietary fiber. Consuming large amounts of fiber from a single food source is not recommended. The popular method of adding large amounts of bran to the diet to increase fiber intake may cause diarrhea, cramping, and other digestive complaints. (1) High intakes of wheat fiber have been associated with decreased absorption of calcium, magnesium, zinc, phosphorous, and iron. (10, 11)

GUIDELINES FOR NUTRITIONAL MANAGEMENT

A wide variety of foods from the four food groups is recommended, with emphasis on whole grains, nuts, seeds, and a variety of fruits and vegetables. Table 22-1 lists foods allowed and foods to avoid for a high-fiber diet.

Adequate fluid is necessary due to the hygroscopic nature of fiber.

NUTRIENT ADEQUACY

Actual nutrient intake depends upon the individual's appetite, preferences, and ability to eat. Provided that the individual consumes a wide variety of foods in adequate amounts, the diet will meet the recommended dietary allowances, 1980. When individuals are under stressful conditions, the recommended dietary allowances may not be adequate to meet nutrient needs.

TABLES

TABLE 22-1. Foods Allowed and Foods to Avoid for a High-Fiber Diet

Food Group	Foods Allowed	Foods to Avoid
Milk and calcium equivalents	All	None
Meat and protein equivalents	All, especially nuts and nut butters, seeds, legumes	None
Fruit and vegetable	All, especially raw and those with skins, seeds, and membranes	None
Grain	Whole grain breads and cereals; bran; brown or wild rice	Refined breads and cereals
Fluid	At least 6 to 8 cups daily	

REFERENCES CITED

1. The Institute of Food Technologists' Expert Panel on Food Safety and Nutrition and the Committee on Public Information. 1979. Dietary fiber. *Food Tech.* 33:35.
2. Plumley, P. F., and Francis, B. 1973. Dietary management of diverticular disease. *J. Am. Dietet. A.* 63:527.
3. Burkitt, D. P.; Walker, A. R. P.; and Painter, N. S. 1974. Dietary fiber and disease. *JAMA* 229:1068.
4. Proceedings of Symposium on Role of Dietary Fiber in Health. 1978. *Am. J. Clin. Nutr.* 31:Supplement.
5. Communication, with W. W. Coon, M.D., professor of surgery, University Hospital, University of Michigan, Ann Arbor, Mich. January 1980.
6. Bogoch, A. 1973. *Gastroenterology,* p. 90. New York: McGraw-Hill.
7. Beyer, P. L., and Flynn, M. A. 1978. Effects of high- and low-fiber diets on human feces. *J. Am. Dietet. A.* 72:271.
8. Kelsay, J. L. 1978. A review of research on effects of fiber intake on man. *Am. J. Clin. Nutr.* 31:142.
9. Goldstein, F. 1972. Diet and colonic disease. *J. Am. Dietet. A.* 60:499.
10. Reinhold, J. G.; Faradji, B.; Abadi, P.; and Ismail-Beigi, F. 1976. Decreased absorption of calcium, magnesium, zinc, and phosphorus by humans due to increased fiber and phosphorus consumption as wheat bread. *J. Nutr.* 106:493.
11. Cummings, J. H. 1978. Nutritional implications of dietary fiber. *Am. J. Clin. Nutr.* 31:S21.

PART V
Energy Modifications

23

Estimating Energy Requirements for the Non-Stressed Adult

Energy requirements are determined by energy expenditure. Energy expenditure is the sum of the basal metabolic rate and the energy expended for activity. Basal metabolic rate varies with sex, age, muscle mass, and state of health and is rarely measured directly. Energy requirements are usually estimated based on estimates of ideal body weight and the energy expended at various levels of activity. The estimated energy requirement is adjusted to produce weight loss, maintenance, or gain.

The methods discussed in this chapter refer to the adult not under stressed conditions. These methods are used primarily for the overweight, diabetic, and hyperlipidemic individual.

Three methods used to estimate ideal body weight

- Estimate ideal body weight using weight allowance for height (Table 23-1).
- Estimate ideal body weight by comparing actual weight for height to table of suggested weights for heights (Table 23-2).
- Determine perceived ideal body weight. Ideal body weight estimated by objective methods should be used to estimate energy requirements but may be inappropriate to use in setting weight goals. The individual may not perceive the estimated ideal body weight as an achievable goal. The body weight that the individual perceives as ideal or desired may be more appropriate to use as a weight goal to encourage compliance. Goals may be reset as the desired weight is achieved.

Three methods used to estimate energy requirement for activity

- For ideal body weight, estimate energy requirement based on activity level (Table 23-3).
- For ideal body weight at various activity levels, estimate energy requirement using food nomogram (Table 23-4).
- Estimate energy requirements by assessing time spent in specific activities (Table 23-5).

Methods used to estimate energy requirement to maintain, lose, or gain weight

- *To maintain present weight,* estimate the energy requirement needed to maintain body weight and add to this 4.0 kcal for each pound above ideal body weight *or* 8.8 kcal for each kilogram above ideal body weight. This adds the approximate cost of maintaining obesity.
- *To lose weight,* the energy intake necessary to maintain present weight is decreased. Each pound of fat is estimated to be 3500 kcal. Decreasing the energy intake necessary to maintain present weight by 500 kcal/day will result in a deficit of 3500 kcal/wk, for a weight loss of approximately 1 lb.

- *To gain weight,* the energy intake necessary to maintain present weight is increased. Increasing the energy intake necessary to maintain present weight by 500 kcal/day will result in an increase of 3500 kcal/wk, for a weight gain of approximately 1 lb.

The procedure for estimating energy requirements is as follows:

Steps	***Example***
1. Review physical data and outcome desired.	SEX: female HEIGHT: 64 in. (163 cm) WEIGHT: 145 lb (66 kg) ACTIVITY LEVEL: Sedentary OUTCOME DESIRED: Weight loss of approximately 1 lb/wk (0.45 kg/wk)
2. Estimate ideal body weight using Table 23-1.	100 lb + (4 in. × 5 lb/in.) = 120 lb
3. For ideal body weight, estimate energy requirement for appropriate activity level using Table 23-3.	120 lb × 13 kcal/lb = 1560 kcal
4. Estimate energy requirement to maintain present weight.	145 lb − 120 lb = 25 lb above ideal body weight 4 kcal/lb above ideal body weight × 25 lb = 100 kcal 1560 kcal + 100 kcal = 1660 kcal
5. Estimate energy intake required to lose weight.	1660 kcal/day − 500 kcal/day = 1160 kcal/day Approximately 1200 kcal/day will result in weight loss of approximately 1 lb/wk (0.45 kg/wk) for this individual.

TABLES

TABLE 23-1. Estimated Weight Allowance for Height

Build	Women	Men
Medium	Allow 100 lb (45.5 kg) for first 5 ft (152 cm) of height, plus 5 lb (2.3 kg) for each additional inch (2.5 cm)	Allow 106 lb (48 kg) for first 5 ft (152 cm) of height, plus 6 lb (2.7 kg) for each additional inch (2.5 cm)
Small	Subtract 10%	Subtract 10%
Large	Add 10%	Add 10%

This table is reprinted from Committees of the American Diabetes Association, Inc. and The American Dietetic Association. 1977. *A guide for professionals: The effective application of exchange lists for meal planning,* p. 17.

TABLE 23-2. Suggested Weights for Heights for Men and Women[1]

Height (without shoes) (in.)	Weight (without clothing) Low	Median (lb)	High	Height (cm)	Weight Low	Median (kg)	High
			MEN				
63	118	129	141	160	54	59	64
64	122	133	145	163	55	60	66
65	126	137	149	165	57	62	68
66	130	142	155	167	59	65	70
67	134	147	161	170	61	67	73
68	139	151	166	173	63	69	75
69	143	155	170	175	65	70	77
70	147	159	174	178	67	72	80
71	150	163	178	180	68	74	81
72	154	167	183	183	70	76	83
73	158	171	188	185	72	77	85
74	162	175	192	188	74	80	87
75	165	178	195	191	75	81	89
			WOMEN				
60	100	109	118	152	45	50	54
61	104	112	121	155	47	51	55
62	107	115	125	157	49	52	57
63	110	118	128	160	50	54	58
64	113	122	132	163	51	55	60
65	116	125	135	165	53	57	61
66	120	129	139	167	55	59	63
67	123	132	142	170	56	60	65
68	126	136	146	173	57	62	66
69	130	140	151	175	59	64	69
70	133	144	156	178	60	65	71
71	137	148	161	180	62	67	73
72	141	152	166	183	64	69	75

Robinson, C. H., and Lawler, M. R. 1977. *Normal and therapeutic nutrition*, p. 677. 15th ed. New York: Macmillan.

[1] Data for heights in inches and weights in pounds taken from Hathaway, M. L., and Foard, E. D.: *Heights and Weights of Adults in the United States.* Home Economics Research Report No. 10, U.S. Department of Agriculture, Washington, D.C., Table 80, p. 111.
Conversions to centimeters and kilograms were rounded off to the nearest whole number.

TABLE 23-3. Estimated Daily Energy Requirement to Maintain Ideal Body Weight at Different Levels of Activity

	Estimated Daily Energy Requirement at Ideal Body Weight	
Activity Level	Per Pound (kcal)	Per Kilogram (kcal)
Basal metabolism	10	22
Sedentary, very light activity	13	29
Moderate, equivalent to 4 hr of walking per day	15	33
Strenuous, heavy manual labor, athletes in training	16–20	35–44

Bassett, D. R. 1974. *Steps in calculating caloric requirements to lose, and to maintain weight.* Ann Arbor, Mich.: Hyperlipidemia Program and Department of Dietetics, University Hospital, University of Michigan.

TABLE 23-4. Nomogram

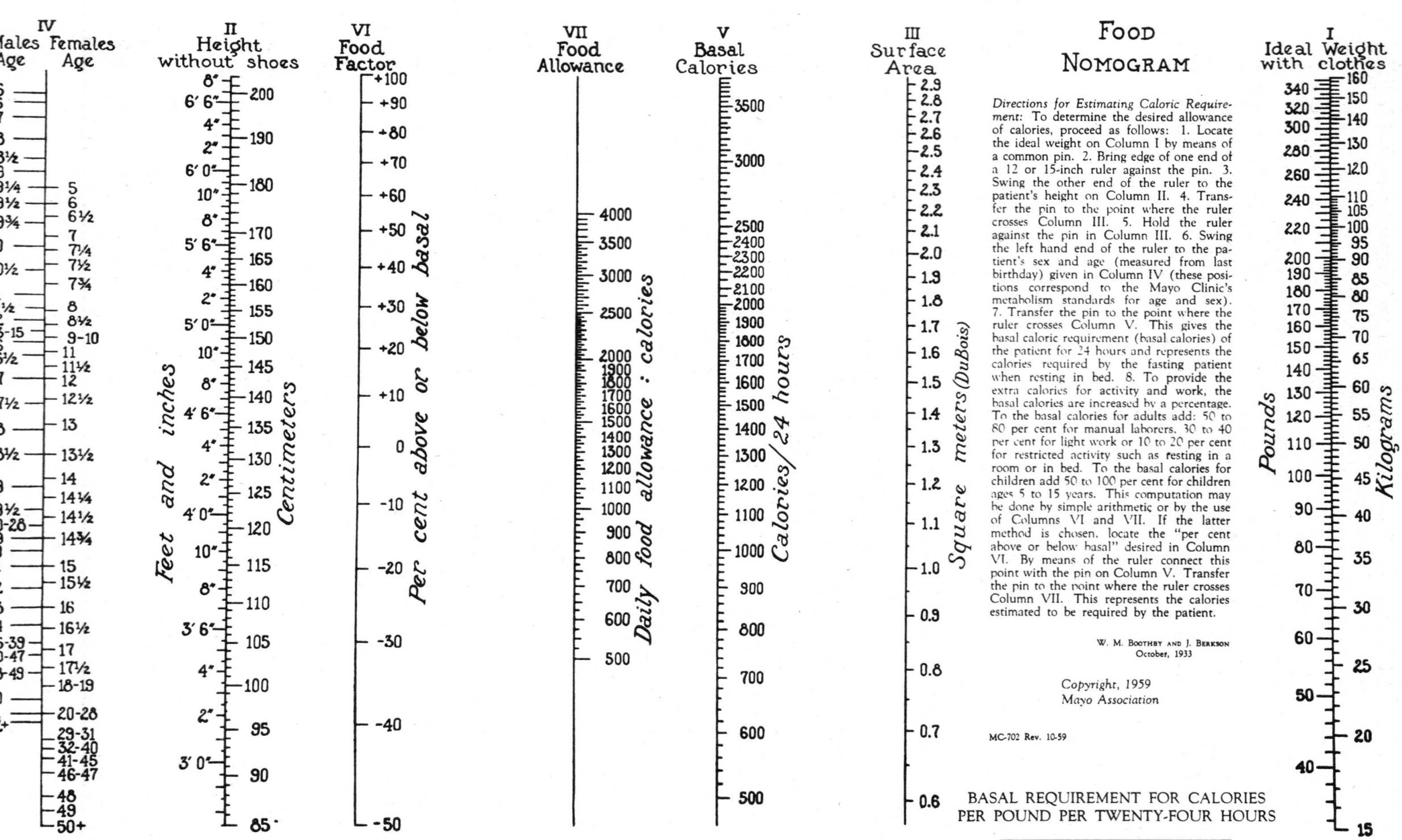

BASAL REQUIREMENT FOR CALORIES PER POUND PER TWENTY-FOUR HOURS

Age	Calories	
	Boys	Girls
6 months	25.0	25.0
1 year	25.5	25.5
2 years	25.0	24.5
3 years	23.5	23.5
4 years	23.0	22.0

For a child less than 5 years of age, the basal caloric requirement for twenty-four hours is computed by multiplying the standard weight for the measured height by the basal requirement for calories per pound per twenty-four hours for the appropriate age (see below Table of "Basal Requirement for Calories per Pound per Twenty-four Hours"). The height is that of the child measured without shoes; the weight to be used is that in the "Woodbury Height-Weight-Age Table" which corresponds to the measured height and age of the child; the age to be used is that of the child to the nearest half year or full year.

TABLE 23-5. Energy Requirement for Specific Activities (kcal/min) at Various Body Weights[1]

Activity	kcal/min/kg	kg 50 lb 110	59 130	68 150	77 170	86 190	95 209
Basketball	0.138	6.9	8.1	9.4	10.6	11.9	13.1
Cycling							
Leisure, 5.5 mph	0.064	3.2	3.8	4.4	4.9	5.5	6.1
Leisure, 9.4 mph	0.100	5.0	5.9	6.8	7.7	8.6	9.5
Eating (sitting)	0.023	1.2	1.4	1.6	1.8	2.0	2.2
Running, horizontal							
11 min, 30 steps/mi	0.135	6.8	8.0	9.2	10.5	11.7	12.9
8 min/mi	0.208	10.8	12.5	14.2	16.0	17.7	19.4
6 min/mi	0.252	13.9	15.6	17.3	19.1	20.8	22.5
Sitting quietly	0.021	1.1	1.2	1.4	1.6	1.8	2.0
Standing quietly	0.027	1.4	1.6	1.8	2.0	2.3	2.5
Tennis	0.109	5.5	6.4	7.4	8.4	9.4	10.4
Swimming							
Crawl, fast	0.156	7.8	9.2	10.6	12.0	13.4	14.8
Crawl, slow	0.128	6.4	7.6	8.7	9.9	11.0	12.2
Side stroke	0.122	6.1	7.2	8.3	9.4	10.5	11.6
Volleyball	0.050	2.5	3.0	3.4	3.9	4.3	4.8
Walking, normal pace	0.080	4.0	4.7	5.4	6.2	6.9	7.6

Excerpted from Katch, F. I., and McArdle, W. D. 1977. *Nutrition, weight control, and exercise*, Boston: Houghton Mifflin.

[1] Refer to the column that comes closest to present body weight. Multiply the number in this column by the number of minutes spent in the activity. If weight is greater than 220 lb (100 kg) use the figure for kcal/min/kg to calculate energy expenditure.

24 Adult Weight Reduction

INDICATIONS FOR USE

Weight reduction is indicated for those individuals who are overweight or obese.

Weight reduction is contraindicated during pregnancy (Chapter 46) and during periods of stress (Chapter 2).

DESCRIPTION

Overweight and obesity are defined as conditions in which there is an excess deposit of body fat. The degree of excess body fat may be determined by measuring skinfold thickness and by underwater weighing. A simpler assessment of overweight is made by comparing actual weight to estimated ideal body weight (Chapter 23). Twenty percent or more above ideal body weight is often considered obese. (1)

Overweight and obesity are associated with increased incidence of many disease states including hypertension, gall bladder disease, adult onset diabetes mellitus, and cardiovascular disease. (1–4) Weight reduction can result in decreased blood pressure even without salt restriction and can improve glucose tolerance. (5, 6)

Successful, lasting weight reduction is important to health and requires a comprehensive weight reduction program. The program should involve health professionals working with the overweight or obese individual to help change behavior, increase energy expenditure, and decrease energy intake. In planning an individualized weight reduction program, several factors must be considered including the individual's motivational level, dietary habits, activity level, support available from family and friends, income, education, and cultural background.

Goals of the weight reduction program are to

- Reach and maintain ideal body weight through safe and practical methods.
- Promote long-range changes in eating habits and other habits that affect weight fluctuations.
- Provide adequate nutrition for maintenance of health.

GUIDELINES FOR A WEIGHT REDUCTION PROGRAM

A weight reduction program designed to meet the goals just cited involves changing behavior, increasing energy expenditure, and decreasing energy intake. Although pharmacologic agents (e.g., anorexic drugs, thyroid hormones, and human chorionic gonadotropin) have been used in the treatment of obesity (7–9), their use *is not recommended.* Reasons are

- potential side effects and, with some, the potential for drug abuse,
- placing the responsibility for change on the drug, not on the individual, and
- frequent resumption of former eating patterns after discontinuation of the drug.

Behavioral Change

The eating habits of an obese individual have been shown to be influenced by external stimuli to a greater degree than by internal appetite-regulating mechanisms. (10, 11) The assumption that eating is a learned response to a stimulus in the environment is the basis for using behavioral change strategies in the treatment of obesity. (12, 13) Therapy is designed to teach the individual to alter external cues or to alter response to external cues to control food intake and body weight.

Behavioral change strategies include four elements (13):

Determination and description of the behaviors to be controlled. A food intake diary is kept for one or two weeks during which time the individual makes no changes in eating behavior. The diary includes recording the amount and type of food eaten, time, location, with whom the food was eaten, and emotional state before and after eating (Table 24-1). The diary is evaluated by a trained health professional with the individual, and behaviors to be changed are identified.

Control of the stimuli preceding eating. Easy availability of high-calorie snacks in the home, television viewing, and opening the refrigerator are examples of stimuli that may precede eating. Limiting the amount of high-calorie foods in the house, having low-calorie snacks prepared, engaging in no other activities while eating, and eating only in one designated place are methods to control stimuli.

Development of tactics to control the act of eating. Examples of tactics to control the act of eating are slowing down eating pace by putting the fork down between bites, counting chews, and not preparing another bite until the preceding has been swallowed.

Establishment of an appropriate reward system. A reward system is developed to provide immediate positive reinforcement to the individual for making appropriate behavioral change. This could be a point system, whereby a given number of points are earned for making positive changes. These points can be redeemed for a tangible reward that the individual values. The rewards must be valued by the individual to be effective.

Making permanent behavioral changes requires dedication and hours of conscientious hard work. Long-term follow-up is needed to determine if behavioral change therapy truly does help individuals to make the permanent changes in eating habits that will enable them to maintain their weight loss. (14) Assistance in making behavioral changes for weight reduction may be obtained from recommended texts, psychiatrists, psychologists, or social workers with training in behavior modification techniques.

Increasing Energy Expenditure

Exercise is an important element in the treatment of obesity. Physiologically, exercise included in weight reduction regimens has been shown to increase weight loss, increase fat loss, decrease loss of lean body weight, decrease energy intake, and possibly increase the caloric cost of food eaten. (15–19) Psychologically, exercise may decrease tension and stress, decrease the desire to eat excessively, and increase self-concept. (19)

Overweight individuals should increase caloric expenditure by increasing their daily activity. They should begin with familiar activities that are pleasurable and do not cause excessive discomfort or fatigue. Examples are walking instead of riding in a car, climbing stairs rather than taking the elevator, and pushing rather than sitting on a lawnmower. Refer to Table 23-5 for the energy expenditures for specific activities.

Before embarking on an exercise program involving major increases in physical activity, sedentary individuals with increased risk factors for coronary heart disease and individuals over age 35 should be evaluated by a physician. (20) The evaluation should include a thorough physical exam and may include a supervised stress test to determine starting and target intensities of the exercise program. (17, 21) If the physician is unable to do exercise stress testing with prescription, referrals can be made to an exercise stress laboratory. For example, at University Hospital exercise stress testing is available at the Center for Fitness and Development, Central Campus Recreation Building, University of Michigan or the Work Performance Laboratory, University Hospital, University of Michigan.

Decreasing Energy Intake

A diet history or food diary is evaluated to determine inappropriate eating behavior. The dietitian and client will identify what changes are needed and how they can be made. A diet pattern is planned considering sound nutritional principles, the individual's current eating habits, and behavioral changes acceptable.

A calorie level is established between the dietitian and the client. The calorie level should be low enough so the individual loses weight but does not become nutrient depleted, ill, or discouraged. A maximum loss of 2 lb/wk is suggested. Calorie-restricted diets should be carefully evaluated for nutrient adequacy. Vitamin and mineral supplements may be indicated, especially for individuals consuming fewer than 1200 kcal/day.

Many different diets may be used for weight reduction. A safe weight reduction diet for adults (22)

- Results in a weight loss of an average of 1–2 lb/wk. Greater weight loss may result in undesirable loss of body fluid and lean muscle mass rather than body fat.
- Contains at least 1200 kcal/day. It is difficult to consume adequate amounts of the essential nutrients on less than 1200 kcal/day.
- Contains a wide variety of foods from the four food groups to ensure an adequate intake of all nutrients.

A safe weight reduction diet *does not*

- Rely on one or two foods or food groups only,
- Make cure-all claims,
- Recommend doses of vitamins or minerals greater than the recommended dietary allowances,
- Recommend self-diagnosis, or
- Use testimonials as the only proof of effectiveness.

Weight reduction diet patterns may be developed utilizing one of the following food systems:

Basic four food groups. The diet pattern is based on the basic four food groups with an emphasis on the lower-calorie and lower-fat foods. Total calories equal about 1200 kcal/day if only the recommended amounts are used (Table 24-2).

Basic four food groups and calorie-counting books. The individual is instructed to use the guidelines of the basic four food groups and to add up the calories so the total day's intake equals a specified calorie level. To ensure the selection of a balanced diet using sound nutritional principles, calorie counting alone is discouraged.

Diabetic food exchange system. Refer to Chapter 25 for guidelines for calculation of the diet and the food exchange system. Table 24-3 lists the exchange value of some combination foods appropriate for use in weight reduction programs.

Weight control food exchange system. The procedure for calculating the diet follows the same steps as the procedure for calculating the diabetic diet (Chapter 25). Careful distribution of food throughout the day is not necessary but may improve adherence to the diet.

NUTRIENT ADEQUACY

Nutrient adequacy of weight reduction diets will depend upon the level of energy restriction and the food choices made by the individual. All energy-restricted diets should be evaluated for nutritional adequacy. Vitamin and mineral supplements are indicated for diets below 1200 kcal/day and may be indicated at higher calorie levels depending upon individual nutrient requirements and food choices.

TABLES

TABLE 24-1. Food Intake Diary to Identify Potential Behavioral Changes

	Food Eaten		Location[2] and Concurrent Activity			Mood[4]	
Time[1]	Item	Amount		With Whom	Physical Position[3]	Before Eating	After Eating

[1] Circle time if food is part of a meal.
[2] Living room, watching TV, etc.
[3] Sitting, standing, lying, etc.
[4] Happy, bored, tired, satisfied, etc.

TABLE 24-2. Guidelines for Use of Basic Four Food Groups in Weight Reduction Diet Programs

Food Group	Servings per Day	Foods Allowed	Foods to Avoid
Milk and calcium equivalents	2 cups	Skim, 1%, or low-fat milk; low-fat plain yogurt; buttermilk	Whole or 2% milk; chocolate milk or cocoa; milkshakes or malts; half and half, cream
Meat and protein equivalents	4 ounces cooked	Lean meat, fish, or poultry; substitutes for 1 ounce of meat are 1 ounce cheese ¼ cup cottage cheese ¼ cup tuna or salmon 1 egg ½ cup cooked dried peas or beans	High-fat meats; bacon, spareribs, sausage, cold cuts; fried meats, poultry, and fish; peanut butter
Fruit and vegetable	4 1 serving: ½ cup cooked or juice 1 cup raw 1 piece medium size whole fruit	Fresh, frozen, or canned items as long as they are not sweetened or served with fats or sauces	Sweetened fruits; vegetables in butter sauce, au gratin, or other sauces; deep-fried vegetables
Grain	4 1 serving: 1 slice bread 1 dinner roll ½ cup rice or noodles ½ cup cereal 1½ cups popcorn	Bread, dinner rolls, bagels, biscuits, plain muffins; rice, noodles, or spaghetti; plain hot or cold cereals; plain popcorn	Sugar-coated cereals; sweet breads; pastries
Other			
Fat	3 1 serving: 1 teaspoon butter, margarine, mayonnaise 1 tablespoon salad dressing	Butter, margarine; salad dressings; oils, shortening (be sure to count all fats used in cooking)	Gravy; rich sauces
Miscellaneous		1 tablespoon per day of catsup, chili sauce, steak sauce, soy sauce, or Worchestershire sauce; sugarless gum; sugar-free pop; sugar-free gelatin	Pie, cake, other desserts; candy; soda pop; other high-sugar and/or high-fat foods

TABLE 24-3. Combination Foods

Food Item	Amount (serving size)	Exchange Group and Value
Beer	12 ounces	1 bread + 2 fat
Biscuit, 2 in. diameter[1]	1	1 bread + 1 fat
Cheese[1]	1 ounce	1 meat + 1 fat
Chili, with beans, beef	½ cup	1 bread + 1 meat
Chow mein noodles[1]	½ cup	1 bread + 1 fat
Chop suey	1 cup	1 bread + 1 meat
Corn bread[1]	2 in. × 2 in. × 1 in.	1 bread + 1 fat
Crackers, round butter[1] type 1½ in. diameter	5	1 bread + 1 fat
Distilled liquors		
80 proof	1½ ounces	2 fats
100 proof	1½ ounces	3 fats
Dried beans and peas, cooked (including garbanzo, kidney, lima, navy, pinto, and soybeans, lentils, split peas)	½ cup	1 bread + 1 meat
French fries (2 in. × 3½ in.)[1]	8	1 bread + 1 fat
Hot dogs[1]	1 ounce	1 meat + 1 fat
Luncheon meats[1]	1 ounce	1 meat + 1 fat
Muffin[1], plain, small	1	1 bread + 1 fat
Pancake, 5½ in. diameter[1]	1	1 bread + 1 fat
Peanut butter	2 tablespoons	1 meat + 2 fat
Pizza[1]	3 in. × 4 in. rectangle	1 bread + 1 fat + 1 meat
Potato chips[1]	12	1 bread + 2 fat
Ice cream[1]	½ cup	1 bread + 2 fat
Ice milk[1]	½ cup	1 bread + 1 fat
Stuffing (dressing)	⅓ cup	1 bread + 1 fat
Sunflower seeds	½ cup	½ bread + 1 meat + 3 fat
Wheat germ	3 tablespoons	1 bread + 1 meat + 1 fat
Wine, dry	3½ ounces	1½ fat

[1] For a prudent diet, limit or omit these food items (Chapter 10).

REFERENCES CITED

1. Van Itallie, T. B. 1979. Obesity: Adverse effects on health and longevity. *Am. J. Clin. Nutr.* 32:2723.
2. Bray, G. A. 1976. The overweight patient. In *Advances in internal medicine,* ed., G. H. Stollerman. Vol. 21, pp. 267–308. Chicago: Yearbook Medical Publisher.
3. Kannel, W. B.; Gordon, T.; and Castelli, W. P. 1979. Obesity, lipids, and glucose intolerance: The Framingham study. *Am. J. Clin. Nutr.* 32:1238.
4. Rimm, A. A.; Werner, L. H.; Van Yserloo, B.; and Bernstein, R. A. 1975. Relationship of obesity and disease in 73,532 weight-conscious women. *Public Health Reports* 90:44.
5. Reisen, E.; Abel, R.; Modan, M.; Silverberg, D. S.; Eliahou, H. E.; and Modan, B. 1978. Effect of weight loss without salt restriction on the reduction of blood pressure in overweight hypertensive patients. *N. Eng. J. Med.* 298:1.
6. Olefsky, J.; Reaven, G. M.; and Farquhar, J. W. 1974. Effects of weight reduction on obesity. *J. Clin. Invest.* 53:64.
7. Bray, G. A. 1976. Drug therapy for the obese patient. In *The obese patient,* pp. 353–410. Philadelphia: W. B. Saunders.
8. Craddock, D. 1976. Anorectic drugs: Use in general practice. *Drugs* 11:378.
9. Sullivan, A. C., and Comai, K. 1978. Pharmacological treatment of obesity. *Int. J. Obesity* 2:167.
10. Schachter, S., and Gross, L. P. 1968. Manipulated time and eating behavior. *J. Personal. and Soc. Psych.* 10:98.
11. Nisbett, R. E. 1968. Taste, deprivation, and weight determinants of eating behavior. *J. Personal. and Soc. Psych.* 10:107.
12. Stuart, R. B., and Davis, B. 1972. *Slim chance in a fat world: Behavior control of obesity.* Champaign, Ill.: Research Press.
13. Stunkard, A. J. 1975. Presidential address—1974: From explanation to action in psychosomatic medicine: The case of obesity. *Psychosom. Med.* 37:195.
14. Mahoney, M. J. 1978. Behavior modification in the treatment of obesity. *Psych. Clinics N. Am.* 1:651.
15. Bray, G. A.; Whipp, B. J.; and Koyal, S. N. 1974. The acute effects of food intake on energy expenditure during cycle ergometry. *Am. J. Clin. Nutr.* 27:254.
16. Johnson, R. E.; Mastropaolo, J. A.; and Wharton, M. A. 1972. Exercise, dietary intake, and body composition. *J. Am. Dietet. A.* 61:399.
17. Kenrick, M. M.; Ball, M. F.; and Canary, J. J. 1972. Exercise and weight reduction in obesity. *Arch. Phys. Med. Rehab.* 53:323.
18. Mayer, J.; Roy, P.; and Mitra, K. P. 1959. Relation between caloric intake, body weight, and physical work: Studies in an industrial male population in West Bengal. *Am. J. Clin. Nutr.* 4:169.
19. Stuart, R. B. 1975. Exercise prescription in weight management: Advantages, techniques and obstacles. *Obesity/Bariatric Med.* 4:16.
20. The Committee on Exercise, American Heart Association. 1972. *Exercise testing and training of apparently healthy individuals. A handbook for physicians.* Dallas, Tex.: American Heart Association.
21. Wilmore, J. H., and Haskell, W. L. 1971. Use of the heart rate–energy expenditure relationship in the individualized prescription of exercise. *Am. J. Clin. Nutr.* 24:1186.
22. Michigan Department of Public Health. 1979. *Want to lose weight? Do it safely.* Lansing, Mich.: Bureau of Personal Health Services, Department of Public Health.

OTHER REFERENCES

Bruch, H. 1973. *Eating disorders. Obesity, anorexia nervosa, and the person within.* New York: Basic Books.

Nash, J. D., and Long, L. O. 1978. *Taking charge of your weight and well-being. Leader's guide.* Palo Alto, Calif.: Bull Publishing.

PAULSEN, B. K.; LUTZ, R. N.; MCREYNOLDS, W. T.; and KOHRS, M. B. 1976. Behavior therapy for weight control: Long-term results of two programs with nutritionists as therapists. *Am. J. Clin. Nutr.* 29:880.

WATSON, D. L., and THARP, R. G. 1977. *Self-directed behavior: Self-modification for personal adjustment.* 2nd ed. Monterey, Calif.: Brooks/Cole Publishing.

RECOMMENDED REFERENCES FOR THE LAY PUBLIC

BEHAVIORAL CHANGE

JORDAN, H. A.; LEVITZ, L. S.; and KIMBRELL, G. M. 1976. *Eating is okay!* New York: Signet.

LINDNER, P. G. 1976. *Mind over platter.* North Hollywood, Calif.: Wilshire Book Co.

NASH, J. D., and LONG, L. O. 1978. *Taking charge of your weight and well-being.* Palo Alto, Calif.: Bull Publishing.

PLOEGER, J. 1977. *Day by day.* Port Huron, Mich.: Slim Living.

STUART, R. B., and DAVIS, B. 1972. *Slim chance in a fat world: Behavior control of obesity.* Champaign, Ill.: Research Press.

STUART, R. B. 1978. *Act thin, stay thin.* New York: W. W. Norton.

INCREASING ENERGY EXPENDITURE

KONISHI, F. 1975. *Exercise equivalents of foods: A practical guide for the overweight.* Carbondale: Southern Illinois U. P.

SMITH, N. J. 1976. *Food for sport.* Palo Alto, Calif.: Bull Publishing.

Adult physical fitness. No. 027G, Consumer Information Catalogue, Spring 1979. Pueblo, Colorado 81009.

Exercise and weight control. No. 029G, Consumer Information Catalogue, Spring 1979. Pueblo, Colorado 81009.

An introduction to physical fitness. No. 032G, Consumer Information Catalogue, Spring 1979. Pueblo, Colorado 81009.

DECREASING ENERGY INTAKE

BERLAND, T., and the editors of *Consumer Guide.* 1979. *Rating the diets.* New York: Beekman House.

Food and your weight. No. 025G, Consumer Information Catalogue, Spring 1979. Pueblo, Colorado 81009.

MAYER, J. 1975. *A diet for living.* New York: Pocket Books.

Michigan Department of Public Health. 1979. *Want to lose weight? Do it safely.* Lansing: Bureau of Personal Health Services, Michigan Department of Public Health.

Metropolitan Life Insurance Company, Health & Welfare Division. *Metropolitan Life's four steps to weight control.* New York: Metropolitan Life.

Weight Watchers International, Inc. Booklets on weight control available from Weight Watchers International, 800 Community Drive, Manhasset, N.Y. 11030.

Tomer, J., and Corvi, P. 1981. *Meal planning for weight control.* Ann Arbor, Mi.: Department of Dietetics, University Hospital, University of Michigan.

WEIGHT REDUCTION ORGANIZATIONS FOR THE LAY PUBLIC

Slim Living, Jo Ann Ploeger, 3605 Strawberry Lane, Port Huron, Mich. 48060

Overeaters Anonymous, World Service Office, 3730 Motor Ave., Los Angeles, Calif. 90034

Weight Watchers International, Inc., 800 Community Drive, Manhasset, N.Y. 11030

TOPS Club, Inc., P.O. Box 07489, Milwaukee, Wisc. 53207

25

Diabetes Mellitus

INDICATIONS FOR USE

This diet is indicated for adults with diabetes mellitus. For individuals under 18 years of age with diabetes mellitus, refer to Chapter 54. Diagnosis is confirmed by fasting plasma glucose levels greater than or equal to 140 mg/100 ml on more than one occasion, or overt diabetic symptoms and hyperglycemia, or an abnormal glucose tolerance test. (1) Diabetes has many causes; in most cases the cause is unknown. Genetic and environmental factors play important roles in the etiology of diabetes. Diabetes may also occur secondary to many conditions including destruction of the pancreas by disease or surgery, certain endocrine disorders, drug administration including steroids and thiazides, and hereditary neuromuscular disorders. (1)

DESCRIPTION

Diabetes mellitus is a disorder of metabolism associated with a relative or absolute insufficiency of insulin and is characterized by hyperglycemia and glycosuria. In the normal individual, the beta cells of the pancreas release insulin in response to the rise in blood glucose levels that follows the digestion and absorption of food. Insulin facilitates the transport of glucose from the blood into the cells where glucose is used as the major source of energy. In diabetes mellitus, a lack of insulin or resistance to the insulin produced causes glucose to accumulate in the blood resulting in hyperglycemia. Glucosuria results when the renal threshold for glucose has been exceeded. The two main types of diabetes mellitus are insulin-dependent diabetes mellitus and noninsulin-dependent diabetes mellitus. These two types are compared in Table 25-1.

Dietary management is necessary for control of all types of diabetes mellitus. Control of plasma glucose levels requires a balance of food intake, insulin, and exercise. Food intake provides glucose from digestion of carbohydrates, protein, and fats; insulin and exercise facilitate glucose removal from the blood into the cells. The goals of diet therapy are to (2)

- Reach and maintain ideal body weight by provision of an appropriate level of energy, including sufficient calories for normal growth and development.
- Prevent hyper- and hypoglycemia by maintaining plasma glucose at a level as near the normal physiologic range as possible.
- Maintain or improve overall health by providing a nutritionally adequate diet.
- Prevent or delay the development or progression of complications of diabetes to the extent that they are related to metabolic control.
- Modify the diet as necessary for the treatment of existing cardiovascular, renal, and other complications of diabetes and for the treatment of associated diseases.

The translation of these goals into recommendations for dietary management requires flexibility. The physician, dietitian, and individual with diabetes must work together to develop a realistic diet plan. (3) Individual personality, life-style, physical condition, and diabetic state must be considered. The diet plan must be reviewed periodically and adjusted for changes in energy requirements, life-style, and physical condition. If renal, cardiovascular, or other complications develop, appropriate changes in diet therapy must be made.

Education of the individual with diabetes and significant family members is essential. Knowledge of the nature of diabetes; the relationship of food to medication, illness, exercise, and health; the nutrient composition of food; food selection and preparation; and the daily meal plan—all are necessary for the individual to take responsibility for his or her own care. *The use of preprinted diet plan handouts does not fulfill the need for individualization and education and is not acceptable.*

GUIDELINES FOR NUTRITIONAL MANAGEMENT

The following guidelines for nutritional management are based on recommendations of the American Diabetes Association (ADA). (2)

General guidelines for dietary management of individuals with diabetes

Composition of the diet. For most individuals with diabetes mellitus, a nutritionally adequate normal diet with the elimination of refined glucose and refined glucose-containing disaccharides (sucrose, lactose) is satisfactory. Protein should be sufficient to meet the recommended dietary allowances and usually contributes 12–20% of total energy intake. Carbohydrate, with emphasis on complex carbohydrate and dietary fiber, should provide approximately 50–60% of total energy intake. The remainder of energy intake comes from fat. A lower carbohydrate intake may be indicated for those individuals with endogenous hypertriglyceridemia, as triglyceride levels may be sensitive to increases in dietary carbohydrate. (4)

Dietary fat. Because of the relationship of diabetes mellitus to hyperlipidemia and atherosclerosis, a diet limited in saturated fat and cholesterol and with increased polyunsaturated fat is recommended. (2, 5) The ADA exchange lists were designed to encourage these modifications. If specific levels of fat and cholesterol are desired, they should be specified by the physician. (6)

Sugars and sweeteners. Refined glucose (dextrose) and refined glucose-containing disaccharides (sucrose, lactose) are restricted in the diet to prevent the peak in blood glucose level that follows glucose ingestion. (2, 7) The long-term effects of fructose, xylitol, sorbitol, and mannitol on plasma glucose control and on metabolism in diabetes have not been well studied. (2, 7) At University Hospital, use of these nutritive sweeteners is restricted; nonnutritive sweeteners are used. This policy may be modified when necessary to comply with further recommendations of the ADA.

Dietary fiber. There is evidence that increased intake of dietary fiber in the diet results in lower postmeal plasma glucose, decreased glycosuria, and decreased insulin requirement. (8, 9) Wherever acceptable to the individual with diabetes, natural foods containing unrefined carbohydrate and dietary fiber should be substituted for highly refined carbohydrates low in dietary fiber. (2) For the individual treated with insulin, where it is important for the composition of the diet to be consistent from day to day, changes in fiber content may require insulin adjustment and should be brought to the attention of the physician.

Alcohol. With the approval of the responsible physician, alcohol may be planned into the diet with the following considerations (3, 6):

- Alcohol should be used only when diabetes is well controlled.
- Alcohol should only be consumed along with food.
- Sweet wines, liquors, and mixed drinks should be avoided.
- Alcohol provides calories without other nutrients and stimulates appetite; thus it may not be appropriate on weight reduction programs.
- In fasting insulin-treated individuals, consumption of large amounts of alcohol may precipitate hypoglycemia. If symptoms are attributed to intoxication, the hypoglycemia will not be recognized.

Guidelines for individuals with diabetes receiving insulin therapy

Daily consistency. A standardized regimen of food intake is necessary for effective insulin treatment. Consistency of energy intake, composition of the diet, and timing of meals on a day-to-day basis are the most important elements of therapy. To best ensure consistency, the diet must be individualized and planned only after a thorough diet history has been obtained.

Energy intake. Total energy intake should be controlled and set at a level to achieve and/or maintain ideal body weight. Sufficient calories for regular exercise should be included in the diet plan. Variations in exercise will require adjustments in energy intake.

Timing of meals. Meals should be planned so that a consistent intake can be achieved on a day-to-day basis. As much as possible, timing of meals should be based on preexisting meal patterns, taking into consideration working hours, scheduled breaks, and family mealtimes. Three well-balanced meals plus scheduled snacks, particularly at bedtime, are encouraged to distribute food intake throughout the day. The wide range of available insulin preparations and treatment programs generally enable the physician to prescribe an insulin program that is individualized to the preexisting life-style. Table 25-2 summarizes the action of various types of insulin.

Exercise. In the patient with diabetes, exercise tends to lower serum glucose levels. To prevent hypoglycemia, the insulin-treated individual should eat a snack before exercise that has not been accounted for in the daily meal pattern. The amount of food that will be required to maintain plasma glucose levels will depend on the individual and the duration and intensity of the exercise.

Diet during illness. When the insulin-treated individual is ill and cannot tolerate solid foods, carbohydrate, generally in liquid form, is provided to prevent hypoglycemic reactions. The amount of carbohydrate planned in the original diet is provided. Refer to Table 25-3 for the carbohydrate content of liquids. Use of foods or fluids containing refined sugars generally not included in the diet may be appropriate to prevent hypoglycemia. (3)

Guidelines for obese individuals with diabetes not receiving insulin therapy

Weight reduction. The primary goal of diet therapy in obese, noninsulin-treated diabetics is the achievement and maintenance of ideal body weight. For obese individuals, reduction in adiposity improves sensitivity to insulin and improves glucose tolerance. (11–13) The composition of the diet and timing of meals are less important than the reduction in total calorie intake. Rate of weight loss is recommended at 1–2 lb (0.5–0.9 kg)/wk. Energy levels of less than 1000 kcal/day should be used only with close medical supervision. The diabetic diet or weight reduction diet (Chapter 24) may be used for meal planning. Exercise is an important element in the weight reduction program as it both increases energy expenditure and improves glucose tolerance. (14)

Calculation of the diabetic diet. The diet is calculated using the diabetic food exchange system listed in Tables 25-4 and 25-5. The current revision of the food exchange system was printed by the American Diabetes Association, the American Dietetic Association, and the National Institutes of Health. *A Guide for Professionals: The Effective Application of "Exchange Lists for Meal Planning"* provides guidelines. (5) At University Hospital the food exchange system has been modified slightly.

The procedure for calculating a diabetic diet is as follows:

Steps	***Example***
1. Review medical history; include Anthropometric data Stage of diabetes Medications, insulin schedule Complications Other diseases present Frequency of insulin reactions Frequency of ketoacidosis	FEMALE: 25 yr old HEIGHT: 66 in. (167 cm) WEIGHT: 130 lb (59 kg) DIABETIC STATE: newly diagnosed, insulin dependent
2. Review life-style and dietary history; include Daily pattern of eating Use of dietary nutrient supplements Work schedule Exercise pattern Sleep habits Dietary and schedule changes on weekends, vacation, special days Use of alcohol Who is responsible for shopping for and preparing food Intake of sugars, sweets, fats	WORK SCHEDULE: sedentary job, 8–5, 1-hr lunch, two 15-min breaks SLEEP SCHEDULE: generally 11:00–6:30, weekends variable EATING PATTERN (simplified from diet history): BREAKFAST: juice, ½ cup; cereal and "low-fat" milk MORNING SNACK: coffee and donut LUNCH: cheese sandwich and fruit AFTERNOON SNACK: coffee SUPPER: meat, potato, and other vegetable or casserole, salad, low-fat milk EVENING SNACK: ice cream or popcorn ALCOHOL: occasional weekend use WEEKENDS: no breakfast, large lunch, supper in restaurant EXERCISE PATTERN: volleyball once a week; walking ½–1 hr/day

3. Determine if individual is at acceptable weight (Chapter 23).

Weight is acceptable

4. Determine energy requirement (Chapter 23).

130 lb × 14 kcal/lb = 1820 kcal

5. Determine approximate distribution of calories among carbohydrate, protein, and fat. Fifty per cent carbohydrate, 20% protein, and 30% fat are used as guidelines. Individual adjustments may be made.

Carbohydrate:
.50 × 1800 kcal = 900 kcal

Protein:
.20 × 1800 kcal = 360 kcal

Fat:
.30 × 1800 kcal = 540 kcal

6. Determine the grams of carbohydrate, protein, and fat to be included in diet:

CARBOHYDRATE, 4 kcal/g
PROTEIN, 4 kcal/g
FAT, 9 kcal/g

Carbohydrate:

$$\frac{900 \text{ kcal}}{4 \text{ kcal/g}} = 225 \text{ g}$$

Protein:

$$\frac{360 \text{ kcal}}{4 \text{ kcal/g}} = 90 \text{ g}$$

Fat:

$$\frac{540 \text{ kcal}}{9 \text{ kcal/g}} = 60 \text{ g}$$

7. Determine the number of exchanges desired from the milk, fruit, and vegetable groups. Identify the milk group as skim, 2% or whole. Determine the carbohydrate contributed by these groups using Table 25-4.

Food Exchange Groups	No. Exchanges	Carbohydrate (g)	Protein (g)	Fat (g)
Milk, skim	2	24	16	—
Fruit	3	30	—	—
Vegetable	2	10	4	—
Bread				
Meat, L–M fat[1]				
Meat, H-fat[2]				
Fat				
Total		64		

[1] L–M = Lean–medium.
[2] H = high.

8. Provide the remainder of the carbohydrate as bread exchanges.

One bread exchange:
15 g carbohydrate

Carbohydrate remaining:
225 g − 64 g = 161 g

$$\frac{161 \text{ g}}{15 \text{ g/exchange}} \cong 11 \text{ Bread exchanges}$$

9. Determine the protein provided by these food groups.

Food Exchange Groups	No. Exchanges	Carbohydrate (g)	Protein (g)	Fat (g)
Milk, skim	2	24	16	—
Fruit	3	30	—	—
Vegetable	2	10	4	—
Bread	11	165	22	—
Meat, L–M fat				
Meat, H-fat				
Fat				
Total		229	42	

10. Provide the remainder of the protein as meat exchanges.

Protein remaining:
90 g − 42 g = 48 g

One meat exchange:
7 g protein

$$\frac{48\text{ g}}{7\text{ g/exchange}} \cong 7 \text{ Meat exchanges}$$

Designate number of exchanges to come from lean–medium and high-fat meat groups.

5 exchanges from lean–medium fat meat group
2 exchanges from high-fat meat group

11. Determine the fat provided by these food groups.

Food Exchange Groups	No. Exchanges	Carbohydrate (g)	Protein (g)	Fat (g)
Milk, skim	2	24	16	—
Fruit	3	30	—	—
Vegetable	2	10	4	—
Bread	11	165	22	—
Meat, L–M fat	5	—	35	25
Meat, H-fat	2	—	14	16
Fat				
Total		229	91	41

12. Provide the remainder of the fat as fat exchanges.

Fat remaining:
60 g − 41 g = 19 g

One fat exchange:
5 g fat

$$\frac{19\text{ g}}{5\text{ g/exchange}} \cong 4 \text{ Fat exchanges}$$

13. Determine if desired carbohydrate, protein, fat, and calorie levels have been achieved. Adjust if necessary.

Food Exchange Groups	No. Exchanges	Carbohydrate (g)	Protein (g)	Fat (g)	kcal
Milk, skim	2	24	16	—	160
Fruit	3	30	—	—	120
Vegetable	2	10	4	—	56
Bread	11	165	22	—	748
Meat, L–M fat	5	—	35	25	365
Meat, H-fat	2	—	14	16	200
Fat	4	—	—	20	180
Total		229	91	61	1829
Diet prescription		225	90	60	1820

14. Distribute food between meals and snacks.

    Suggested:
    2/10–4/10 at each meal; 1/10 at snacks. (5)

Food Exchange Groups	Total for Day	Breakfast	sn[1]	Lunch	Supper	sn
Milk, skim	2	1			1	
Fruit	3	1		2		
Vegetable	2				2	
Bread	11	2	1	3	3	2
Meat, L–M fat	5				4	1
Meat, H-fat	2			2		
Fat	4			1	2	1

sn[1] = Snack.

NUTRIENT ADEQUACY

Actual nutrient intake depends upon the calorie level of the diet and the individual's appetite, preferences, and ability to eat. At calorie levels planned for weight reduction, the diet will need to be assessed for nutritional adequacy. Vitamin and mineral supplements may be indicated.

University Hospital procedures

Establishing nutritional care. When an individual has been identified as having diabetes mellitus, the dietitian will see that person as soon as possible to obtain a diet history and assess nutritional status, activity level, and living schedule. From this information, a desirable level of caloric intake and an individualized diet pattern are established together with the physician and the patient.

Prior to the dietitian's contact with the individual, meals will be provided according to the following criteria:

1. *"House diabetic" diet prescribed.* For individuals receiving insulin, a 1500 kcal diet is provided; carbohydrate is divided between three meals and an evening snack in a 3/10 : 3/10 : 3/10 : 1/10 distribution.

   For individuals not receiving insulin, a 1500 kcal diet is provided; carbohydrate is divided among three meals in a 1/3 : 1/3 : 1/3 distribution.

2. *Specific calorie level prescribed.* For individuals receiving insulin, a diet at the prescribed calorie level; initially carbohydrate is provided; carbohydrate is divided between three meals and an evening snack in a 3/10 : 3/10 : 3/10 : 1/10 distribution.

   For individuals not receiving insulin; a diet at the prescribed calorie level is provided; initially carbohydrate is divided between three meals in a 1/3 : 1/3 : 1/3 distribution.

3. *Liquid diets.* When a clear liquid diet is ordered for the diabetic patient, a clear liquid meal is provided with a carbohydrate content equal to the glucose equivalents calculated for that meal in the diet pattern. Refer to Table 25-3 for carbohydrate content of liquids.

   Glucose equivalents are the approximate percentages of the nutrients that are expected to be converted to glucose after digestion. They are (15)

carbohydrate	100%
protein	50%
fat	10%

Example:

Planned meal	Glucose equivalents
70 g carbohydrate × 100%	70 g
32 g protein × 50%	16 g
30 g fat × 10%	3 g
Total	89 g

A meal of clear liquids would be planned containing approximately 89 g carbohydrate.

When a full liquid diet is ordered, a liquid meal is provided with carbohydrate, protein, and fat content equal to the equivalent meal in the diet plan.

When the individual receiving insulin is to be on a liquid diet for an extended period of time, adjustment of insulin dosage and diet pattern may be necessary.

Monitoring and replacement of food intake. All diabetic inpatients receiving insulin are monitored for food intake following each meal. If more than 7 g of carbohydrate is not eaten at any one meal it is replaced with an equivalent amount of carbohydrate in a form acceptable to the individual. If significant amounts of protein and fat also remain uneaten, foods such as milk or custard, which contain protein and fat along with the carbohydrate, are offered as replacements. The nutrient intake is recorded daily in the medical record.

TABLES

TABLE 25-1. Comparison of Insulin-Dependent Diabetes Mellitus and Noninsulin-Dependent Diabetes Mellitus (1)

Characteristics	Insulin-Dependent Diabetes Mellitus	Noninsulin-Dependent Diabetes Mellitus
Age at onset	Usually in youth but may occur at any age	Usually over 40 but may occur at any age
Type of onset	Abrupt	Gradual
Nutritional status at onset	Generally recent weight loss	60–90% are obese
Symptoms	Polyuria, polydypsia, ketonuria, weight loss	Minimal or none
Defect	Lack of insulin	May be hyperinsulinemic and insulin resistant
Ketosis prone	Yes	No
Treatment	Insulin and diet	Diet; diet and oral hypoglycemic drugs; diet and insulin for control of hyperglycemia

TABLE 25-2. Summary of Action of Insulins (10)

Type	Action	Peak Action (hr)	Duration (hr)
Regular	Rapid	1–2	5–6
Semilente[R]	Rapid	1–2	12–16
NPH	Intermediate	2–8	24–28
Lente[R]	Intermediate	2–8	24–28
Ultralente[R1]	Long acting	8–14	36
Protamine Zinc[1]	Long acting	8–14	36

[1] Less frequently used.

TABLE 25-3. Carbohydrate Content of Liquids Used During Illness That Precludes Ingestion of Solid Foods

Food Item	Amount (serving size)	Carbohydrate (g)
Carbonated beverage, regular, not diet	½ cup	10
Orange juice	½ cup	10
Apple or pineapple juice	⅓ cup	10
Grape or prune juice	¼ cup	10
Milk	1 cup	12
Ice cream, vanilla	½ cup	15
Cereal, cooked	½ cup	15
Jello, regular	½ cup	20
Sherbet	½ cup	30
Popsicle	1	30
Sugar	1 teaspoon	5
Coffee, tea, bouillon, broth	1 cup	0
Soup, thin cream	1 cup	15
Soup, thick cream	1 cup	30
Fruit exchange	See exchange group	10
Bread exchange	See exchange group	15

TABLE 25-4. Nutrient Content of One Exchange, Diabetic Food Exchange System

Food Exchange Group	Carbohydrate (g)	Protein (g)	Fat (g)	kcal
Milk				
Skim	12	8	—	80
2%	12	8	5	125
Whole	12	8	10	170
Vegetable	5	2	—	28
Fruit	10	—	—	40
Bread	15	2	—	68
Meat				
Lean–medium fat	—	7	5	73
High fat	—	7	8	100
Fat				
Unsaturated	—	—	5	45
Saturated	—	—	5	45
Free	—	—	—	—

TABLE 25-5. Diabetic Food Exchange System

Group	Food Item		One Exchange (serving size)
Milk	Skim milk, nonfat milk		1 cup
	Buttermilk made from skim milk		1 cup
	Skim milk powder		$\frac{1}{3}$ cup
	Evaporated skim milk, before adding water		$\frac{1}{2}$ cup
	Milk, $\frac{1}{2}$% butterfat		1 cup
	Milk, 1% butterfat		1 cup
	Milk, 2% butterfat		1 cup
	Yogurt, plain, lowfat		1 cup
	Whole milk		1 cup
	Buttermilk, made from whole milk		1 cup
	Evaporated whole milk, before adding water		$\frac{1}{2}$ cup
	Yogurt, plain		1 cup
Vegetable	Alfalfa sprouts	Mushrooms	$\frac{1}{2}$ cup cooked or raw
	Artichoke	Okra	
	Asparagus	Onions	
	Bamboo shoots	Pea pods	
	Bean sprouts	Pepper, green and pimiento	
	Beans, string, green, or wax	Pickles, unsweetened	
	Beets	Rhubarb	
	Broccoli	Rutabaga	
	Brussels sprouts	Sauerkraut	
	Cabbage	Squash, summer	
	Carrots	Tomatoes	
	Cauliflower	Tomato juice	
	Celery	Tomato sauce, unsweetened	
	Chard	Turnips	
	Cucumber	Vegetable juice	
	Eggplant	Zucchini	
	Kohlrabi		
	Greens: beet, collard, dandelion, kale, mustard, spinach, turnip		
Miscellaneous vegetables	Mixed vegetables		$\frac{1}{3}$ cup
	Tomato catsup		1 tablespoon
	Tomato paste		2 tablespoons
	Tomato puree		$\frac{1}{4}$ cup
	Water chestnuts		4
Free vegetables	Chicory	Lettuce	As desired
	Chinese cabbage	Parsley	
	Chives	Radishes	
	Endive	Romaine	
	Escarole	Watercress	

[*Continued*]

TABLE 25-5. Diabetic Food Exchange System [*Continued*]

Group	Food Item	One Exchange (serving size)
Fruit	Apple	½ large or 1 small, 2 in.
	Apple juice, cider	⅓ cup (3 ounces)
	Applesauce	½ cup
	Apricots, fresh	2 medium
	Apricots, dried or canned	4 halves
	Banana	3 in. long (½ small)
	Berries	
	Blackberries	½ cup
	Blueberries	½ cup
	Raspberries	½ cup
	Strawberries	¾ cup
	Cantaloupe, 6 in. diameter	¼
	Cherries	10 large or 15 small
	Dates	2 small
	Figs, fresh or dried	1
	Fruit cocktail	½ cup
	Grapefruit	½
	Juice	½ cup (4 ounces)
	Sections	½ cup
	Grapes	12
	Grape juice	¼ cup (2 ounces)
	Guava	½ medium
	Honeydew melon, 6 in. diameter	⅛
	Lemon	1 large
	Lime	1 medium
	Mango	½ small
	Nectarine	1 small
	Orange	1 small
	Juice	½ cup (4 ounces)
	Sections	½ cup
	Papaya	¾ cup
	Peach	1 medium
	Halves	2
	Slices	½ cup
	Pear	½ large or 1 small
	Halves	2 small
	Persimmon	1 medium
	Pineapple	½ cup or 1½ rings
	Juice	⅓ cup (3 ounces)
	Plums	2 medium
	Prunes, dried	2 medium
	Prune juice	¼ cup (2 ounces)
	Raisins	½ ounce or 2 tablespoons
	Rhubarb	1 cup
	Tangerine	1 medium
	Tomato juice	1 cup (8 ounces)
	Watermelon, 3 in. × ½ in. slice	1
	Diced	1 cup

TABLE 25-5. Diabetic Food Exchange System [*Continued*]

Group	Food Item	One Exchange (serving size)
Bread	Breads	
	White	1 slice
	Wheat: whole, cracked	1 slice
	Rye or pumpernickle	1 slice
	Raisin	1 slice
	Other breads	
	Bagel	½
	Bread crumbs, dried	3 tablespoons
	Bread sticks, 8½ in. long	2
	Buns, hamburger or weiner	½ bun
	English muffin, 2 ounces	½ small
	Flat bread, Middle East, 6 in.	½
	Plain roll, bread	1
	Tortilla, 6 in. baked	1
	Crackers	
	Animal	10
	Arrowroot	3
	Graham, 2½ in. square	2
	Matzo, 4 in. × 6 in.	½
	Melba toast	4 slices
	Oyster	20
	Rye wafers, 2 in. × 3½ in.	3
	Saltines, 2 in. square	6
	Soda, 2½ in. square	4
	Cereals, ready-to-eat	
	Bran, bud type	⅓ cup
	Bran Flakes	½ cup
	Grapenuts	¼ cup
	Puffed cereals, unsweetened	1 cup
	Shredded Wheat biscuit	1 large
	Wheat germ (omit 1 fat exchange for each bread exchange used)	¼ cup
	Other "ready-to-eat" unsweetened cereals	¾ cup
	Cereals, cooked	
	Barley, cornmeal, grits, rice, wheat, oatmeal	½ cup
	Flours and thickening agents	
	Arrowroot	2 tablespoons
	Cornmeal, dry	2 tablespoons
	Cornstarch	2 tablespoons
	Flour	2½ tablespoons
	Tapioca, dry	2 tablespoons
	Grains	
	Macaroni, noodles, spaghetti, cooked	½ cup
	Popcorn, popped, no fat added, large kernel	3 cups
	Popcorn, popped, no fat added, regular kernel	1½ cups
	Rice, cooked	½ cup

TABLE 25-5. Diabetic Food Exchange System [*Continued*]

Group	Food Item	One Exchange (serving size)
	Starchy vegetables	
	Corn	$\frac{1}{3}$ cup
	Corn on cob	3 inch ear
	Dried beans and peas, cooked, includes garbanzo, kidney, lima, navy, pinto, soybeans, lentils, and split peas (omit 1 lean–medium fat meat exchange for each bread exchange used)	$\frac{1}{2}$ cup
	Parsnips	$\frac{2}{3}$ cup
	Peas, green	$\frac{1}{2}$ cup
	Potato, white, 2 in. (baked or boiled)	1 small
	Potato, white, mashed	$\frac{1}{2}$ cup
	Pumpkin	$\frac{3}{4}$ cup
	Squash, winter (acorn, butternut)	$\frac{1}{2}$ cup
	Yam or sweet potato	$\frac{1}{4}$ cup
Bread (high fat)[1]	Biscuit, 2 in. diameter	1
	Chow mein noodles	$\frac{1}{2}$ cup
	Corn bread, 2 in. × 2 in. × 1 in.	1 square
	Crackers, round butter type, 1½ in. diameter	5
	Muffin, plain or cornmeal, 2 in. diameter	1
	Potato, French fried, 2 in. to 3½ in. in length	8 pieces
	Pancake, 5 in. × ½ in.	1
	Waffle, 5 in. × ½ in.	1
Meat (lean–medium fat)	Dried beans and peas, cooked (omit 1 bread exchange for each meat exchange used)	$\frac{1}{2}$ cup
	Lean meat: beef, lamb, pork, poultry, veal, wild game	1 ounce
	Cottage cheese	$\frac{1}{4}$ cup
	Egg[2]	1
	Egg substitute, low cholesterol	$\frac{1}{4}$ cup
	Fish	1 ounce or $\frac{1}{4}$ cup
	Oysters, shrimp[2], clams	5 small or 1 ounce
	Organ meats[2]: liver, heart, kidney, sweetbread (thymus gland)	1 ounce
	Peanut butter (omit 2 fat exchanges for each meat exchange used)	2 tablespoons
	Sardines, drained	3
	Tofu	3 ounces
	Wild game: bear, elk, deer, rabbit	1 ounce
Meat (high fat)[2]	Cheese	1 ounce
	Cold cuts	1 ounce
	Frankfurter or hot dog	1
	Sausage	2 links
	Sausage, Vienna	3
Fat (unsaturated)	Avocado, 4 in. diameter	$\frac{1}{8}$
	Margarine, made from vegetable oils[3]	1 teaspoon
	Nuts (regular or dry roasted)	
	Almonds	10 whole
	Cashews	4 whole

TABLE 25-5. Diabetic Food Exchange System [*Concluded*]

Group	Food Item	One Exchange (serving size)
	Peanuts, Spanish	20 whole
	Peanuts, Virginia	10 whole
	Pecans	3 whole
	Other nuts	6 small
	Chopped nuts	1 tablespoon
	Oil, vegetable, especially corn, safflower, sunflower, soybean[3]	1 teaspoon
	Olives	5 small or 3 large
	Salad dressings	
	Blue cheese	2 teaspoons
	French	1 tablespoon
	Italian	1 tablespoon
	Mayonnaise	1 teaspoon
	Miracle Whip	2 teaspoons
	Thousand Island	2 teaspoons
	Tartar sauce	2 teaspoons
Fat (saturated)	Bacon, crisp	1 slice
	Butter, lard, bacon fat	1 teaspoon
	Cream	
	Coffee (20%)	2 tablespoons
	Half and half (12%)	3 tablespoons
	Sour (20%)	2 tablespoons
	Whipping (30%), unwhipped	1 tablespoon
	Cream cheese	1 tablespoon
	Salt pork	$\frac{3}{4}$ in. cube
Free	Coffee, tea, unsweetened sugar-free carbonated beverages	As desired
	Fat-free broths and bouillons	
	Free vegetables	
	Horseradish	
	Lemon juice[4]	
	Lime juice[4]	
	Mustard	
	Rennet tablets	
	Spices and herbs	
	Unsweetened cranberries	
	Unsweetened gelatin	
	Vinegar	

[1] These higher-fat items may be used. Omit one fat exchange for each bread exchange used.
[2] These items are high in cholesterol. Omit or limit to decrease cholesterol intake.
[3] Two oils, coconut and palm, contain saturated fatty acids and should be omitted.
[4] Limit to 2 tablespoons per day.

REFERENCES CITED

1. National Diabetes Data Group. 1979. Classification and diagnosis of diabetes mellitus and other categories of glucose intolerance. *Diabetes* 28:1039.
2. American Diabetes Association. 1979. Principles of nutrition and dietary recommendations for individuals with diabetes mellitus: 1979. *Diabetes Care* 2:520.
3. West, K. M. 1979. Diabetes mellitus. In *Nutritional support of medical practice,* eds., H. A. Schneider, C. E. Anderson, and D. B. Coursin, pp. 278–296. New York: Harper & Row.
4. Committee on Food and Nutrition. 1971. Principles of nutrition and dietary recommendations for patients with diabetes mellitus. *Diabetes* 20:633.
5. Arky, R. A. 1978. Current principles of dietary therapy of diabetes mellitus. *Med. Clinics N. Am.* 62: 655.
6. American Diabetes Association, Inc. and The American Dietetic Association. 1977. *A guide for professionals: The effective application of "exchange lists for meal planning."* Chicago: American Dietetic Association.
7. Brunzell, J. D. 1978. Use of fructose, sorbitol, or xylitol as a sweetener in diabetes mellitus. *J. Am. Dietet. A.* 73:499.
8. Trowell, H. 1978. Diabetes mellitus and dietary fiber of starchy foods. *Am. J. Clin. Nutr.* 31:S53.
9. Anderson, J. W., and Ward, K. 1979. High-carbohydrate, high-fiber diets for insulin-treated men with diabetes mellitus. *Am. J. Clin. Nutr.* 32:2312.
10. Skillman, T. G., and Tzagournis, M. 1970. *Diabetes mellitus,* p. 20. The Upjohn Company.
11. Kalkhoff, R. K.; Kim, H. J.; Cerletty, J.; and Ferrou, C. A. 1971. Metabolic effects of weight loss in obese subjects. *Diabetes* 20:83.
12. Olefsky, J.; Reaven, G. M.; and Farquhar, J. W. 1974. Effects of weight reduction on obesity. *J. Clin. Invest.* 53:64.
13. Salans, L. B.; Knittle, J. L.; and Hirsch, J. 1968. The role of adipose cell size and adipose tissue insulin sensitivity in the carbohydrate intolerance of human obesity. *J. Clin. Invest.* 47:153.
14. West, K. M. 1976. Diet and diabetes. *Postgrad. Med.* 60:209.
15. Robinson, C. H., and Lawler, M. R. 1977. *Normal and therapeutic nutrition,* p. 67. 15th ed. New York: Macmillan.

REFERENCES FOR THE LAY PUBLIC

MAGAZINES

Diabetes Forecast, 2 Park Avenue, New York, N.Y. 10016

Diabetes Care, 2 Park Avenue, New York, N.Y. 10016

Diabetes in the News, Ames Company, Division Miles Laboratory, Inc., P.O. Box 70, Elkhart, Indiana 46515

BOOKS

Bennett, M. 1968. *The peripatetic diabetic.* New York: Hawthorn Books.

Biermann, J., and Toohey, B. 1974. *The diabetes question and answer book.* New York: Two Continents Publishing Group.

Biermann, J., and Toohey, B. 1977. *The diabetic's sports and exercise book: How to play your way to better health.* Philadelphia: J. B. Lippincott.

Bloom, A. 1972. *Diabetes explained.* Baltimore, Md.: University Park Press.

Corvi, P.; Grills, N.; Lasichak, A.; Templeton, C.; and Valentine, J. 1980. *Meal planning: Diabetes mellitus.* Ann Arbor, Mi. Department of Dietetics, University Hospital, University of Michigan.

Goodman, J. I., and Watts Biggers, W. 1979. *Diabetes without fear.* New York: Arbor House.

Middleton, K., and Hess, M. A. 1979. *The art of cooking for the diabetic.* New York: New American Library.

PART VI
Protein Modifications

Renal Failure

INDICATIONS FOR USE

This diet is indicated for individuals who have renal failure. Nutritional management will depend on the type and stage of the disease, whether the individual is on dialysis, and the type of dialysis.

DESCRIPTION

The primary function of the kidneys is to excrete end products of metabolism and to regulate the composition and volume of body fluids. When renal function is impaired, dietary treatment is essential and will vary with the individual and the degree of impairment. To establish the initial degree of impairment, the glomerular filtration rate (GFR) is measured. Serum creatinine levels are used to determine further changes in renal function. Depending upon the degree of renal impairment, the following factors must be considered in planning nutritional management:

Protein. Protein intake must be carefully monitored. Inadequate protein intake, lower than 40 g/day, results in malnutrition with accompanying negative nitrogen balance. (2, 3) Excessive protein intake results in increased nitrogenous waste products in the blood. These nitrogenous wastes are not cleared adequately by the defective kidney and uremic symptoms may result. There is considerable controversy regarding when to restrict protein for the patient who has not yet started dialysis. One theory maintains that early reduction of dietary protein will delay onset of uremic symptoms. The other maintains that, since reduction of dietary protein will not slow down the course of renal deterioration, restriction is unnecessary until the patient presents with uremic symptoms.

At University Hospital, protein is generally not restricted until the individual exhibits overt symptoms of uremia, the GFR falls below 25 ml/min (4), or the blood urea nitrogen (BUN) is greater than 80–100 mg/100 ml. When the GFR is below 4–5 ml/min, dietary protein restriction usually will not prevent uremic symptoms. (1) The level of protein in the diet is lowered and established at a level to maintain neutral to slightly positive nitrogen balance and to minimize the symptoms of uremia. (5) The appropriate level of protein in the diet will depend on stage of the disease, whether or not dialysis is being used, the type of dialysis, body size, and requirements for growth and development. Foods with relatively high concentrations of essential amino acids are used to provide the allowed protein in the diet. At least one and one-half times the minimum daily requirement of each essential amino acid is needed. (6) The high percentage of essential amino acids helps to increase the utilization of urea nitrogen to form nonessential amino acids, thereby reducing blood urea levels. (7)

Individuals undergoing regular hemodialysis usually require 1.0–1.2 g protein per kilogram body weight per day, with at least half of the protein being of high biological value. (4) Individuals undergoing regular peritoneal dialysis may require 1.2–1.5 g protein per kilogram body weight per day as protein is lost in the peritoneal dialysis process. (8) Whether or not dialysis is used, diets are planned with a minimum of 40 g protein to prevent tissue catabolism. (3)

Sodium. Sodium restriction is based on the GFR and the presence of complications such as edema, hypertension, or congestive heart failure. A GFR below 4–10 ml/min usually requires a sodium restriction. (4) In the nonoliguric phase of chronic renal failure, sodium is generally not restricted.

Fluids. Fluid restriction is based on GFR and urine output. A GFR below 2–5 ml/min requires a fluid restriction. (4) The amount of fluid allowed is determined by the insensible water loss, normally 400–500 ml/day (1), plus the 24 hr urine output from the previous day. Patients undergoing dialysis are encouraged to limit fluid so that no more than 1–2 kg of body weight is gained between dialysis sessions.

Potassium. A potassium restriction is usually not required until the urine volume falls to approximately 1000 ml/day. (4) When urinary output falls below 500–1000 ml/day, serum potassium levels may rise to very high levels without careful control of dietary potassium. (9)

Energy. Adequate energy intake is essential. Due to the restrictive diets and the lack of appetite from disease symptoms, individuals with renal disease often consume a very-low-calorie diet resulting in catabolism of body protein and negative nitrogen balance. (2) Diets high in carbohydrate and fat are used to spare protein. Diet prescriptions for effective dietary management of individuals with chronic renal failure contain 70–100 g fat and 150–400 g carbohydrate (10, 11), supplying an energy intake high enough to maintain lean body mass and prevent protein catabolism.

Vitamins. There is little documentation for the specific vitamin requirements for individuals with renal disease. The requirements would be expected to be different from those for the normal individual due to alterations in vitamin metabolism, renal absorption and excretion, and vitamin loss through dialysate fluid.

Evidence indicates that, with the exception of vitamin D, the dietary intake of fat-soluble vitamins is usually adequate and the amount lost in dialysis is minimal. There have been no reported deficiencies of vitamins A, K, or E (12), although low plasma levels of vitamin E have been reported. (13)

Vitamin D poses a special problem. The kidney is the sole site of the synthesis of the active form of vitamin D, 1,25-dihydroxycholecalciferol. In the normal individual, vitamin D_3 and 25-hydroxycholecalciferol are converted to the active form that functions to stimulate intestinal absorption of calcium and the mobilization of bone calcium. (14) In chronic renal failure, 1,25-dihydroxycholecalciferol is not produced and severe bone and calcium disorders result. The active form of vitamin D is now available and is distributed through Hoffman-LaRoche Inc.

The intake of water-soluble vitamins is often inadequate due to restriction of foods rich in water-soluble vitamins, altered vitamin metabolism, recurrent anorexia and illness, vitamin loss via dialysis, and cooking practices that, designed to leach potassium from foods, also remove vitamins. (15) Supplementation of water-soluble vitamins to the level of the recommended dietary allowances is probably adequate.

Presence of other nutrition-related disorders. Modifications in energy and intakes of other nutrients are necessary for obese individuals and those with diabetes and/or hyperlipidemia.

Anemia in individuals with chronic renal failure may be due to blood loss, iron deficiency, hemolysis, decreased erythropoietin production, or deficiency of certain vitamins or protein. (16) Each patient must be individually evaluated for the cause of anemia. Treatment may include androgen therapy, iron supplementation, daily doses of folic acid or other vitamins, and/or blood transfusions.

GUIDELINES FOR NUTRITIONAL MANAGEMENT

The dietary prescription is based on the individual's renal function, clinical status, medical therapy, and nutrient needs and is determined by the physician and dietitian. The diet may be restricted in protein, sodium, potassium, and fluid or any combination of these nutrients. Phosphorus may also be restricted (Chapter 39). To facilitate meal planning, three food exchange systems were developed: one for diets restricted in protein, one for diets restricted in protein and sodium, and one for diets restricted in protein, sodium, and potassium. Other nutrient restrictions can be built into these food exchange systems. Refer to Tables 26-1 and 26-2, Tables 26-3, 26-4, and 26-5, and Tables 26-6, 26-7, and 26-8, respectively.

Two different calculation methods can be used to meet the diet prescription. One method most suitable for the hospitalized patient requires daily calculation of nutrients from the food items the patient selects. Adjustments often must be made in portion sizes to meet specific dietary restrictions. This method is very time consuming for a technician or dietitian, but it allows the patient greater choice of foods and encourages intake of calories needed to maintain nitrogen balance.

The other method, illustrated in the following example, requires obtaining a complete diet history and establishing with the patient a daily meal pattern from the appropriate food exchange system. This method is often more practical for the ambulatory patient.

The procedure for calculating a protein-, sodium-, and potassium-controlled diet is as follows:

Steps	*Example*
1. Review medical history.	Male, 38 yr old Laboratory values: serum creatinine 15.0 mg/100 ml urea nitrogen 140 mg/100 ml potassium 5.4 mEq/l 24 hr urine output: 500 ml Patient not as yet on dialysis Diagnosis: chronic renal failure
2. Review diet prescription and diet history.	Diet prescription: 40 g protein 920 mg (40 mEq)[1] sodium (Na) 1560 mg (40 mEq) potassium (K) Summary from diet history: Milk: 1 cup/day Eggs: 1/day Meat: likes beef, poultry Fruits and vegetables: prefers fresh Breads, fats: uses regular, salted Beverages: 3 cups coffee/day

3. Use Tables 26-5 and 26-6. Calculate the number of servings to come from the milk and meat food groups. These food groups are included in amounts to provide at least 50% of the protein allowance as they provide protein of high biological value.

Food Group	No. Servings	Protein (g)	Sodium (mg)	Potassium (mg)
Milk	1	4	60	170
Meat	3	21	30	110
Total		25	90	280

4. Calculate the protein, sodium, and potassium to be provided by the remaining food groups.

Protein:
40 g − 25 g = 15 g

Sodium:
920 mg − 90 mg = 830 mg

Potassium:
1560 mg − 280 mg = 1280 mg

5. Calculate the number of servings allowed from the other food groups. Adjust amounts so that the total from all food groups meets the diet prescription.

Food Group	No. Servings	Protein (g)	Sodium (mg)	Potassium (mg)
Fruit I	2	1.0	—	200
Fruit II	1	0.5	—	150
Vegetable I	1	1.5	10	150
Vegetable II	1	1.5	25	250
Bread, salted	5	10.0	600	250
Fat, salted	4	—	200	—
Beverage	3	—	—	300
Subtotal		14.5	835	1300
Milk and meat group total		25.0	90	280
Total		39.5	925	1580
Diet prescription		40.0	920	1560

6. Provide foods from the free food group to meet caloric requirements.

[1] Refer to Table A.7-4.

NUTRIENT ADEQUACY

Actual requirements for vitamins and minerals are unknown for individuals with renal disease. A diet restricted in protein, sodium, potassium, and fluid will be inadequate in calcium, iron, water-soluble vitamins, especially ascorbic acid, and the active form of vitamin D in comparison with the recommended dietary allowances for healthy individuals. (12, 17) Routine supplementation of fat-soluble vitamins is not recommended with the exception of the active form of vitamin D for children. Supplementation of water-soluble vitamins is recommended at levels to meet the RDA. Due to decreased renal excretion, the potential for excess intakes of water-soluble vitamins with toxic side effects must be considered and supplementation administered accordingly. (18)

TABLES

TABLE 26-1. Protein Content of One Exchange (Serving), Protein Food Exchange System

Food Group	Average Content of One Exchange Protein (g)
Milk	4.0
Meat I	9.0
Meat II	7.0
Fruit	0.5
Vegetable	1.5
Bread	2.0

Table 26-2. Protein Food Exchange System

Group	Food Item	Description	Serving Size: Household Measure	Serving Size: Weight (g)	Avoid
Milk (4 g protein/serving)	Cream	Light	½ cup	120	
		Heavy	¾ cup	180	
		Sour	½ cup	125	
		Half and half	½ cup	120	
	Ice cream		¾ cup	100	
	Ice milk		¾ cup	100	
	Cream cheese		3 tablespoons	42	
	Milk	Butter	½ cup	120	
		Chocolate	½ cup	125	
		Evaporated	¼ cup	57	
		Skim	½ cup	125	
		2%	½ cup	125	
		Whole	½ cup	125	
Meat I (9 g protein/serving)	Beef	Cooked	1 ounce	30	
	Canadian bacon	Cooked	1 ounce	30	
	Cheese				
	American	Cheese spread	2 ounces	60	
	Mozzarella	Low moisture, part skim	1 ounce	30	
	Parmesan	Grated	¼ cup	20	
	Swiss		1 ounce	30	
	Chicken	Cooked	1 ounce	30	
	Codfish	Cooked	1 ounce	30	
	Peanut butter		2 tablespoons	33	
	Rabbit	Cooked	1 ounce	30	
	Salmon	Cooked	1 ounce	30	
	Tuna	Cooked	¼ cup	40	
	Turkey	Cooked	1 ounce	30	
	Veal	Cooked	1 ounce	30	
	Venison	Cooked	1 ounce	30	
Meat II (7 g protein/serving)	Bacon		3 strips	21	
	Cheese				
	American		1 ounce	30	
	Brick		1 ounce	30	
	Cheddar		1 ounce	30	
	Colby		1 ounce	30	
	Cottage		2 tablespoons	55	
	Gouda		1 ounce	30	
	Monterey		1 ounce	30	
	Muenster		1 ounce	30	
	Parmesan	Grated	3 tablespoons		
	Swiss	Processed	1 ounce	30	
	Clams	Soft, large	2	50	
	Crab	Cooked	1 ounce	30	
	Duck	Cooked	1 ounce	30	
	Egg	Medium	1	50	
	Finfish	Cooked	1 ounce	30	
	Ham	Cooked	1 ounce	30	
	Lamb	Cooked	1 ounce	30	
	Liver	Cooked	1 ounce	30	

TABLE 26-2. Protein Food Exchange System [*Continued*]

Group	Food Item	Description	Serving Size: Household Measure	Serving Size: Weight (g)	Avoid
	Lobster	Cooked	1 ounce	30	
	Lunchmeat		1 slice (1 ounce)	30	
	Pheasant	Cooked	1 ounce	30	
	Pork	Cooked	1 ounce	30	
	Scallops	Cooked	1 ounce	30	
	Shrimp	Raw	1 ounce	30	
	Tongue	Cooked	1 ounce	30	
Fruit (0.5 g protein/serving)	Apple	Large	1	200	
	Applesauce		$\frac{3}{4}$ cup	225	
	Apple juice		2 cups	480	
	Apricots	Fresh, medium	1	50	
		Canned	3 halves	100	
		Nectar	$\frac{3}{4}$ cup	180	
	Banana	Small	$\frac{1}{2}$	50	
	Berries				
	Blueberries	Raw	$\frac{1}{2}$ cup	80	
	Blackberries	Raw	$\frac{1}{3}$ cup	55	
	Boysenberries	Canned	$\frac{1}{2}$ cup	75	
	Gooseberries	Raw	$\frac{1}{2}$ cup	75	
	Raspberries	Red	$\frac{1}{3}$ cup	40	
	Strawberries		$\frac{3}{4}$ cup	75	
	Blended juice	Orange/grapefruit	$\frac{1}{3}$ cup	80	
	Cantaloupe		$\frac{1}{3}$ cup	80	
	Cherries	Sweet, canned	$\frac{1}{3}$ cup	65	
		Sweet, raw	$\frac{1}{4}$ cup	50	
		Sour, raw	$\frac{1}{4}$ cup	50	
		Sour, canned	$\frac{1}{3}$ cup	65	
	Cranberries	Raw	1 cup	100	
		Sauce	$1\frac{1}{2}$ cups	480	
		Juice	2 cups	480	
	Dates	Medium	2	20	
	Figs	Fresh, large	1	50	
		Canned, medium	3	100	
		Dried, small	1	10	
	Fruit cocktail		$\frac{2}{3}$ cup	133	
	Grapefruit	Fresh	$\frac{1}{2}$	100	
		Canned	$\frac{1}{2}$ cup	100	
		Juice	$\frac{1}{2}$ cup	125	
	Grapes	Medium	20	80	
	Grapejuice		1 cup	250	
	Honeydew melon		$\frac{1}{8}$	50	
	Lemon juice		$\frac{1}{2}$ cup	125	
	Lemonade		2 cups	480	
	Lime juice		$\frac{1}{2}$ cup	125	
	Melon balls	Frozen	$\frac{1}{2}$ cup	100	
	Nectarine	Large	1	75	
	Orange	Fresh, small	$\frac{1}{2}$	50	
		Sections	$\frac{1}{3}$ cup	83	
		Juice	$\frac{1}{3}$ cup	80	

TABLE 26-2. Protein Food Exchange System [*Continued*]

Group	Food Item	Description	Serving Size: Household Measure	Serving Size: Weight (g)	Avoid
	Papayas	Medium	1/3	100	
	Peach	Fresh, small	1	75	
		Canned	2 halves	100	
		Nectar	1 cup	250	
	Pears	Fresh, small	1/2	100	
		Canned	3 halves	150	
		Nectar	3/4 cup	185	
	Pineapple	Fresh	1 cup	125	
		Canned, small slices	2	125	
		Juice	1/2 cup	125	
	Plums	Fresh, medium	2	100	
		Canned	4	133	
	Pomegranate	Medium	1	100	
	Prunes	Dried, large	2	20	
	Raisins		2 tablespoons	20	
	Rhubarb	Cooked	1/3 cup	88	
	Sherbet		1/2 cup	50	
	Tangerine	Small	1	50	
	Tomato juice		1/4 cup	63	
	Vegetable juice		1/4 cup	63	
	Watermelon		1/2 cup	100	
Vegetable (1.5 g protein/serving)	Asparagus	Cooked	1/2 cup	75	Dried beans
	Beans, green or wax	Cooked	1 cup	100	Dried peas
	Bean spouts	Cooked	1/2 cup	50	Lima beans
	Beets	Cooked	3/4 cup	125	Nuts
	Broccoli	Cooked	1/3 cup	50	
	Brussels sprouts	Cooked	1/4 cup	38	
	Cabbage	Raw	1 cup	100	
		Cooked	3/4 cup	125	
	Carrots	Raw, large	1	100	
		Cooked	1 cup	250	
	Cauliflower	Cooked	1/2 cup	57	
		Raw	1/2 cup	50	
	Celery	Raw, diced	1 1/2 cups	150	
		Cooked	1 1/2 cups	150	
	Collard greens	Cooked	1/4 cup	50	
	Corn	Cooked	1/3 cup	50	
		On cob	2 in.	50	
	Cucumber	Large	1	150	
	Eggplant	Cooked	3/4 cup	150	
	Escarole/endive	Raw	17 leaves	85	
	Green pepper	Cooked or raw, large	1	100	
	Kale	Cooked	1/4 cup	33	
	Kohlrabi	Cooked	1/2 cup	75	
	Lettuce		2 cups	120	
	Mushrooms	Raw, large	3	66	
	Mustard greens	Cooked	1/3 cup	67	
	Okra	Cooked	6–7 pods	75	
	Onions	Raw, small	1	100	
		Cooked	1/2 cup	100	

Table 26-2. Protein Food Exchange System [*Continued*]

Group	Food Item	Description	Serving Size: Household Measure	Serving Size: Weight (g)	Avoid
	Parsley	Fresh	½ cup	33	
	Parsnips	Cooked	½ cup	100	
	Peas	Cooked	¼ cup	38	
	Pickles	Large	2	200	
	Potato	Baked, small	½	50	
		Boiled, small	½	50	
		Mashed	⅓ cup	66	
		French fries	8	40	
		Hash browns	¼ cup	50	
	Pumpkin	Cooked	⅔ cup	165	
	Radishes	Small	15	150	
	Rutabaga	Cooked	¾ cup	150	
	Sauerkraut		1 cup	150	
	Spinach	Cooked	¼ cup	50	
		Raw	1 cup	50	
	Squash	Summer, cooked	¾ cup	150	
		Winter, baked	⅓ cup	65	
		Winter, boiled	½ cup	125	
	Sweet potato	Baked, small	1	100	
		Boiled, small	1	100	
	Swiss chard	Cooked	½ cup	85	
	Tomato	Cooked	½ cup	100	
		Raw, medium	1	125	
		Puree	¼ cup	66	
	Tomato juice		¾ cup	185	
	Turnips	Cooked	1 cup	150	
	Turnip greens	Cooked	½ cup	75	
Bread (2.0 g protein/serving)	Bread	White	1 slice	20	
		Wheat	1 slice	20	
		Rye	1 slice	20	
	Biscuit		½	17	
	Bun		½	15	
	Cereal				
	Cheerios		½ cup	16	
	Corn Chex		⅔ cup	19	
	Cornflakes		1 cup	24	
	Puffed Rice		2 cups	26	
	Puffed Wheat		1 cup	12	
	Rice Chex		2 cups	56	
	Rice Krispies		½ cup	14	
	Shredded Wheat	Biscuit	1	22	
		Spoon size	½ cup	25	
	Sugar Crisp		¾ cup	24	
	Wheat Chex		⅓ cup	30	
	Cream of Rice	Cooked	1 cup	240	
	Cream of Wheat	Cooked	½ cup	120	
	Farina	Cooked	½ cup	120	
	Oatmeal	Cooked	⅓ cup	83	
	Corn bread	2 in. square	½	22	
	Cornmeal	Dry	3 tablespoons	28	

TABLE 26-2. Protein Food Exchange System [*Concluded*]

Group	Food Item	Description	Serving Size: Household Measure	Serving Size: Weight (g)	Avoid
	Crackers				
	Animal		17		
	Graham squares		3		
	Oyster		30	21	
	Saltines		6		
	Rye wafers		6		
	Cupcakes	Small	1	50	
	Flour	All purpose	2 tablespoons	15	
	Macaroni products	Cooked	⅓ cup	44	
	Melba toast	Slices	4	13	
	Muffin		½	17	
	Pancakes	4 in. diameter	1		
	Pie crust	Double 9 in.	⅛	35	
	Popcorn	Popped	1 cup	16	
	Rice	Cooked	⅔ cup	100	
	Roll		½	17	
	Rusk		1	12	
	Tortilla shell	6 in. diameter	1	30	
	Vanilla wafers		12	39	
Free food	Butter				Chocolate
	Candy, hard				
	Carbonated beverages				
	Catsup				
	Chewing gum				
	Coffee				
	Cool Whip				
	Dream Whip				
	Hawaiian Punch				
	Honey				
	Koolaid				
	Margarine				
	Marshmallows				
	Mayonnaise				
	Mustard				
	Popsickle				
	Salad dressings				
	Seasonings				
	Sugar				
	Syrup				
	Tea				
	Vegetable oil				
	Vinegar				

TABLE 26-3. Protein and Sodium Content of One Exchange (Serving), Protein–Sodium Food Exchange System

Food Group	Average Content of One Exchange: Protein (g)	Average Content of One Exchange: Sodium (mg)
Milk	4.0	60
Meat I	9.0	30
Meat II	7.0	30
Fruit	0.5	—
Vegetable	1.5	20
Bread, unsalted	2.0	10
Bread, salted	2.0	120
Fats, salted	—	50
Variable	0–14	60–765

TABLE 26-4. Protein–Sodium Food Exchange System

Group	Food Item	Description	Serving Size: Household Measure	Serving Size: Weight (g)	Avoid
Milk (4 g protein, 60 mg sodium/ serving)	Cream	Light	½ cup	120	
		Heavy	¾ cup	180	
		Sour	½ cup	125	
	Half and half		½ cup	120	
	Ice cream		⅔ cup	88	
	Ice milk		⅔ cup	88	
	Milk	Chocolate	½ cup	125	
		Evaporated	¼ cup	57	
		Skim	½ cup	125	
		2%	½ cup	125	
		Whole	½ cup	125	
Meat I (9 g protein, 30 mg sodium/ serving)	Beef	Cooked	1 ounce	30	Clams
	Chicken	Cooked	1 ounce	30	Crab
	Codfish	Cooked	1 ounce	30	Lobster
	Rabbit	Cooked	1 ounce	30	Oysters
	Salmon	Fresh or low sodium, canned	1 ounce	30	Scallops Shrimp
	Tuna	Water packed, no salt	¼ cup	40	
	Turkey	Cooked	1 ounce	30	
	Veal	Cooked	1 ounce	30	
	Venison	Cooked	1 ounce	30	
Meat II (7 g protein, 30 mg sodium/ serving)	Cheese	Low sodium	1 ounce	30	
	Duck	Cooked	1 ounce	30	
	Egg	Medium	1	50	
	Finfish	Cooked	1 ounce	30	
	Hamburger	Cooked	1 ounce	30	
	Lamb	Cooked	1 ounce	30	
	Liver	Cooked	1 ounce	30	
	Pheasant	Cooked	1 ounce	30	
	Pork	Cooked	1 ounce	30	
	Tongue	Cooked	1 ounce	30	
Fruit (0.5 g protein, negligible sodium/ serving)	Apple	Large	1	200	
	Apple juice		2 cups	480	
	Applesauce		¾ cup	225	
	Apricots	Fresh, medium	1	50	
		canned	3 halves	100	
	Apricot nectar		½ cup	125	
	Banana	Small	½	50	
	Berries				
	Blueberries	Raw	½ cup	80	
	Blackberries	Raw	⅓ cup	55	
	Boysenberries	Canned	½ cup	75	
	Gooseberries	Raw	½ cup	75	
	Raspberries	Red	⅓ cup	40	
		Black	⅓ cup	50	
	Strawberries	Frozen	½ cup	130	
		Fresh	¾ cup	75	
	Blended juice	Orange/grapefruit	⅓ cup	80	
	Cantaloupe		⅓ cup	80	
	Cherries	Sweet, fresh	¼ cup	50	
		Sweet, canned	⅓ cup	60	
		Sour, fresh	¼ cup	50	
	Cranberries	Raw	1 cup	100	
		Sauce	1 cup	320	
		Juice	2 cups	480	
	Dates	Medium	2	20	

TABLE 26-4. Protein–Sodium Food Exchange System [*Continued*]

Group	Food Item	Description	Serving Size: Household Measure	Serving Size: Weight (g)	Avoid
	Figs	Fresh, large	1	50	
		Canned medium	3	100	
		Dried, small	1	10	
	Fruit cocktail		⅔ cup	133	
	Grapes	Medium	20	80	
	Grape juice		1 cup	250	
	Grapefruit	Fresh	½	100	
		Canned	½ cup	100	
		Juice	½ cup	125	
	Honeydew melon		⅛	50	
	Lemonade		2 cups	480	
	Lemon juice		½ cup	125	
	Lime juice		½ cup	125	
	Melon balls	Frozen	½ cup	100	
	Nectarine	Large	1	75	
	Orange	Fresh, small	½	50	
		Sections	⅓ cup	83	
		Juice	⅓ cup	80	
	Papayas	Medium	⅓ cup	100	
	Peach	Fresh, small	1	75	
		Canned	2 halves	100	
		Nectar	1 cup	250	
	Pear	Fresh, small	½	100	
		Canned	3 halves	150	
		Nectar	¾ cup		
				185	
	Pineapple	Fresh, diced	1 cup	125	
		Canned, sliced	1 large	100	
		Juice	½ cup	125	
	Plantain	Small	½	50	
	Plums	Fresh, medium	2	100	
		Canned, medium	4	133	
	Pomegranate	Medium	1	100	
	Prunes	Dried, large	2	20	
	Raisins		2 tablespoons	20	
	Rhubarb	Cooked	⅓ cup	88	
	Sherbet		½ cup	50	
	Tangerine	Small	1	50	
	Tomato juice	Unsalted	½ cup	63	
	Watermelon		½ cup	100	
Vegetable (1.5 g protein, 20 mg sodium/ serving)	Asparagus	Cooked	½ cup	75	Dried beans
	Beans, wax or green	Cooked	1 cup	100	Dried peas
	Bean sprouts	Cooked	½ cup	50	Lima beans
	Beets	Cooked	¼ cup	50	
	Broccoli	Cooked	⅓ cup	50	
	Brussels sprouts	Cooked	¼ cup	38	
	Cabbage	Raw	1 cup	100	
		Cooked	1 cup		
	Carrots	Raw, large	½	50	
		Cooked	¼ cup	60	
	Cauliflower	Raw	½ cup	50	
		Cooked	½ cup	57	
	Celery	Raw	¼ cup	25	
		Cooked	¼ cup	30	
	Collard greens	Cooked	¼ cup	50	
	Corn		⅓ cup	50	

TABLE 26-4. Protein–Sodium Food Exchange System [*Continued*]

Group	Food Item	Description	Serving Size: Household Measure	Serving Size: Weight (g)	Avoid
	Corn on cob		2 in. ear	50	
	Cucumber	Medium	1	100	
	Eggplant	Cooked	¾ cup	150	
	Escarole/endive	Raw	17 leaves	85	
	Green pepper	Raw or cooked	1 large	100	
	Kohlrabi	Cooked	½ cup	75	
	Kale	Cooked	¼ cup	33	
	Lettuce	Raw	2 cups	120	
	Mushrooms	Large, raw	3	66	
	Mustard greens	Cooked	⅓ cup	67	
	Okra	Cooked	6–7 pods	75	
	Onions	Raw, small	1	100	
		Cooked	½ cup	100	
	Parsley	Fresh	½ cup	33	
	Parsnips	Cooked	½ cup	100	
	Peas	Cooked	¼ cup	38	
	Potato	Baked, small	½	50	
		Boiled, small	½	50	
		Mashed	⅓ cup	66	
		French fries	8	40	
		Hash browns	¼ cup	50	
	Pumpkin	Cooked	⅔ cup	165	
	Radishes	Small	15	150	
	Rutabaga	Cooked	¾ cup	150	
	Spinach	Raw	¾ cup	36	
		Cooked	¼ cup	50	
	Squash	Summer	¾ cup	150	
		Winter, baked	⅓ cup	65	
		Winter, boiled	½ cup	125	
	Sweet potato	Baked, small	½	50	
		Boiled, small	1	100	
	Swiss chard	Cooked	¼ cup	40	
	Tomato	Cooked	½ cup	100	
		Raw, small	1	100	
		Puree, low sodium	¼ cup	66	
	Turnips	Cooked	½ cup	75	
	Turnip greens	Cooked	⅓ cup	50	
Unsalted bread, (2.0 g protein, 10 mg sodium/ serving)	Bread	Low sodium	1 slice	23	
	Cereal				
	Puffed Rice		1½ cups	20	
	Puffed Wheat		1 cup	12	
	Shredded Wheat	Biscuit	1	22	
		Spoon size	½ cup	25	
	Sugar Crisp		¾ cup	24	
	Cream of Rice	Cooked	1 cup	240	
	Cream of Wheat	Cooked	½ cup	120	
	Farina	Cooked	½ cup	120	
	Oatmeal	Cooked	⅓ cup	83	
	Cornmeal	Dry	3 tablespoons	28	
	Crackers	Unsalted	6		
	Flour	All purpose	2 tablespoons	15	
	Gelatin	Low sodium	½ cup		
	Macaroni products	Cooked	⅓ cup	44	
	Melba toast	Unsalted	4	13	
	Pie crust	No salt	⅛ of 9 in. double crust	35	
	Popcorn	Popped	1 cup	16	
	Rice	Cooked	⅔ cup	100	
	Rusk		1	12	
	Tortilla shell	6 in. diameter		30	

TABLE 26-4. Protein–Sodium Food Exchange System [*Concluded*]

Group	Food Item	Description	Serving Size: Household Measure	Serving Size: Weight (g)	Avoid
Salted Bread, (2.0 g protein, 120 mg sodium/ serving)	Bread				
	White		1 slice	20	Salted crackers
	Wheat		1 slice	20	Salted popcorn
	Rye		1 slice	20	Pretzels
	Biscuit		½	17	
	Bun		½	15	
	Cereal				
	Cheerios		½ cup	16	
	Corn Chex		⅓ cup	19	
	Cornflakes		½ cup	12	
	Rice Chex		½ cup	14	
	Rice Krispies		½ cup	14	
	Wheat Chex		¼ cup	11	
	Corn bread	2 in. square	½	22	
	Crackers				
	Animal		17		
	Graham	Squares	3		
	Rye wafers		6		
	Cupcake	Small	1	50	
	Muffin		½	20	
	Pancake	4 in. diameter	1		
	Roll		½	18	
	Vanilla wafers		12	39	
Fat, salted (negligible protein, 50 mg sodium/ serving)	Butter	Regular	1 teaspoon	5	
	Margarine	Regular	1 teaspoon	5	
	Mayonnaise	Regular	2 teaspoons	10	
	Salad dressing	Mayonnaise type	2 teaspoons	10	
Free foods	Butter, unsalted				Baking soda or powder
	Catsup, low sodium				Bouillon
	Chewing gum				Broth
	Coffee				Carob
	Cool Whip				Celery salt
	Corn syrup				Chocolate, cocoa
	Dream Whip				Garlic salt
	Hard candy				Meat extracts (Kitchen Bouquet)
	Honey				Meat tenderizers
	Jelly beans				Molasses
	Koolaid				MSG (monosodium glutamate, Accent)
	Life Savers				Onion salt
	Maple syrup				Salt
	Marshmallows				Salt substitute
	Margarine, unsalted				Softened water
	Mayonnaise, unsalted				Soups, canned or dried
	Oil				Soy sauce
	Popsicle				Steak sauce
	Salad dressing, unsalted				Worchestershire sauce
	Spices				
	Sugar				
	Tang				
	Tea				
	Vinegar				

TABLE 26-5. Variable Food Group, Protein–Sodium Food Exchange System

Group	Food Item	Description	Serving Size: Household Measure	Serving Size: Weight (g)	Protein (mg)	Sodium (mg)
Variable	Bacon	Cooked	1 strip	7	2	70
	Buttermilk		½ cup	120	4	155
	Canadian bacon	Cooked	1 ounce	30	8	765
	Catsup	Regular	1 teaspoon	6	0	60
	Cheese					
	American	Pasteurized, processed	1 ounce	30	7	430
		Cheese spread	1 ounce	30	5	400
	Brick	Natural	1 ounce	30	7	170
	Cheddar	Natural	1 ounce	30	7	210
	Colby		1 ounce	30	7	180
	Cottage	Creamed, regular	¼ cup	110	14	450
	Cream		3 tablespoons	42	3	125
	Gouda		1 ounce	30	7	245
	Monterey		1 ounce	30	7	160
	Mozzarella		1 ounce	30	6	110
	Mozzarella	Low moisture, part skim	1 ounce	30	8	160
	Muenster		1 ounce	30	7	190
	Parmesan	Grated	1 tablespoon	5	2	95
	Swiss	Natural	1 ounce	30	8	80
		Pasteurized, processed	1 ounce	30	7	410
	Coconut	Shredded, dried	2 tablespoons	15	0.5	115
	Frankfurter	Average	1	50	7	540
	Ham	Cooked	1 ounce	30	7	270
	Lunchmeat		1 slice (1 oz)	30	5	370
	Mustard	Regular	1 teaspoon	5	0	60
	Peanut butter	Regular	2 tablespoons	33	8	200
	Pork sausage	Links, cooked	2 (1½ oz)	40	7	385
	Salad dressings	Regular				
	Blue cheese		2 tablespoons	28	1	310
	French		1 tablespoon	14	0	190
	Italian		1 tablespoon	14	0	295
	Tomato juice	Regular	½ cup	125	1	250
	Tuna	Oil packed	¼ cup	40	10	320

TABLE 26-6. Protein, Sodium, and Potassium Content of One Exchange (Serving), Protein–Sodium–Potassium Food Exchange System

Food Group	Average Content of One Exchange		
	Protein (g)	Sodium (mg)	Potassium (mg)
Milk	4.0	60	170
Meat	7.0	30	110
Fruit I	0.5	—	100
Fruit II	0.5	—	150
Vegetable I	1.5	10	150
Vegetable II	1.5	25	250
Bread, unsalted	2.0	10	50
Bread, salted	2.0	120	50
Fats, salted	—	50	—
Beverages	—	—	100
Variable	0–14	0–765	0–215

TABLE 26-7. Protein–Sodium–Potassium Food Exchange System

Group	Food Item	Description	Serving Size: Household Measure	Serving Size: Weight (g)	Avoid
Milk (4 g protein, 60 mg sodium, 170 mg potassium/serving)	Cream	Light	½ cup	120	Chocolate-flavored dairy products
		Heavy	¾ cup	180	
		Sour	½ cup	125	
		Half and half	½ cup	120	
	Ice cream	Vanilla	⅔ cup	88	
	Ice milk	Vanilla	⅔ cup	88	
	Milk	Evaporated	¼ cup	57	
		Skim	½ cup	125	
		2%	½ cup	125	
		Whole	½ cup	125	
Meat (7 g protein, 80 mg sodium, 110 mg potassium/serving)	Beef	Cooked	1 ounce	30	Clams
	Chicken	Cooked	1 ounce	30	Crab
	Cheese	Low sodium	1 ounce	30	Lobster
	Duck	Cooked	1 ounce	30	Oysters
	Egg	Medium	1	50	Scallops
	Finfish	Cooked	1 ounce	30	Shrimp
	Lamb	Cooked	1 ounce	30	
	Liver	Cooked	1 ounce	30	
	Pheasant	Cooked	1 ounce	30	
	Pork	Cooked	1 ounce	30	
	Rabbit	Cooked	1 ounce	30	
	Salmon	Fresh or low sodium canned	1 ounce	30	
	Tongue	Cooked	1 ounce	30	
	Turkey	Cooked	1 ounce	30	
	Veal	Cooked	1 ounce	30	
	Venison	Cooked	1 ounce	30	
Fruit I (0.5 g protein, negligible sodium, 100 mg potassium/serving)	Apple juice		⅓ cup	125	
	Applesauce		½ cup	150	
	Berries				
	Blueberries	Raw	¾ cup	120	
	Boysenberries	Canned	¾ cup	112	
	Gooseberries	Raw	½ cup	75	
	Raspberries	Red, raw	½ cup	66	
		Red, frozen	½ cup	100	
	Strawberries	Raw	½ cup	50	
		Sliced, frozen	⅓ cup	80	
	Blended juice	Orange/grapefruit	¼ cup	62	
	Cherries	Sweet, raw	¼ cup	50	
	Cranberries	Raw	1 cup	100	
	Grapes	Thompson seedless	14	58	
	Grape juice	Frozen, diluted	1 cup	250	
	Grapefruit juice	Canned	¼ cup	62	
	Lemon juice		¼ cup	62	
	Lime juice		⅓ cup	33	
	Mango	Medium	¼	50	
	Melon balls	Frozen	¼ cup	50	
	Orange	Fresh, small	½	50	
	Orange juice		¼ cup	62	
	Peach nectar		½ cup	125	
	Pears	Canned	½ cup	100	
	Pear nectar		1 cup	250	
	Pineapple	Frozen or syrup packed	1 large slice	100	
		Canned			
		Fresh	¾ cup	66	
	Pineapple juice		¼ cup	62	
	Watermelon		½ cup	100	
	Raisins		1 tablespoon	10	

TABLE 26-7. Protein–Sodium–Potassium Food Exchange System [*Continued*]

Group	Food Item	Description	Serving Size: Household Measure	Serving Size: Weight (g)	Avoid
Fruit II (0.5 g protein, negligible sodium, 150 mg potassium/serving)	Apple	Raw, medium	1	150	Avocado
	Berries				
	Blackberries	Raw	½ cup	80	Apricots
	Loganberries	Raw	½ cup	75	Bananas
	Raspberries	Black, raw	½ cup	75	Dates
	Cantaloupe		¼ cup	60	Papayas
	Cherries	Sour, fresh	⅓ cup	66	Rhubarb
		Sweet, canned	½ cup	100	
	Figs	Fresh, small	2	66	
		Canned, medium	3	100	
		Dried, medium	1	20	
	Fruit cocktail	Canned	½ cup	100	
	Grape juice	Bottled	½ cup	125	
	Grapefruit	Medium	½	100	
		Canned	½ cup	100	
	Honeydew melon		⅛	75	
	Mandarin oranges		⅓ cup	133	
	Nectarine	Small	1	50	
	Orange sections		½ cup	66	
	Pear	Fresh, small	½	100	
		Canned, juice pack	2 halves	100	
	Peach	Fresh, small	1	75	
		Canned	2 halves	100	
	Pineapple	Canned, juice pack	1 large slice	100	
	Plums	Fresh, medium	1	50	
		Fresh, medium prune-type	3	100	
	Plums	Canned	3	100	
	Pomegranate	Medium	½	50	
	Prunes	Dried	2	20	
	Tangerine	Large	1	100	
	Tomato juice	Unsalted	¼ cup	63	
Vegetable I (1.5 g protein, 10 mg sodium, 150 mg potassium/serving)	Asparagus	Cooked	½ cup	75	
	Beans, green or wax	Cooked	1 cup	100	
	Beets	Cooked	⅓ cup	55	
	Bean sprouts	Cooked	½ cup	50	
	Broccoli	Cooked	⅓ cup	50	
	Cabbage	Raw	½ cup	50	
		Cooked	½ cup	84	
	Carrots	Cooked	½ cup	125	
	Cauliflower	Raw or cooked	½ cup	50	
	Celery	Raw	⅓ cup	33	
		Cooked	½ cup	63	
	Collard greens	Cooked	¼ cup	50	
	Corn	Cooked	⅓ cup	56	
		On cob	2 in. ear	50	
	Cucumber	Medium	1	100	
	Eggplant	Cooked	½ cup	100	
	Kale	Cooked	½ cup	66	
	Lettuce		1½ cups	90	
	Mustard greens	Cooked	⅓ cup	67	
	Okra	Cooked	6–7 pods	75	
	Onion	Raw, medium	1	100	
		Cooked	⅔ cup	133	
	Parsley		¼ cup	15	
	Pepper, green	Raw, large	½	50	
		Cooked	½ cup		
	Peas	Cooked	¼ cup	40	

TABLE 26-7. Protein–Sodium–Potassium Food Exchange System [*Continued*]

Group	Food Item	Description	Serving Size: Household Measure	Serving Size: Weight (g)	Avoid
	Potato	Boiled, small	½	50	
	Rutabaga	Cooked	½ cup	100	
	Spinach	Cooked	¼ cup	45	
	Squash	Summer, cooked	½ cup	100	
	Swiss chard	Cooked	¼ cup	42	
	Turnips	Cooked	½ cup	75	
	Turnip greens	Cooked	⅔ cup	100	
Vegetable II (1.5 g protein, 25 mg sodium, 250 mg potassium/serving)	Brussels sprouts	Cooked	½ cup	75	Artichokes
	Carrots	Raw, medium	1	75	Lima beans
	Escarole/endive	Raw	17 leaves	85	Pinto beans
	Kohlrabi	Cooked	½ cup	75	Kidney beans
	Mushrooms	Raw	3 large or 7 small	66	Sauerkraut
	Parsnips	Cooked	⅓ cup	66	Baked sweet potato
	Potato	Baked, small	½	50	Bamboo shoots
		French fries	6	30	Lentils
		Hash browns	¼ cup	50	Pickles
		Mashed	½ cup	100	Olives
	Pumpkin	Canned, unsalted	⅓ cup	83	
	Radishes	Raw, small	8	80	
	Spinach	Raw	1 cup	50	
		Cooked	⅓ cup	60	
	Squash	Winter, baked	¼ cup	50	
		Winter, boiled	⅓ cup	83	
	Sweet potato	Boiled, small	1	100	
	Tomato	Raw, small	1	100	
		Cooked	⅓ cup	66	
	Tomato puree	Low sodium	¼ cup	66	
Bread, unsalted (2 g protein, 10 mg sodium, 50 mg potassium/serving)	Bread	Unsalted	1 slice	23	
	Cereal				
	Puffed Rice		1 cup	13	
	Puffed Wheat		1 cup	12	
	Shredded Wheat		½ cup spoon size or 1 biscuit	22	
	Sugar Crisp		¾ cup	24	
	Oatmeal	Cooked	⅓ cup	80	
	Farina	Cooked	½ cup	120	
	Cream of Rice	Cooked	1 cup	240	
	Cream of Wheat	Cooked	½ cup	120	
	Cornmeal	Dry	3 tablespoons	28	
	Crackers	Unsalted	3	21	
	Flour	All purpose	¼ cup	29	
	Macaroni products	Cooked	⅓ cup	44	
	Melba toast	Unsalted, thin slice	4	15	
	Piecrust	Unsalted, double	⅙ of 9 in.	45	
	Popcorn	Popped	1 cup	16	
	Rice	Cooked	⅔ cup	100	
	Rusk		1	11	
	Tortilla shell	6 in. diameter	1	30	
	Gelatin	Low sodium	½ cup	62	
Bread, salted (2 g protein, 120 mg sodium, 50 mg potassium/serving)	Biscuit		½	17	Pretzels
	Bread		1 slice	20	Salted crackers
	Bun	Hamburger or weiner	½	15	
	Cake	Angel food	$\frac{1}{10}$ average	45	
		Cupcake	1 small	50	
	Cereal				
	Cornflakes		½ cup	12	
	Corn Chex		½ cup	14	

TABLE 26-7. Protein–Sodium–Potassium Food Exchange System [*Concluded*]

Group	Food Item	Description	Serving Size: Household Measure	Serving Size: Weight (g)	Avoid
	Rice Chex		½ cup	14	
	Rice Krispies		½ cup	14	
	Corn bread	1 in. square	1	22	
	Crackers				
	Animal		20	40	
	Graham		2 squares	15	
	Jello		½ cup	62	
	Pancakes	4 in. diameter	1	45	
	Sherbet		½ cup	50	
	Vanilla wafers		12	39	
Fat, salted (negligible protein, 50 mg sodium, negligible potassium/ serving)	Butter	Regular	1 teaspoon	5	
	Margarine	Regular	1 teaspoon	5	
	Mayonnaise	Regular	2 teaspoons	10	
	Salad dressing	Mayonnaise type	2 teaspoons	10	
Beverages (negligible protein and sodium, 100 mg potassium/ serving)	Coffee	Instant	1 cup	240	
	Postum		¾ cup	180	
	Tea		1 cup	240	
Free foods	Butter, unsalted				Baking soda or powder
	Cool Whip				Bouillon
	Cranberry juice, cocktail				Broth
	Dream Whip				Carob
	Hard candy				Celery salt
	Honey				Chocolate
	Jelly beans				Cocoa
	Koolaid				Garlic salt
	Lemonade				Meat extracts (Kitchen Bouquet)
	Maple syrup				Meat tenderizers
	Margarine, unsalted				Molasses
	Marshmallows				MSG (monosodium glutamate, Accent)
	Oil				Onion salt
	Sugar, granulated or powdered				Salt
	Vinegar (limit 2 tablespoons/day)				Salt substitute
					Softened water
					Soups, canned or dried
					Soy sauce
					Steak sauce
					Worcestershire sauce

TABLE 26-8. Variable Food Exchange Group, Protein–Sodium–Potassium Food Exchange System

Group	Food Item	Description	Serving Size: Household Measure	Serving Size: Weight (g)	Protein (g)	Sodium (mg)	Potassium (mg)
Variable	Bacon	Cooked	1 strip	7	2	70	15
	Brown sugar		1 tablespoon	14	0	5	50
	Buttermilk		½ cup	120	4	155	170
	Canadian bacon	Cooked	1 ounce	30	8	765	130
	Catsup	Regular	1 teaspoon	6	0	60	20
	Cheese						
	American	Pasteurized processed	1 ounce	30	7	430	50
		Processed cheese spread	1 ounce	30	5	400	70
	Brick	Natural	1 ounce	30	7	170	40
	Cheddar	Natural	1 ounce	30	7	210	25
	Colby		1 ounce	30	7	180	40
	Cottage	Creamed, regular	¼ cup	110	14	450	95
	Cream		3 tablespoons	42	3	125	50
	Gouda		1 ounce	30	7	245	35
	Monterey		1 ounce	30	7	160	25
	Mozzarella		1 ounce	30	8	160	30
	Mozzarella	Low moisture, part skim	1 ounce	30	6	110	20
	Muenster		1 ounce	30	7	190	40
	Parmesan	Grated	1 tablespoon	5	2	95	5
	Swiss	Natural	1 ounce	30	8	80	35
		Pasteurized, processed	1 ounce	30	7	410	65
	Cranberry sauce		¼ cup	80	0	0	25
	Frankfurter	Average	1	50	7	540	110
	Ham	Cooked	1 ounce	30	7	270	95
	Lunch meat	Sliced	1 ounce	30	5	370	65
	Mustard		1 teaspoon	5	0	60	5
	Peanut butter	Regular	2 tablespoons	33	8	220	215
	Pork sausage	Links	2 (1½ oz)	40	7	385	110
	Salad dressings						
	Blue cheese		1 tablespoon	14	0.5	155	5
	French	Regular	1 tablespoon	14	0	190	10
	Italian	Regular	1 tablespoon	14	0	295	0
	Tomato juice	Regular	¼ cup	63	0.5	125	145
	Tuna	Oil packed	¼ cup	40	10	320	120
		Unsalted, water packed	¼ cup	40	11	15	110

REFERENCES CITED

1. Kerr, D. N. S. 1975. Chronic renal failure. In *Cecil–Loeb textbook of medicine,* eds., P. B. Beeson and W. McDermott. 14th ed. Philadelphia: W. B. Saunders.
2. Giovannetti, S., and Maggiore, Q. 1964. A low-nitrogen diet with proteins of high biological value for severe chronic uraemia. *Lancet* 1:1000.
3. Kopple, J. D., and Coburn, J. W. 1973. Metabolic studies of low protein diets in uremia. I. Nitrogen and potassium. *Medicine* 52:583.
4. Kopple, J. D. Nutritional management of chronic renal failure. *Postgrad. Med.* 64:135.
5. Kopple, J. D.; Shinaberger, J. H.; Coburn, J. W.; Sorensen, M. K.; and Rubini, M. E. 1969. Evaluating modified protein diets for uremia. *J. Am. Dietet. A.* 54:481.
6. Kopple, J. D.; Sorensen, M. K.; Coburn, J. W.; Gordon, S.; and Rubini, M. E. 1968. Controlled comparison of 20-g and 40-g protein diets in the treatment of chronic uremia. *Am. J. Clin. Nutr.* 21:553.
7. Scott, R. B., ed. 1978. *Price's textbook of the practice of medicine.* 12th ed. Oxford: Oxford University Press.
8. Blumenkrantz, M. J.; Roberts, C. E.; Card, B.; Coburn, J. W.; and Kopple, J. D. 1978. Nutritional management of the adult patient undergoing peritoneal dialysis. *J. Am. Dietet. A.* 73:251.
9. Isselbacher, K. J.; Adams, R. D.; Braunwald, E.; Petersdorf, R. G.; and Wilson, J. D., eds. 1978. *Harrison's principles of internal medicine.* 9th ed. New York: McGraw-Hill.
10. Merrill, A. J. 1956. Nutrition in chronic renal failure. *Am. J. Clin. Nutr.* 4:497.
11. Merrill, A. J. 1960. Nutrition in chronic renal failure. *JAMA* 173:125.
12. Kopple, J. D., and Swendseid, M. E. 1975. Vitamin nutrition in patients undergoing maintenance hemodialysis. *Kidney Int.* 7 (Suppl. 2) :79.
13. Ito, T.; Niwa, T.; and Matsui, E. 1971. Vitamin B_2 and vitamin E in long-term hemodialysis. *JAMA* 217:699.
14. DeLuca, H. F. 1975. The kidney as an endocrine organ involved in the function of vitamin D. *Am. J. Med.* 58:39.
15. Tsaltas, T. T. 1969. Dietetic management of uremic patients. I. Extraction of potassium from foods for uremic patients. *Am. J. Clin. Nutr.* 22:490.
16. Roberts, C. E. 1979. Anemia in patients with chronic renal failure. *Dialysis and Transplantation.* 8:547.
17. Sullivan, J. F., and Eisenstein, A. B. 1972. Ascorbic acid depletion during hemodialysis. *JAMA* 220:1697.
18. Kopple, J. D.; Swendseid, M. E.; Holliday, M. A.; Alfrey, A. C.; and Gulyassy, P. F. 1975. Recommendations for nutritional evaluation of patients on chronic dialysis. *Kidney Int.* 7 (Suppl. 2) :249.

OTHER REFERENCES

Association of Michigan Nephrology Dietitians. 1975. *Diet instruction manual.* Ann Arbor, Mich.: Kidney Foundation of Michigan.

Nephrotic Syndrome

INDICATIONS FOR USE

This diet is indicated for individuals who have nephrotic syndrome. It should be used until hyperproteinuria diminishes and nitrogen balance is restored. If glomerular filtration rate decreases and uremic symptoms develop, the diet for renal failure is indicated.

DESCRIPTION

The goals of diet therapy for nephrotic syndrome are to replenish body nitrogen stores, maintain nitrogen balance, control edema, and control blood lipid values. Nutrition therapy may include modifications in protein, energy, sodium, fluid, and/or fat content of the diet.

Protein. In nephrotic syndrome the renal glomeruli are abnormally permeable to protein, resulting in urinary excretion of large amounts of plasma proteins, primarily albumin. (1, 2) The proteinuria produces negative nitrogen balance that, if untreated, leads to catabolism of tissue protein. A high-protein diet will improve nitrogen balance and protect body nitrogen stores. (2, 3) A therapeutic level of dietary protein is determined by urinary nitrogen loss and the degree of protein depletion already present. (3) A protein intake of 120 g/day has been shown to produce positive nitrogen balance in most adults with nephrotic syndrome. (4) Some individuals may require higher levels of dietary protein to achieve positive nitrogen balance. Refer to Table 1-4 to calculate nitrogen balance and to Table A.7-2 to estimate grams of protein lost.

Energy. Individuals who have nephrotic syndrome are in a catabolic state, and an energy intake of 50–60 kcal per kilogram of ideal body weight is recommended. (2) If patients lose weight, kilocalories per kilogram should be increased.

Sodium/Fluid. Albumin contributes 80% of the colloid osmotic pressure of normal plasma. When the albumin level drops, the colloid osmotic pressure is reduced, causing a net loss of fluid from plasma, through the capillaries, into the interstitial space. The resulting edema may be treated with a combination of diuretics, fluid restriction, and/or a low-sodium diet. When edema is severe, a strict sodium restriction, 10 mEq (230 mg) per day may be necessary. (2, 3) As edema decreases, sodium intake should be liberalized to improve palatability and other nutrient intake. (3)

Fat. Hyperlipoproteinemia, generally Types II, IV, or V, and an increased incidence of coronary heart disease are associated with the nephrotic syndrome. (3–5) Measures to control the hyperlipidemia should be instituted. (3–5)

GUIDELINES FOR NUTRITIONAL MANAGEMENT

The dietary prescription should meet the following criteria:

- Provide a minimum of 120 g of protein per day.
- Provide 50–60 kcal per kilogram of ideal body weight.

- Provide sodium at the level required to control edema. Low-sodium milk or high-protein, low-sodium supplements may be necessary to provide adequate protein and calories when sodium restriction is severe (Chapter 3).
- Control hyperlipidemia by appropriate dietary modifications (Chapter 32).

The meal plan is established with the patient to meet the calorie, protein, sodium, fat, and/or fluid restrictions necessary to control symptoms. Appropriate food exchange systems or tables of nutrient values may be used. Table 27-1 lists some appropriate food tables. Small, frequent meals with supplements (Chapters 2 and 3) may be necessary to provide for the high protein and energy requirements of the diet. Patients may be nauseated, with little appetite, and need encouragement to eat.

NUTRIENT ADEQUACY

Nutrient adequacy of the diet for an individual with nephrotic syndrome can only be determined by ongoing assessment of nutrient intake and nutritional status.

TABLES

TABLE 27-1. Food Exchange Systems Appropriate for Nephrotic Syndrome

Diet Prescription	Food Exchange Systems	Tables
High protein, high calorie	Diabetic Hyperlipoproteinemia	25-4, 25-5 32-5, 32-6
High protein, high calorie, low sodium	Protein–sodium	26-3, 26-4, 26-5
High protein, high calorie, low cholesterol, increased polyunsaturated/saturated fat ratio	Hyperlipoproteinemia	32-5, 32-6

REFERENCES CITED

1. Earley, L. E., and Forland, M. 1979. Nephrotic syndrome. In *Strauss and Welt's diseases of the kidney.* eds., L. E. Earley and C. W. Gottschalk, pp. 765–813. 3rd ed. Boston: Little, Brown.
2. Kark, R. M., and Oyama, J. H. 1980. Nutrition, hypertension and kidney diseases. In *Modern nutrition in health and disease,* eds., R. S. Goodhart, and M. E. Shils, pp. 998–1044. 6th ed. Philadelphia: Lea & Febiger.
3. Squire, J. R. 1956. Nutrition and the nephrotic syndrome in adults. *Am. J. Clin. Nutr.* 4:509.
4. Blainey, J. D. 1954. High protein diets in the treatment of the nephrotic syndrome. *Clin. Sci.* 13:567.
5. Chopra, J. S., Mallick, N. P., and Stone, M. C. 1971. Hyperlipoproteinaemias in nephrotic syndrome. *Lancet* 1:317.
6. Alexander, J. H., Schapel, G. J., and Edwards, K. D. G. 1974. Increased incidence of coronary heart disease associated with combined elevation of serum triglyceride and cholesterol concentrations in the nephrotic syndrome in man. *Med. J. Austr.* 2:119.

Cirrhotic Liver Disease

INDICATIONS FOR USE

This diet is indicated for use with individuals with cirrhotic liver disease. Nutritional management will depend on the disease state and concurrent medical therapy.

DESCRIPTION

The cirrhotic liver is characterized by abnormal cell structure that interferes with the normal hepatic blood flow and filtration system. Nutrition therapy for cirrhosis may include protein, sodium, fluid, potassium, and energy modifications. The degree of modification is determined by the individual's clinical symptoms and blood levels of sodium, potassium, and ammonia. Symptoms and blood levels change as the disease and treatment progress. The individual's nutritional needs must be continually reevaluated and the diet adjusted appropriately.

Protein. For individuals with liver disease, a high-protein intake may lead to hepatic encephalopathy. The exact cause of the encephalopathy is under investigation. The high blood levels of ammonia have been implicated. (1, 2) Other researchers have linked a disordered amino acid pattern in the blood, increased levels of the aromatic amino acids, and decreased levels of the branched-chain amino acids to the encephalopathy. (3–6) At present, acute encephalopathy is treated by removal of protein from the diet. As mental status improves, protein is added back to the diet beginning with 20–30 g/day. The use of oral or infused solutions specially formulated to contain low concentrations of aromatic amino acids and high concentrations of branched-chain amino acids is being studied and requires further investigation to substantiate effectiveness. (3, 4, 6, 7)

Sodium. Ascites and edema are often present with cirrhosis. Ascites result from the combination of low serum colloid osmotic pressure and portal hypertension. Serum colloid osmotic pressure is reduced due to defective synthesis of albumin. Portal hypertension results from the obstruction of venous blood flow through the liver. The increased venous pressure results in leakage of fluid from the circulatory system into the interstitial space producing ascites. The kidney attempts to compensate for the loss of circulatory fluid by conserving fluid and sodium. (8) When ascites and edema are severe, sodium intake may need to be restricted below 500 mg (9, 10) As edema and ascites lessen, sodium intake may be slowly liberalized up to 2500 mg if body weight does not increase and edema and ascites do not recur. (9)

Fluid. With persistent fluid retention, fluid intake should be restricted to equal the previous day's urinary output plus insensible losses.

Potassium. Serum potassium levels must be monitored. Serum potassium may fall due to decreased intake and losses from vomiting, diarrhea, and diuretic therapy. (9) Serum potassium may rise if renal impairment is present.

Energy. Adequate calorie intake is essential but is often difficult to attain because of necessary protein and sodium restrictions. The failure to ingest sufficient calories results in catabolism of body protein. (11) Caloric intake should be great enough to prevent loss of lean body mass.

GUIDELINES FOR NUTRITIONAL MANAGEMENT

The dietary prescription is determined by the physician and dietitian based on the individual's hepatic function, clinical status, medical therapy, and nutrient needs.

The diet is generally modified in protein, sodium, and fluid. To facilitate meal planning, foods have been divided into groups depending on their protein and sodium content. Table 26-3 lists the average protein and sodium content of one serving from each of the food groups in the protein–sodium food exchange system. Table 26-4 lists the specific foods in each of the food groups and their serving sizes.

The diet prescription can be met using two calculation methods. One method suitable for the hospitalized patient requires daily calculation of the protein and sodium content of the food items that the patient selects and adjustment of portion sizes to meet the specific requirements. The other method requires calculation of a daily meal pattern from the food groups. (Refer to Chapter 26 for a sample calculation, omitting the procedure for potassium restriction unless a potassium restriction is indicated.)

Because of the difficulty in providing adequate calories while the protein intake is severely restricted, low-protein supplements are often necessary. These may be in the form of supplementary beverages (Chapter 3), butterballs (Table 28-1), or low-protein, specially manufactured baked products.

NUTRIENT ADEQUACY

Nutrient adequacy of the diet is dependent on the degree of protein restriction. A diet severely restricted in protein will be deficient in calories, vitamins, and minerals.

TABLES

TABLE 28-1. Recipe: Butterballs[1]

Ingredients	Weight (g)	Household Measure[2]
Butter, unsalted	115	½ cup
Sugar, powdered	350	2¾ cups
Flavoring (lemon juice/ vanilla)	15	1 tablespoon

[1] Butterballs should be kept frozen. Recipe makes 32, 15-g balls. Total nutrients in recipe are protein, 1 g; fat, 90 g; carbohydrate, 350 g; calories, 2200; sodium, 13 mg; potassium, 12 mg.
[2] Household measures approximately equal the gram weight.

REFERENCES CITED

1. Harper, H. A. 1961. Protein intake in liver disease. *J. Am. Dietet. A.* 38:350.
2. Lockwood, A. H.; McDonald, J. M.; Reiman, R. E.; Gelbard, A. S.; Laughlin, J. S.; Duffy, T. F.; and Plum, F. 1979. The dynamics of ammonia metabolism in man. Effects of liver disease and hyperammonemia. *J. Clin. Invest.* 63:449.
3. Freund, H.; Yoshimura, N.; and Fischer, J. E. 1979. Chronic hepatic encephalopathy. Long-term therapy with a branched-chain amino-acid-enriched elemental diet. *JAMA* 242:347.
4. Fischer, J. E.; Funovics, J. M.; Aguirre, A.; James, J. H.; Keane, J. M.; Wesdorp, R. I. C.; Yoshimura, N.; and Westman, T. 1975. The role of plasma amino acids in hepatic encephalopathy. *Surgery* 78:276.
5. Fischer, J. E.; Rosen, H. M.; Ebeid, A. M.; James, J. H.; Keane, J. M.; and Soeters, P. E. 1976. The effects of normalization of plasma amino acids on hepatic encephalopathy in man. *Surgery* 80:77.
6. Rosen, H. M.; Yoshimura, N.; Hodgman, J. M.; and Fischer, J. E. 1977. Plasma amino acid patterns in hepatic encephalopathy of differing etiology. *Gastroenterology* 72:483.
7. Baker, A. L. 1979. Amino acids in liver disease: A cause of hepatic encephalopathy? *JAMA* 242:355.
8. Editorial. 1978. Management of hepatic ascites. *Lancet* 1:311.
9. Gabuzda, G. J. 1970. Nutrition and liver disease. Practical considerations. *Med. Clinics N. Am.* 54:1455.
10. Davidson, C. S. 1980. Diseases of the liver. In *Modern nutrition in health and disease,* eds., R. S. Goodhart and M. E. Shils, pp. 962–976. 6th ed. Philadelphia: Lea & Febiger.
11. Borst, J. G. G. 1948. Protein catabolism in uremia. Effects of protein-free diet, infections, and blood transfusions. *Lancet* 1:824.

PART VII
Fat Modifications

Low Fat

INDICATIONS FOR USE

A low-fat diet may be indicated in the treatment of gallbladder disease or malabsorption syndromes. (1) Treatment of disorders involving fat intolerance or malabsorption is focused on the underlying cause and may involve surgery (e.g., cholecystectomy), drug therapy, or enzyme replacements.

DESCRIPTION

A fat-restricted diet is used to reduce symptoms related to fat ingestion. In gallbladder disease, fat restriction has been used prior to surgery to prevent stimulation of contractions of the gallbladder through release of cholecystokinin. In malabsorption states as may occur with pancreatic disease or short bowel, fat restriction may decrease diarrhea and nutrient losses. Medium-chain triglycerides may be useful. Medium-chain fatty acids are absorbed more efficiently than are long-chain fatty acids in pancreatic enzyme or bile salt deficiency and in other malabsorption syndromes. When steatorrhea is present, absorption of fat-soluble vitamins and other nutrients may be impaired. (1, 2)

GUIDELINES FOR NUTRITIONAL MANAGEMENT

Restrict fat to 50 g/day unless otherwise indicated by diet prescription. The level of fat may need to be adjusted to control symptoms of steatorrhea.

Medium-chain triglycerides are not considered part of the total fat restriction and may be used as desired (refer to Chapter 3 for information regarding use and nutrient content of MCT oil).

Provide protein in amounts at least equal to the recommended dietary allowances. Adequate protein intake may be difficult to achieve when fat intake is severely restricted as protein and fat occur together in many foods. Skim milk, nonfat cottage cheese, egg whites, and nonfat protein supplements may be useful in meeting protein requirements.

The diet is planned using the diabetic (Chapter 25) or the hyperlipoproteinemia (Chapter 32) food exchange systems.

The procedure for calculating a low-fat diet is as follows:

Steps	*Example*
1. Obtain diet history. Establish an appropriate calorie level and minimum protein requirement.	Calories: 2000 kcal/day Minimum protein: 44 g/day
2. Identify total grams of fat allowed per day as defined by diet prescription.	Diet prescription: 20 g/day

3. Identify food groups that contribute fat and calculate the number of exchanges allowed from each of the fat-containing food groups to provide the fat allowance (diabetic food exchange groups used, Table 25-4).

Food Exchange Group	No. Exchanges	Protein (g)	Fat (g)
Milk, nonskim	0	—	—
Meat, lean–medium fat	3	21	15
Meat, high fat	0	—	—
Fat	1	—	5
Total		21	20

4. Calculate minimum number of exchanges necessary to meet minimum protein requirement from food groups that contribute protein but no fat.

Food Exchange Group	No. Exchanges	Protein (g)	Fat (g)
Totals from food groups contributing fat		21	20
Milk, skim	2	16	—
Fruit	As desired		
Vegetable	As desired		
Bread	4	8	—
Total		45	20

5. Provide remainder of caloric requirement from food groups that do not contribute fat, other foods with negligible fat content (Table 29-1), and MCT oil, which contains 8.3 kcal/g (116.2 kcal per tablespoon).

Food Exchange Group or Food Item	No. Exchanges or Total Amount	Protein (g)	Fat (g)	kcal
Meat, lean–medium fat	3	21	15	219
Fat	1	—	5	45
Milk, skim	2	16	—	180
Fruit	6	—	—	240
Vegetable	2	4	—	56
Bread	10	20	—	680
MCT oil	4 tablespoons	—	—	465
Jelly	2 tablespoons	—	—	98
Total		61	20	1983

NUTRIENT ADEQUACY

Nutrient adequacy will depend on the level of dietary fat restriction and the individual's food choices. At very low levels of fat intake, protein requirements may not be met if adequate quantities of skim milk or other high-protein, low-fat foods are not consumed.

Nonfat protein supplements and vitamin–mineral supplements may be indicated. If fat malabsorption is present, fat-soluble vitamins should be supplemented in adequate amounts to meet deficiencies and compensate for fecal fat losses. (1) Supplementation should be done on an individual basis.

Fat-free diets or diets extremely low in fat may be deficient in essential fatty acids. Use of small amounts of polyunsaturated oil should supply the essential fatty acid requirement, 1–2% of total calories. (3)

TABLES

TABLE 29-1. Food of Negligible Fat Content

Food Item	Serving Size	Weight (g)	kcal
Cake, angel food	$\frac{1}{12}$ of medium cake	60	161
Candy			
Hard	1 ounce	28	109
Marshmallow	1 large	7	23
Carbonated beverage			
Cola-type	12 fluid ounces	369	144
Fruit-flavored	12 fluid ounces	372	171
Cottage cheese, dry curd	1 cup packed	200	172
Egg white	1 medium	29	15
Gelatin dessert	$\frac{1}{2}$ cup	120	71
Honey	1 tablespoon	21	64
Jam	1 tablespoon	20	54
Jelly	1 tablespoon	18	49
Lemonade	8 fluid ounces	248	107
Syrup, maple	1 tablespoon	20	50
Sugar, granulated	1 tablespoon	12	46
Sherbet	$\frac{1}{2}$ cup	97	130

REFERENCES CITED

1. Council on Foods and Nutrition. 1962. The regulation of dietary fat. *JAMA* 181:411.
2. Goodhart, R. S., and Shils, M. F., eds. 1980. *Modern nutrition in health and disease,* pp. 1301–1304. 6th ed. Philadelphia: Lea & Febiger.
3. Food and Nutrition Board. 1980. *Recommended dietary allowances,* pp. 33–35. 9th rev. ed. Washington, D.C.: National Academy of Sciences.

Intestinal Lymphangiectasia

INDICATIONS FOR USE

This diet is indicated for individuals with intestinal lymphangiectasia.

DESCRIPTION

Intestinal lymphangiectasia is a disorder of the intestinal lymphatics resulting in a protein-losing enteropathy. (1, 2) It is characterized by albumin losses, enteric protein losses, and morphologic changes in the small bowel biopsy. Edema and mild gastrointestinal symptoms are common. (1–3) Severe diarrhea and steatorrhea, nausea, vomiting, abdominal pain, chylous effusions, hypoalbumenemia, hypogammaglobulinemia, and lymphocytopenia may be present. (3)

The goal of nutritional management is to reduce symptoms of the disease by decreasing dietary fat. (1) Dietary fat stimulates lymphatic flow in the gut. (1) The increased intestinal lymphatic pressure with dilation of the vessels is thought to result in discharge of lymphatic fluid into the bowel and loss of plasma proteins. (3) Restriction of dietary fat has been effective in treatment. (2, 4)

Medium-chain triglycerides are absorbed directly into the portal vein without utilizing the lymphatic system and do not result in lacteal engorgement. (2) Medium-chain triglycerides are useful in dietary treatment. They increase the caloric content and palatability of the diet.

A high-protein intake is recommended to alleviate hypoproteinemia. (2)

GUIDELINES FOR NUTRITIONAL MANAGEMENT

Restrict dietary fat to a level to control symptoms. Less than 5 g fat/day may be necessary. (2, 4)

Medium-chain triglycerides are not considered part of the fat allowance and may be used as desired (refer to Chapter 3 for information regarding use and nutrient content of MCT oil).

Increase dietary protein and carbohydrate to allow for adequate caloric intake to reach weight goals.

Follow the guidelines in Chapter 29 for calculation of the diet.

NUTRIENT ADEQUACY

Refer to Chapter 29 for nutrient adequacy of a low-fat diet.

REFERENCES CITED

1. Halpern, S. L. 1979. *Quick reference to clinical nutrition,* p. 180. Philadelphia: J. B. Lippincott.
2. Vardy, P. A.; Lebenthal, E.; and Shwachman, H. 1975. Intestinal lymphangiectasia: A reappraisal. *Pediatrics* 55:842.
3. Broitman, S. A., and Zamchek, N. 1980. Nutrition in diseases of the gastrointestinal tract. B. Nutrition in diseases of the intestines. In *Modern nutrition in health and disease.* eds., R. S. Goodhart and M. E. Shils, p. 932. 6th ed. Philadelphia: Lea & Febiger.
4. Jeffries, G. H.; Chapman, A.; and Sleisenger, M. H. 1964. Low-fat diet in intestinal lymphangiectasia. *N. Eng. J. Med.* 270:761.

Hyperlipoproteinemia, I

INDICATIONS FOR USE

This diet is indicated for individuals with Type I hyperlipoproteinemia. The term hyperlipoproteinemia is often abbreviated to hyperlipidemia. The two words are used interchangeably throughout the manual.

DESCRIPTION

Type I hyperlipoproteinemia (hyperchylomicronemia) is found in individuals who have a genetically determined deficiency of lipoprotein lipase, resulting in an inability to clear chylomicrons from the blood. Plasma triglyceride levels are very high, 1000–4000 mg or higher per 100 ml, following a 12 hour fast. Plasma very-low-density (pre-beta) lipoprotein level is normal. Lipemia retinalis, hepatosplenomegaly, eruptive xanthomas, abdominal pain, and pancreatitis may result. (1)

The goal of nutritional management is to reduce chylomicron formation by decreasing dietary fat. Medium-chain triglycerides may be substituted for long-chain fatty acids since medium-chain triglycerides are absorbed directly into the portal vein and do not form chylomicrons. (1)

GUIDELINES FOR NUTRITIONAL MANAGEMENT

Restrict dietary fat to approximately 0.5 g/kg body weight. This restriction applies to both saturated and polyunsaturated fatty acids. (1)

Medium-chain triglyceride oil is not considered part of the fat allowance and may be used as desired (refer to Chapter 3 for information regarding use and nutrient content of MCT oil).

Follow the guidelines in Chapter 29 for calculation of the diet.

NUTRIENT ADEQUACY

Refer to Chapter 29 for nutrient adequacy of a low-fat diet.

REFERENCES CITED

1. Brown, W. V.; Baginsky, M. L.; and Ehnholm, C. 1977. Primary type I and type V hyperlipoproteinemia. In *Hyperlipidemia: Diagnosis and therapy,* eds., B. M. Rifkind and R. I. Levy, pp. 93–112. New York: Grune and Stratton.

Hyperlipoproteinemia, II–IV

INDICATIONS FOR USE

The hyperlipidemia diet is indicated for individuals with a definitive diagnosis of one of the five phenotypes of hyperlipoproteinemia (HLP) as defined by Frederickson et al. (1), the World Health Organization (2), and Gotto et al. (3) Hyperlipoproteinemia phenotype is determined by measurement of fasting plasma (or serum) cholesterol and triglyceride concentration and by lipoprotein electrophoresis. To obtain a representative lipoprotein electrophoretic profile, an individual should have maintained a stable weight on a normal mixed diet for several weeks. The blood sample should be drawn after the individual has fasted 12 hours from food (4) and 24 hours from alcohol. (5)

Lipoprotein electrophoretic patterns obtained up to eight weeks following myocardial infarction may not be accurate. Plasma cholesterol levels may be depressed and plasma triglyceride levels may be elevated during this period. (6)

Hyperlipoproteinemia often occurs secondary to another disease. Treatment should be directed toward the primary disease rather than toward the hyperlipoproteinemia. (7) Table 32-1 lists disease states that may result in secondary hyperlipoproteinemia.

DESCRIPTION

Lipoproteins, synthesized by the liver, are vehicles for extrahepatic transport of triglyceride, cholesterol, and phospholipid to the tissues. Four principal lipoprotein particles have been identified. They can be classified two ways: on the basis of electrical charge by lipoprotein electrophoresis or on the basis of density by lipoprotein ultracentrifugation.

Table 32-2 identifies the four lipoprotein particles on the basis of each system of classification and identifies their characteristic protein and lipid composition.

Hyperlipoproteinemia Types II-V are described in the following paragraphs and are summarized in Table 32-3. Refer to Chapter 31 for information regarding type I.

Type II (Hypercholesterolemia). Plasma cholesterol and low-density (beta) lipoprotein levels are elevated in Type IIA familial hypercholesterolemia. A deficiency of low-density lipoprotein receptors on the cell membrane, preventing normal uptake by the cell, is believed to be the primary defect. (9)

When very-low-density (pre-beta) lipoprotein levels are also elevated, the classification is Type IIB.

Type III (Remnant Removal, "Broad-Beta" Disease). Type III is a familial condition, occurring infrequently. Both plasma triglyceride and cholesterol levels are elevated, in the range of 350–800 mg/100 ml. Defective conversion of very-low-density (pre-beta) lipoprotein to low-density (beta) lipoprotein results in a lipoprotein of abnormal composition. This abnormal lipoprotein appears as a broad beta band upon electrophoresis.

Type IV (Endogenous Hypertriglyceridemia). Plasma triglycerides and very-low-density (pre-beta) lipoproteins are elevated in Type IVA. Chylomicrons are absent after fasting, and low-density (beta) lipoproteins are normal. The classification Type IVB is made when plasma cholesterol levels are also elevated. Type IV responds well to dietary modifications.

Type V (Mixed Hypertriglyceridemia). Plasma triglyceride levels range from 1000–6000 mg/100 ml. Chylomicrons are present in fasting plasma, and very-low-density (pre-beta) lipoproteins are elevated.

Hypercholesterolemia is a primary risk factor in coronary heart disease; hypertriglyceridemia is an associated risk factor. (10) The goals of nutrition therapy are to reduce plasma cholesterol and triglyceride levels by the following means:

Reduce to ideal body weight. Weight reduction alone can significantly reduce both plasma triglyceride and cholesterol levels in individuals with hyperlipoproteinemia. The lipid-lowering effect of weight reduction appears to be related to decreased production of very-low-density (pre-beta) lipoproteins by the liver. (11)

Reduce saturated fat intake. Reduction of saturated fat in the diet has the greatest cholesterol-lowering effect of all dietary modifications currently reported. (12) Animal fats and coconut oil are comprised primarily of saturated fat.

Increase polyunsaturated fat intake. An increase of polyunsaturated fat in the diet is the second most effective dietary modification currently reported to lower plasma cholesterol levels. (12) The maximum cholesterol-lowering effect of a high-polyunsaturated-fat diet can only be achieved with a concomitant reduction in saturated fat intake. The cholesterol-elevating effect of saturated fat is approximately two times greater than the cholesterol-lowering effect of polyunsaturated fatty acids. (13)

For type II, in which elevated cholesterol levels are the major lipid defect, two times as much polyunsaturated as saturated fat (P : S ratio of 2 : 1) is planned in the diet to give a maximum cholesterol-lowering effect.

For types III, IV, and V, in which the lipoprotein defect involves primarily triglyceride-rich particles, it is recommended that an equal amount of polyunsaturated and saturated fat be consumed (P : S ratio 1 : 1).

Serum triglyceride levels are also lowered by diets with a high ratio of polyunsaturated to saturated fatty acids. (14)

Restrict cholesterol intake. As dietary cholesterol intake increases from 0 mg/day to 600 mg/day, plasma cholesterol levels increase. (15)

Control carbohydrate and fat intake. Triglyceride synthesis in the liver is stimulated by diets high in free or refined fructose and sucrose; such diets result in elevated plasma triglyceride levels in some persons with abnormal lipoprotein metabolism. (16) Restriction of these refined sugars reduces triglyceride levels. (17)

Diets that control fat intake at 30–40% of calories and carbohydrate intake at 40–50% of calories can significantly lower serum triglyceride levels even in the absence of weight loss. (18)

Restrict alcohol intake. Alcohol ingestion can induce hypertriglyceridemia (19, 20) especially in the presence of a high-fat diet. (19) The alcohol-induced elevation of serum triglyceride is greater in persons with hypertriglyceridemia than in those with normal lipids. (19)

Other considerations. Low mean plasma lipid levels have been seen in populations consuming predominantly vegetarian diets. (21) Differences in protein source, amount of fiber, and kinds of fat consumed may all contribute to the lipid-lowering effect.

Conclusive statements about the effect of dietary fiber on lipid levels cannot be made at this time. (22, 23) Diets adequate in fiber may be of benefit for weight reduction due to their high satiety value and low caloric density.

Consuming two thirds to three fourths of the day's calories in one meal may contribute to hyperlipidemia. Distribution of food intake into three or more meals per day is recommended.

The following factors should be considered when evaluating research about the effects of dietary modification on plasma lipid levels:

Research subjects
- normo- or hyperlipidemic
- degree of physical fitness
- degree of adiposity or leanness
- change in weight during course of study
- presence of insulin resistance

Study diet
- iso-, hypo-, or hypercaloric
- quantitative and qualitative fat, protein, and carbohydrate composition
- fiber content

Other factors
- neuroendocrine factors influencing lipid and carbohydrate metabolism (stress, degree of adiposity)

The relationship of these multiple variables to lipid metabolism has not been thoroughly investigated.

GUIDELINES FOR NUTRITIONAL MANAGEMENT

Table 32-4 summarizes guidelines for nutritional management of hyperlipoproteinemias. Food exchange systems were developed to enable calculations of the dietary modifications required for control of hyperlipidemia. Table 32-5 lists the average nutrient composition of one exchange for each food group. The foods contained in each food group are listed in Tables 32-6 and 32-7. Table 32-8 is a worksheet used at University Hospital for calculating a diet using these food groups. When alcoholic beverages are used, refer to Table A.8-3.

The procedure for calculating a hyperlipoproteinemia diet is as follows:

Steps	***Example***
1. Review medical history.	MALE: 45 years old HEIGHT: 72 in. (183 cm) WEIGHT: 209 lb (95 kg) LIPOPROTEIN ELECTROPHORESIS: ↑ pre-beta plasma triglycerides: 418 mg percent plasma total cholesterol: 262 mg percent plasma HDL cholesterol: 33 mg percent DIAGNOSIS: type IV HLP; overweight

2. Obtain diet history.

FINDINGS:
Meat: eats mainly beef
Milk: 8 ounces whole milk per day
Cheese: 2 ounces per day
Eggs: 6 per week
Fruit: eats occasionally
Alcohol: 3, 12 ounce beers per day
Activity: moderately active

3. Determine approximate ideal body weight. Refer to Table 23-2.

Approximate ideal body weight: 167 lb (76 kg)

4. Determine kilocalories needed to maintain present weight. Refer to Chapter 23.

(167 lb × 14 kcal/lb) + [(209 lb − 167 lb)(4 kcal/lb)] = 2506 kcal

5. Subtract 500 kcal to give a weight loss of 1 lb/wk.

2500 kcal/day to maintain present weight
−500 kcal
2000 kcal/day to lose 1 lb/wk

6. Determine percentage of kilocalories to come from carbohydrate (CHO), protein, fat, and alcohol and the P:S ratio and cholesterol content of the diet. Consult Table 32-4 for the type of HLP being treated.

Type IVB HLP:
alcohol: no more than 5% of kcal
carbohydrate: 40%
protein: 20%
fat: 40%
(carbohydrate, protein, fat: of non-alcohol kcal)
P:S ratio: 1:1
cholesterol: less than 300 mg/day

7. Determine total grams of alcohol allowed per day.

Daily kcal allowance × % kcal to come from alcohol ÷ 7 kcal/g alcohol = grams of alcohol allowed per day.

$$\frac{(2000 \text{ kcal/day})(.05)}{7 \text{ kcal/g alcohol}} = 14 \text{ g alcohol/day}$$

8. Calculate number of nonalcohol kilocalories remaining.

Daily kcal allowance − kcal from alcohol = nonalcohol kcal remaining.

2000 kcal/day − 100 kcal from alcohol = 1900 kcal remaining

9. Calculate total grams of carbohydrate allowed per day from nonalcohol kilocalories.

Nonalcohol kcal × % kcal to come from CHO ÷ 4 kcal/g CHO = grams of CHO allowed per day.

$$\frac{(1900 \text{ kcal})(.40)}{4 \text{ kcal/g CHO}} = 190 \text{ g CHO/day}$$

10. Calculate total grams of protein allowed per day from nonalcohol kilocalories.

    Nonalcohol kcal × % kcal to come from protein ÷ 4 kcal/g protein = grams of protein allowed per day.

    $$\frac{(1900 \text{ kcal})(.20)}{4 \text{ kcal/g protein}} = 95 \text{ g protein/day}$$

11. Calculate total grams of fat allowed per day from nonalcohol kilocalories.

    Nonalcohol kcal × % kcal to come from fat ÷ 9 kcal/g fat = grams of fat allowed per day.

    $$\frac{(1900 \text{ kcal})(.40)}{9 \text{ kcal/g fat}} = 84 \text{ g fat/day}$$

12. Determine the number of exchanges to come from carbohydrate-containing foods based on preferences obtained during the diet history. Use Table 32-5. Also include the carbohydrate from alcoholic beverages (Table A.8-3). No more than 40% carbohydrate should come from fruit exchanges.

Food Group	No. Exchanges	Carbohydrate (g)	Protein (g)	Fat (g)	Polyunsaturated Fat (g)	Saturated Fat (g)	Cholesterol (mg)	Alcohol (g)
Milk, skim	1	12	8					
Vegetable	2	10	4					
Fruit	3	30						
Bread	9	135	18					
Beer (12 oz)	1	14						13
Subtotal		201	30					13

13. Determine the grams of protein remaining in the daily total to come from meat.

    Total grams protein − grams of protein from CHO-containing exchanges = grams of protein coming from meat.

    95 g − 30 g = 65 g of protein to come from meat

14. Determine the number of exchanges to come from meat. Divide among groups A, B, and C. Meat A choices, the lowest in fat, may always be used in place of meat B or C choices.

    Grams of protein to come from meat ÷ grams of protein per meat exchange = number of meat exchanges.

    $$\frac{65 \text{ g protein from meat}}{8 \text{ g protein per meat exchange}} \cong 8 \text{ meat exchanges}$$

Food Group	No. Exchanges	Carbohydrate (g)	Protein (g)	Fat (g)	Polyunsaturated Fat (g)	Saturated Fat (g)	Cholesterol (mg)	Alcohol (g)
CHO-containing groups, subtotal		201	30					13
Meat A								
Meat B	7		56	21	0.7	8.4	210	
Meat C	1		8	8	0.2	5.4	20	
Subtotal		201	94	29	0.9	13.8	240	13

15. Determine the number of egg exhanges allowed per week.

Total cholesterol allowed per day − cholesterol already planned ÷ amount of cholesterol per egg exchange = number of egg exchanges per week.

$$\frac{\text{300 mg cholesterol/day} - \text{240 mg cholesterol}}{\text{40 mg cholesterol/egg exchange}} = \text{1.5 or 1 egg exchange per week}$$

16. Determine the number of exchanges to come from fat.

Total grams fat − grams fat already used ÷ 5 g fat per fat exchange = number of fat exchanges.

$$\frac{\text{84 g fat/day} - \text{30 g fat used}}{\text{5 g fat per fat exchange}} \cong \text{10 fat exchanges}$$

Divide between groups A and B to achieve the desired P:S ratio. Fat A choices higher in polyunsaturated fat may always be used in place of fat B choices. One or more of the following manipulations may also be necessary to achieve the designated ratio.

a. Specify a calculated number of meat and/or fat exchanges from the A groups.
b. Use a lower-fat milk.
c. Omit choices from meat C group.

Food Group	No. Exchanges	Carbohydrate (g)	Protein (g)	Fat (g)	Polyunsaturated Fat (g)	Saturated Fat (g)	Cholesterol (mg)	Alcohol (g)
CHO-containing and meat groups, subtotal		201	94	29	0.9	13.8	240	13
Egg	1		1	1	0.1	0.3	40	
Fat A								
Fat B	10			50	19.0	8.0		
Total		201	95	80	20.0	22.1	280	13

17. Determine that prescribed P:S ratio has been met.

P:S ratio = Grams polyunsaturated fat ÷ Grams saturated fat.

$$\frac{\text{20.0 g polyunsaturated fat}}{\text{22.1 g saturated fat}} \cong 1:1$$

18. Determine that diet prescription has been met.

Diet Prescription: 2000 kcal
Alcohol: no more than 5% of kcal
Carbohydrate: 40%
Protein: 20%
Fat: 40%
} of nonalcohol kcal
P:S: 1:1
Cholesterol: less than 300 mg/day
Diet calculation:

Food Group	No. Exchanges	Carbohydrate (g)	Protein (g)	Fat (g)	Polyunsaturated Fat (g)	Saturated Fat (g)	Cholesterol (mg)	Alcohol (g)
Milk, skim	1	12	8					
Vegetable	2	10	4					
Fruit	3	30						
Bread	9	135	18					
Meat B	7		56	21	0.7	8.4	210	
Meat C	1		8	8	0.2	5.4	30	
Egg per week	1		1	1	0.1	0.3	40	
Fat B	10			50	19.0	8.0		
Beer (12 oz)	1	14						13
Total		201	95	80	20.0	22.1	280	13

Total kcal: 1995
Alcohol: 5% of kcal
Carbohydrate: 42%
Protein: 20%
Fat: 38%
} of nonalcohol kcal
P:S: 1:1
Cholesterol: 280 mg

Diet prescription is adequately met.

Sample Menu for 2000 Calorie type IV hlp Diet

Breakfast
Orange juice, 4 ounces
Puffed wheat, 1 ounce
Toast, whole wheat, 2 slices
Cottage cheese, ¼ cup
Polyunsaturated margarine, 2 teaspoons
Skim milk, 8 ounces
Coffee or tea
Sugar substitute

Lunch
Tuna, 3 ounces
Mayonnaise, 1 tablespoon
Polyunsaturated margarine, 1 teaspoon
Bread, whole wheat, 2 slices
Asparagus cuts, ½ cup
Fresh peach
Coffee or tea
Sugar substitute
Salt and pepper

Dinner
Roast beef, 3 ounces
Baked potato, medium
Green beans, ½ cup
Shredded lettuce with tomato wedge
French dressing, 2 tablespoons
Dinner roll
Polyunsaturated margarine, 2 teaspoons
Unsweetened applesauce, ½ cup
Coffee or tea
Sugar substitute
Salt and pepper

Evening snack
Cheddar cheese, 1 ounce
Saltine crackers, 6
Beer, 12 ounces

NUTRIENT ADEQUACY

Types II–V hyperlipidemia diets can be planned to meet the recommended dietary allowances, 1980, provided that a variety of foods is consumed in adequate amounts. Vitamin and mineral supplementation may be necessary when calories are restricted.

TABLES

TABLE 32-1. Disease States That May Result in Secondary Hyperlipoproteinemia (7)

Disease	Secondary Hyperlipoproteinemia
Dysgammaglobulinemia	Type I
Dysgammaglobulinemia Hypothyroidism Acute intermittent porphyria	Type II
Diabetes mellitus Hypothyroidism Dysgammaglobulinemia	Type III
Diabetes mellitus Nephrosis Chronic renal failure Dysgammaglobulinemia Hypothyroidism Alcohol excess Glycogen storage disease Idiopathic hypercalcemia Progeria Addison's disease Cushing's disease Sepsis	Types IV, V

Adapted from Rifkind, B. M., and Levy, R. I., eds. 1977. *Hyperlipidemia: Diagnosis and Therapy*. New York: Grune and Stratton. Used by permission of the publisher.

TABLE 32-2. Classification of Lipoprotein Particles and Their Characteristic Protein and Lipid Composition (8)

Classifications		Composition (percentage)			
Ultracentrifugation	Electrophoresis	Protein	Cholesterol	Triglyceride	Phospholipid
Chylomicrons		0.5–1.0	2–5	85	3–6
VLDL[1]	pre-beta	5–15	10–20	50–70	10–20
LDL[2]	beta	25	40–45	5–10	20–25
HDL[3]	alpha	45–55	18	2	30

[1] VLDL are very-low-density lipoproteins.
[2] LDL are low-density lipoproteins.
[3] HDL are high-density lipoproteins.

TABLE 32-3. Summary of Plasma Lipid Characteristics of Hyperlipoproteinemias

Hyperlipo-proteinemia	Character of Lipoprotein Abnormality	Total Plasma Cholesterol (mg/dl)	Total Plasma Triglycerides (mg/dl)
II			
A	LDL (beta) ↑ or ↑↑	>250	Normal
B	LDL (beta) ↑ or ↑↑ VLDL (pre-beta) ↑	>250	>150
III	VLDL (pre-beta) and LDL (beta) of abnormal composition	>250	>150
IV			
A	VLDL (pre-beta) ↑ or ↑↑	Normal	>150
B	VLDL (pre beta) ↑ or ↑↑	>250	>150
V	Chylomicrons ↑↑ VLDL (pre-beta) ↑ or ↑↑	≥250	1000–6000

↑Mild elevation.
↑↑Moderate elevation.

TABLE 32-4. Summary of Nutrition Management for Hyperlipoproteinemias, II–V

	Percentage of Calories						
Classsifications	Carbohydrate	Protein	Fat	Alcohol[1]	P:S Ratio	Cholesterol (mg/100 ml)	Carbohydrate Modifications
II							
A	50	20	30	≤5	2:1	200	Avoid refined sugars
B	40	20	40	≤5	2:1	200	Avoid refined sugars
III	40	20	40	≤5	1:1	300	Avoid refined sugars
IV							
A	40	20	40	≤5	1:1	400	Avoid refined sugars
B	40	20	40	≤5	1:1	300	Avoid refined sugars
V	50	20	30	Avoid	1:1	400	Avoid refined sugars

[1] Alcohol should comprise no more than 5% of total calories in the diets. The number of calories to come from alcohol should be calculated first. The amount of protein, fat, and carbohydrate to be included in the diet should be calculated from the remaining calories (nonalcohol calories) using the proportions listed. Refer to Table A.8-3 for the alcohol content of some beverages.

TABLE 32-5. Nutrient Content of One Exchange, Hyperlipoproteinemia Food Exchange System

	Nutrients in One Exchange						
Food Exchange Group	Carbohydrate (g)	Protein (g)	Fat (g)	Polyunsaturated Fat (g)	Saturated Fat (g)	Cholesterol (mg)	kcal
Milk							
Skim	12	8			0.3	5	80
2%	12	8	5	0.2	2.9	20	125
Vegetable	5	2					28
Fruit	10						40
Bread	15	2					68
Meat							
A		8	1	0.4	0.6	25	41
B		8	3	0.1	1.2	30	59
C		8	8	0.2	5.4	30	104
Fat							
A			5	3.3	0.5		45
B			5	1.9	0.8		45
Egg		1	1	0.1	0.3	40	13

TABLE 32-6. Hyperlipoproteinemia Food Exchange System

Group	Food Item	One Exchange (serving size)	Foods to Avoid
Milk	Milk, skim	1 cup	Whole milk; whole milk beverages; evaporated whole milk; condensed whole milk; eggnog; malted beverage mixes; instant beverage drinks; flavored yogurt; 2% milk (unless planned into the diet)
	Buttermilk	1 cup	
	Powdered skim milk, dry	$\frac{1}{3}$ cup	
	Evaporated skim milk, undiluted	$\frac{1}{2}$ cup	
	2% milk (must be planned into the diet)		
Vegetable	Use vegetable groups in the diabetic food exchange system. Table 25-5	Varies	None
Fruit	Use fruit group in the diabetic food exchange system, Table 25-5	Varies	Avocados; coconut; syrup-packed fruit
Bread	Use bread group in the diabetic food exchange system, Table 25-5, except for dried peas and beans and wheat germ. For serving sizes, refer to Table 32-7, vegetarian meat group	Varies	Products made with butter, lard, egg yolks Biscuits; corn bread; muffins; pancakes; waffles unless made with allowed ingredients[1]
			Animal crackers; chow mein noodles; butter-type crackers; French fried potatoes
Meat A	Chicken	1 ounce	Bacon; duck; frankfurters; goose; ground meats (unless made from trimmed lean meat); lunch meats; meat fat; poultry skin
	Crab		
	Fish		
	Lobster		
	Skim milk cheese		
	Tuna, water packed		
	Turkey		
	Clams	$1\frac{1}{2}$ ounces	
	Oysters	$1\frac{1}{2}$ ounces	
	Scallops	$1\frac{1}{2}$ ounces	
	Low-fat cottage cheese	$\frac{1}{4}$ cup	Heart, liver, shrimp, and sweetbreads unless used as egg exchanges
	Egg whites	2	
Meat B	Beef	1 ounce	
	Ham		
	Lamb		
	Pork		
	Salmon, canned		
	Tuna, oil packed, drained		
	Veal		
	Wafer sliced meats		
	Wild game		
	Tofu	3 ounces	
	Regular cottage cheese	$\frac{1}{4}$ cup	

[*Continued*]

TABLE 32-6. Hyperlipoproteinemia Food Exchange System [*Concluded*]

Group	Food Item	One Exchange (serving size)	Foods to Avoid
Meat C	Whole milk cheese	1 ounce	
Fat A	Corn oil	1 teaspoon	Coconut oil; cottonseed oil; olive oil; palm oil; peanut oil
	Safflower oil	1 teaspoon	
	Sunflower seed oil	1 teaspoon	
	Walnuts	6 halves	
Fat B	Margarines made with liquid corn, safflower, sunflower seed oil and/or with a P:S ratio of at least 2:1	1 teaspoon	Bacon drippings; butter; cashews; cream cheese; cream sauces; whipping cream, sour cream, imitation sour cream substitutes; French-fried foods; gravies; lard; macadamia nuts; margarines that list the first ingredient as hardened, partially hardened, hydrogenated, or partially hydrogenated; diet margarines; diet mayonnaise; olives
	Mayonnaise	2 teaspoons	
	Salad dressings	2 teaspoons	
	Blue cheese		
	Italian		
	Thousand Island		
	Miracle Whip		
	Tartar sauce		
	French dressing	1 tablespoon	Pistachios; salt pork; whipped toppings
	almonds	9 whole	
	pecans	6 halves	
Egg	Egg	1 whole	
	Kidney	1 ounce	
	Sweetbreads	1 ounce	
	Liver	2 ounces	
	Heart[2]	3 ounces	
	Shrimp[2]	5 ounces	
Free	Artificial sweeteners	As desired	Barbecue sauce; steak sauce; sugar; jam, jelly; honey; molasses
	Sugar-free diet pop		
	Club soda		
	Bouillon or clear broth		
	Decaffeinated coffee		
	Free vegetables		
	Gelatin, unsweetened		
	Mustard		
	Pepper		
	Salt		
	Spices		
	Vinegar		
	Coffee[3]		
	Tea[3]		
	Lemon juice[4]		
	Lime juice[4]		
	Soy sauce		

[1] Subtract 1 fat B exchange for each serving used.
[2] Subtract 2 meat A exchanges for each serving used.
[3] These beverages may be limited for some patients.
[4] Limit to 2 tablespoons per day.

TABLE 32-7. Hyperlipoproteinemia Vegetarian Meat Exchange Group

Food Item	One Exchange (serving size)	Food Group Equivalent	Foods to Avoid
Garbanzo beans	½ cup cooked	1 Meat A + 2 Bread	Beans, canned or homemade with bacon, molasses, or sugar added
Pinto beans	½ cup cooked	1 Meat A + 2 Bread	
Kidney beans	¾ cup cooked	1 Meat A + 2 Bread	
Lima beans	¾ cup cooked	1 Meat A + 2 Bread	
Navy beans	¾ cup cooked	1 Meat A + 2 Bread	
Split peas	¾ cup cooked	1 Meat A + 2 Bread	
Lentils	1 cup cooked	1 Meat A + 2 Bread	
Wheat germ	¼ cup	1 Meat B + 1 Bread	
Soybeans	½ cup cooked	1 Meat B + 1 Bread	
Peanut butter	2 tablespoons	1 Meat B + 2 Fat B	
Peanuts	¼ cup	1 Meat B + 3 Fat B	
Sunflower seeds	¼ cup	1 Meat B + 3 Fat A	
Yogurt			
Plain	¾ cup	1 Meat B + 1 Fruit	Sweetened, flavored yogurt
Low-fat	¾ cup	1 2% milk	

TABLE 32-8. Hyperlipoproteinemia Diet Calculation Sheet

Name ____________________

DIET PRESCRIPTION ____________________

FOOD GROUP		DAILY TOTAL	CHO g	PRO g	FAT g	SAT g	POLY g	CHOL mg	ETOH g	MEAL 1	SNACK 1	MEAL 2	SNACK 2	MEAL 3	SNACK 3
MEAT	A			8	1	0.6	0.4	25							
	B			8	3	1.2	0.1	30							
	C			8	8	5.4	0.2	30							
FAT	A				5	0.5	3.3								
	B				5	0.8	1.9								
EGGS/WEEK				1	1	0.3	0.1	40							
MILK	SKIM		12	8		0.3		5							
	2%		12	8	5	2.9	0.2	20							
VEGETABLE			5	2											
FRUIT			10												
BREAD			15	2											
ALCOHOL															
TOTAL										TOTAL CARBOHYDRATE PER MEAL OR SNACK					
DIET ORDER															

Carbohydrate, protein, and total fat are rounded to the nearest 1; SAT/POLY are rounded to the nearest 0.1; cholesterol is rounded to the nearest 5

Department of Dietetics, University Hospital — University of Michigan

REFERENCES CITED

1. Fredrickson, D. S.; Levy, R. I.; and Lees, R. S. 1967. Fat transport in lipoproteins—An integrated approach to mechanisms and disorders. *N. Eng. J. Med.* 276:273.
2. World Health Organization. 1972. Classification of hyperlipidemias and hyperlipoproteinemias. *Circulation* 45:501.
3. Gotto, A. M., Jr.; Shepherd, J.; Scott, L. W.; and Manis, E. 1979. Primary hyperlipoproteinemia and dietary management. In *Nutrition, lipids, and coronary heart disease,* eds., R. Levy, B. Rifkind, B. Dennis, and N. Ernst, pp. 247–283. New York: Raven Press.
4. Tzagournis, M. 1978. Triglycerides in clinical medicine. A review. *Am. J. Clin. Nutr.* 31:1437.
5. Standard procedure. Hyperlipidemia Clinic, University Hospital, University of Michigan, Ann Arbor, Mich., 1980.
6. Fredrickson, D. S. 1969. The role of lipids in acute myocardial infarction. *Circulation* 39–40 (Suppl. 4): 99.
7. LaRosa, J. C. 1977. Secondary hyperlipoproteinemia. In *Hyperlipidemia: Diagnosis and therapy,* eds., B. M. Rifkind and R. I. Levy, pp. 205–216. New York: Grune and Stratton.
8. Stare, F. J., ed. 1974. *Atherosclerosis.* New York: Medcom; Baltimore, Md.: William & Wilkins.
9. Brunzell, J. D.; Chait, A.; and Bierman, E. L. 1978. Pathophysiology of lipoprotein transport. *Metabolism* 27:1109.
10. Glueck, C. J.; Mattson, F.; and Bierman, E. L. 1978. Diet and coronary heart disease: Another view. *N. Eng. J. Med.* 298:1471.
11. Kudchodkar, B. J.; Sodhi, H. S.; Mason, D. T.; and Borhani, N. O. 1977. Effects of acute caloric restriction on cholesterol metabolism in man. *Am. J. Clin. Nutr.* 30:1135.
12. Anderson, J. T.; Grande, F.; and Keys, A. 1973. Cholesterol-lowering diets. *J. Am. Dietet. A.* 62:133.
13. Keys, A.; Anderson, J. T.; and Grande, F. 1965. Serum cholesterol response to changes in the diet. 1. Iodine value of dietary fat versus 2S-P. *Metabolism* 14:747.
14. Grundy, S. M. 1975. Effects of polyunsaturated fats on lipid metabolism in patients with hypertriglyceridemia. *J. Clin. Invest.* 55:269.
15. Conner, W. R.; Stone, D. B.; and Hodges, R. E. 1964. The interrelated effects of dietary cholesterol and fat upon human serum lipid levels. *J. Clin. Invest.* 43:1691.
16. Nikkila, E. A., and Kekki, M. 1972. Effects of dietary fructose and sucrose on plasma triglyceride metabolism in patients with endogenous hypertriglyceridemia. *Acta Med. Scand.* 542 (Suppl.) :221.
17. Roberts, A. M. 1973. Effects of a sucrose-free diet on the serum-lipid levels of men in Antarctica. *Lancet* 1:1201.
18. Lampman, R. M.; Santinga, J. T.; Hodge, M. F.; Block, W. D.; Flora, J. D.; and Bassett, D. R. 1977. Comparative effects of physical training and diet in normalizing serum lipids in men with type IV hyperlipoproteinemia. *Circulation* 55:652.
19. Ginsberg, H.; Olefsky, J.; Farquhar, J. W.; and Reaven, G. M. 1974. Moderate ethanol ingestion and plasma triglyceride levels. *Ann. Intern. Med.* 80:143.
20. Ostrander, L. D., Jr.; Lamphiear, D. E.; Block, W. D.; Johnson, B. C.; Ravenscroft, C.; and Epstein, F. H. 1974. Relationship of serum lipid concentrations to alcohol consumption. *Arch. Intern. Med.* 134:451.
21. Sacks, F. M.; Castelli, W. P.; Donner, A.; and Kass, E. H. 1975. Plasma lipids and lipoproteins in vegetarians and controls. *N. Eng. J. Med.* 292:1148.
22. Kritchevsky, D. 1978. Fiber, lipids, and atherosclerosis. *Am. J. Clin. Nutr.* 31:S65.
23. Zilversmit, D. B. 1979. Dietary fiber. In *Nutrition, lipids, and coronary heart disease,* eds., R. Levy, B. Rifkind, B. Dennis, and N. Ernst, pp. 149–174. New York: Raven Press.

RECOMMENDED REFERENCES FOR THE LAY PUBLIC

BOSSCHER, M.; BYL, L.; CURREY, J.; GRILLS, N.; and REILLY, M. F. 1979. *Meal planning: Hyperlipidemia.* Ann Arbor, Mich.: Department of Dietetics, University Hospital, University of Michigan.

CONNOR, W. E.; CONNOR, S. L.; FRY, M. M.; and WARNER, S. L. 1976. *The alternative diet book.* Iowa City: University of Iowa Press.

ROBERTSON, L.; FLINDERS, C.; and GODFREY, B. 1976. *Laurel's kitchen: A handbook for vegetarian cookery and nutrition.* Petaluma, Calif.: Nilgiri Press.

PART VIII
Carbohydrate Modifications

33

Dumping Syndrome

INDICATIONS FOR USE

This diet is indicated for individuals who have dumping syndrome. Dumping syndrome may occur following surgical procedures such as subtotal gastric resection, vagotomy, pyloroplasty, and gastroenterostomy. (1–3) An early and late dumping syndrome have been described. (2–5)

Symptoms of early dumping syndrome occur during or shortly after eating. Symptoms of late dumping syndrome (alimentary hyperinsulinism), a rare condition, occur approximately one and one-half to three hours after a meal.

Early dumping syndrome is associated with gastrointestinal symptoms such as epigastric fullness, churning stomach, intestinal cramps, diarrhea, and, in some cases, nausea and vomiting. (2–5) Both early and late dumping syndrome are associated with vasomotor symptoms, such as rapid onset of weakness, fainting, and dizziness, and cardiovascular symptoms, such as sweating, tachycardia, and palpitations. (2–5)

The period of time that the individual must remain on the diet depends upon the presence of symptoms. As symptoms subside, the individual may be advanced gradually to an unrestricted diet.

Late dumping syndrome may be treated with the diet for reactive functional hypoglycemia (Chapter 34).

DESCRIPTION

Dietary treatment of dumping syndrome is directed to avoiding osmotically active foods, decreasing the rapid transit of food through the stomach, and providing a nutritionally adequate diet.

Hypertonic solutions of sodium chloride, amino acids, and glucose can precipitate dumping syndrome. (6) Fluids consumed with a meal can dissolve the ingredients possessing osmotic properties and yield a hypertonic solution capable of producing symptoms. (6) Consumption of solids and consumption of liquids are separated to avoid putting solid foods into solution and to help delay transit of the solid food through the stomach. (2, 4, 6, 7) Highly emulsified fats such as mayonnaise and homogenized milk are rapidly hydrolyzed in the small intestine and may also be poorly tolerated. (7)

To provide a nutritionally adequate diet, multiple small feedings high in protein and fat may be necessary as calorie requirements are often high and tolerance for large meals is low. (4, 7) During hospitalization, the patient should be monitored daily to evaluate the effectiveness of the diet.

GUIDELINES FOR NUTRITIONAL MANAGEMENT

The following criteria are used when planning a diet to decrease symptoms of dumping:

- Avoid foods with high concentrations of mono- and disaccharides such as honey, sugar, syrups, sweetened fruits, beverages, and desserts. (4–6)
- Avoid solutions of free amino acids or protein hydrolysates such as elemental diets. (6)

- Provide solids and liquids separately. Provide liquids 30 to 45 minutes before or after meals of solid foods. (8)
- Plan six or more small meals each day. (4, 7, 8) Lying down after a meal may help decrease the incidence of symptoms. (4)
- Provide foods high in fat and protein such as peanut butter, cheese, and meats with each meal of solid food. (8–10)
- Tolerance to milk varies. (1, 7, 9) Individuals who demonstrate intolerance to homogenized milk may be able to consume warmed milk (11), skim milk, buttermilk, or scalded milk. (9) Avoid any sweetened milk product such as milkshakes and sweetened eggnog.
- The following may not be tolerated by all persons. Restrict them only when the individual demonstrates symptoms:

  finely emulsified fats such as mayonnaise (7)
  raw fruits and vegetables (4)
  spicy foods (4)

  caffeine (4)
  tobacco (4)

  foods of very hot or very cold temperature (10)

Individuals may progress toward a less rigid eating pattern as symptoms subside. If hypertonic substances are avoided, many individuals eventually adapt to fewer and larger meals. (7) Achievement of a more normalized eating pattern will vary with the individual.

NUTRIENT ADEQUACY

Actual nutrient intake depends upon the individual's appetite, preferences, and ability to eat. Provided that the individual consumes a wide variety of foods in adequate amounts, the diet will meet the recommended dietary allowances, 1980. When individuals are under stressful conditions, the recommended dietary allowances may not be adequate to meet nutrient needs.

REFERENCES CITED

1. Lieber, H. 1961. The jejunal hyperosmolic syndrome (dumping) and its prophylaxis. *JAMA* 176:108.
2. Woodward, E. R., and Bushkin, F. L. 1976. The early postprandial dumping syndrome: Prevention and treatment. In *Postgastrectomy syndromes,* eds., F. L. Bushkin and E. R. Woodward, pp. 14–27. Philadelphia: W. B. Saunders.
3. Woodward, E. R., and Neustein, C. L. 1976. The late postprandial dumping syndrome. In *Postgastrectomy syndromes,* eds., F. L. Bushkin and E. R. Woodward, pp. 28–33. Philadelphia: W. B. Saunders.
4. French, A. B. 1965. Treatment of postgastrectomy malabsorption. *Mod. Treatment* 2:335.
5. Woodward, E. R. 1976. The early postprandial dumping syndrome: Clinical manifestations and pathogenesis. In *Postgastrectomy syndromes,* eds., F. L. Bushkin and E. R. Woodward, pp. 1–13. Philadelphia: W. B. Saunders.
6. Machella, T. E. 1949. The mechanism of the post-gastrectomy "dumping" syndrome. *Ann. Surg.* 130:145.
7. Randall, H. T. 1975. Enteric feeding. In *American College of Surgeons, Committee on Pre- and Postoperative Care: Manual of surgical nutrition,* p. 277. Philadelphia: W. B. Saunders.
8. American College of Surgeons, Committee on Pre- and Postoperative Care. 1975. *Manual of surgical nutrition,* pp. 463–466. Philadelphia: W. B. Saunders.
9. Pittman, A. C., and Robinson, F. W. 1962. Dietary management of the "dumping" syndrome. *J. Am. Dietet. A.* 40:108.
10. Pittman, A. C., and Robinson, F. W. 1958. Dumping syndrome—Control by diet. *J. Am. Dietet. A.* 34:596.
11. Lewis, M. N.; Murray, M. A.; and Zollinger, R. M. 1954. Dietary regimen following partial gastric resection. *J. Am. Dietet. A.* 30:852.

OTHER REFERENCES

Alexander, H. C. 1975. A protein dietary supplement for the severe dumping syndrome. *Surg. Gynecol. Obstet.* 141:863.

Willis, M. T., and Postlewait, R. W. 1962. Dietary problems after gastric resection. *J. Am. Dietet. A.* 40:111.

Reactive Functional Hypoglycemia

INDICATIONS FOR USE

This diet is indicated for individuals with reactive functional hypoglycemia. Three main types are recognized: reactive hypoglycemia of mild noninsulin-dependent diabetes, alimentary hyperinsulinism in gastrointestinal dysfunction, and idiopathic functional hypoglycemia. Reactive functional hypoglycemia is characterized by transient subnormal blood glucose levels occurring one to four hours after consumption of a carbohydrate-containing meal. (3) The fasting blood glucose is normal. (3, 4)

Symptoms are divided into two categories, the adrenergic and the neuroglycopenic. Adrenergic symptoms usually predominate and are caused by the hyperepinephrinemia occurring in response to a rapid fall in blood glucose to subnormal levels. Anxiety, hunger, inward trembling, nervousness, nausea and vomiting, palpitations, shaking, sweating, and tachycardia may be present. Neuroglycopenic symptoms occur after a prolonged, severe fall in blood glucose to subnormal levels. Uptake of glucose and utilization of oxygen by the brain are decreased. Headaches, blurred vision, diplopia, mental dullness, confusion, incoherent speech, restlessness, and coma or unconsciousness may occur. (2, 4)

In addition to the history of symptoms, a glucose tolerance test is necessary to establish the diagnosis of reactive functional hypoglycemia. (3) The test is 5 hours long; blood samples are obtained at the onset (fasting), at each 30 minute interval, and whenever symptoms occur. (1) Plasma glucose levels below 45 mg/100 ml coinciding with symptoms confirm the diagnosis of reactive functional hypoglycemia. (3) During the oral glucose tolerance test, plasma glucose levels may, in normal individuals, decrease to 45–50 mg/100 ml without the occurrence of any hypoglycemic symptoms. (4)

This diet is not indicated for individuals with other forms of hypoglycemia that occur in the fasting state, such as that seen in patients with insulin-producing tumors of the pancreas.

This diet may be contraindicated for pregnant women due to its low carbohydrate content that promotes ketone production (Chapter 46).

DESCRIPTION

Symptoms usually occur in response to ingestion of carbohydrates. Total daily carbohydrate intake is limited and divided evenly into three to six meals. (4) Limiting the types of carbohydrate used to those types recommended for the diabetic diet appears to be effective in the dietary treatment. (2) Because of the low carbohydrate content of the diet, protein, fat, and cholesterol content will be high. The role of alcohol and caffeine restriction in the treatment of hypoglycemia is controversial. (1, 2)

GUIDELINES FOR NUTRITIONAL MANAGEMENT

The following criteria are used when planning a diet to control symptoms of reactive functional hypoglycemia:

- Limit daily carbohydrate intake to 75–125 g divided evenly among three to six meals. (3, 4) When this diet is used for late dumping syndrome (alimentary hyperinsulinism), initially limit carbohydrate intake to 50 g/day. Carbohydrate content may be increased slowly, as long as symptoms are controlled.
- Avoid *refined* fructose and *refined* glucose-containing disaccharides (lactose and sucrose).
- Provide remainder of calories in the diet from protein and fat.
- For individuals who are not at ideal body weight, calculate a diet pattern based on the diabetic or hyperlipoproteinemia food exchange systems (Chapters 25 and/or 32). For individuals at ideal body weight, counting grams of carbohydrate-utilizing exchange lists and product labels is an adequate alternative to the use of a strict diet pattern.
- Limit alcohol and caffeine in the diet when the individual demonstrates symptoms related to their ingestion.

NUTRIENT ADEQUACY

Actual nutrient intake depends upon the individual's appetite, preferences, and ability to eat. Provided that the individual consumes a wide variety of foods in adequate amounts, the diet will meet the recommended dietary allowances, 1980. When individuals are under stressful conditions, the recommended dietary allowances may not be adequate to meet nutrient needs.

REFERENCES CITED

1. Hofeldt, F. D. 1975. Reactive hypoglycemia. *Metabolism* 24:1193.
2. Permutt, M. A. 1976. Postprandial hypoglycemia. *Diabetes* 25:719.
3. Floyd, J. C., Jr. 1979. Practical perspectives on reactive functional hypoglycemia. In *Family practice review,* April 16–20, pp. 98–100. Ann Arbor, Mich.: The Towsley Center for Continuing Medical Education, The University of Michigan.
4. Fajans, S. S., and Floyd, J. C., Jr. 1973. Hypoglycemia: How to manage a complex disease. *Mod. Med.* 41:24.

OTHER REFERENCES

Marks, V., and Guildford, U. K. 1974, 1976. The metabolism of blood glucose and the definition of hypoglycemia. In European Symposium on Hypoglycemia, First, Rome, 1974, *Proceedings.* Stuttgart: Georg Thieme.

REFERENCES RECOMMENDED FOR LAY PUBLIC

Arehart-Treichel, J. 1973. The great medical debate over low blood sugar. *Sci. News* 103:172.

Nolen, W. A. 1975. Low blood sugar—What it means. *McCall's* 103 (2):92.

PART IX
Mineral Modifications

Calcium Restricted (400 mg Calcium)

INDICATIONS FOR USE

A calcium-restricted diet is indicated for individuals with hypercalcemia or hypercalciuria resulting from the following:

Hypervitaminosis D. Vitamin D increases calcium absorption from the intestine and calcium withdrawal from the bone. (1–3)

Hyperparathyroidism. A low-calcium diet may be used when surgery is not indicated. (2, 4)

Idiopathic hypercalciuria (absorptive hypercalciuria type). Calcium restriction is indicated for idiopathic hypercalciuria caused by primary intestinal overabsorption of calcium. (2, 4)

Sarcoidosis. The hypercalcemia and hypercalciuria observed in sarcoidosis may be cyclic, increasing in the summer months, and appears to be caused by elevated circulating levels of vitamin D, resulting in increased calcium absorption from the gut. (5–7)

Excess calcium intake. Some individuals appear to be more sensitive to increased calcium intake than others. The following contribute to excessive calcium loads and may increase hypercalcemia or hypercalciuria (8–10):

- Use of large amounts of dairy products and/or antacid (alkali) products containing calcium carbonate.
- Use of large amounts of noncalcium-containing antacids such as Maalox and Amphogel that bind phosphate in the gut, increasing the percentage of calcium absorbed.

CONTRAINDICATIONS FOR USE

A calcium-restricted diet is not effective in the treatment of hypercalcemia or hypercalciuria resulting from the following:

Idiopathic hypercalciuria (renal leak type). The primary defect in this condition is in renal-tubular calcium conservation. (4)

Metastatic carcinoma. Parathyroid hormone or a similar substance is known to be produced by certain carcinomas of the kidney, breast, lung, cervix, ovary, colon, and other organs. Commonly responsible for hypercalcemia, the breast carcinoma produces a potent osteolytic substance that causes mobilization of calcium from the bone. Restriction of dietary calcium has little or no effect on the hypercalciuria, and drug therapy is the treatment of choice. (4, 11)

DESCRIPTION

Prolonged hypercalcemia may result in permanent renal, heart, and aortic damage. (1) Drug therapy may be necessary along with dietary restriction of calcium to reduce serum calcium levels to normal.

Hypercalciuria is associated with renal stone formation. (2, 12) Calcium in the form of calcium oxalate or calcium phosphate is the major cation present in renal stones. (12) Although the cause of renal calcium stones is not fully understood, supersaturation of the urine with these calcium compounds appears to be a major factor. (2, 13) Therapy includes reducing dietary calcium and increasing fluid intake. (2, 10, 12) Low-calcium diets in the range of 250–600 mg/day have been effective in reducing urinary calcium excretion. (12, 14) An adequate fluid intake to maintain urine volume above 2500 ml/24 hr is important, in conjunction with a low-calcium diet in controlling stone formation. (12)

GUIDELINES FOR NUTRITIONAL MANAGEMENT

Restrict dietary calcium to 400 mg/day unless otherwise designated by diet prescription. A low-calcium intake is achieved by restriction of milk and dairy products, fish with fine bones, dark green, leafy vegetables, and other foods containing appreciable amounts of calcium. The diet is planned using food groups. Average calcium content per serving from each food group is listed in Table 35-1. Foods included in the food groups and serving sizes are listed in Table 35-2. Foods should be weighed or measured to ensure correct serving size.

For individuals with hypercalciuria, encourage fluid intake of 250–300 ml of fluid hourly while awake and 250–300 ml of fluid each time upon rising to void during the night. At least 50% of this fluid should be water. (12)

Include the calcium content of water consumed as part of the daily calcium allowance. For calcium restrictions less than or equal to 400 mg, the use of distilled water may be recommended. The calcium content of the water supply varies with geographical area; contact the local public health department for information. For example, Ann Arbor city water contains approximately 28 mg calcium per liter.

NUTRIENT ADEQUACY

A 400 mg calcium diet, which provides 50% of the RDA for calcium, may not meet the recommended dietary allowance for riboflavin and thiamin and may not meet the recommended dietary allowance for iron for the premenopausal woman.

TABLES

TABLE 35-1. Average Calcium Content of One Serving (Exchange), Calcium-Restricted Food Exchange System

Food Group	Calcium: Average Per Serving (mg)	Calcium: Range in Group (mg)
Milk and calcium equivalents	149	146–151
Meat and protein equivalents	4	2–11
Egg	28	28
Nut	17	Trace–27
Fruit	12	2–31
Vegetable	16	3–37
Grain	11	2–26
Other		
Beverage	3	Trace–5
Fat	2	0–4
Sweet	8	0–30

TABLE 35-2. Calcium-Restricted Food Exchange Group

Food Group	Foods Allowed/ Description	Serving Sizes: Weight (g)	Serving Sizes: Household Measure	Calcium (mg)	Foods to Avoid
Milk	Whole milk	120	½ cup	146	Milk, large amounts
	Low-fat milk	120	½ cup	150	Milk beverages
	Skim milk	120	½ cup	151	Cheese, all kinds
					Ice cream
					Sherbet made with milk
					Yogurt
					Puddings and custards
Meat	Beef, cooked	28	1 ounce	4	Fish with fine bone
	Lamb, cooked	28	1 ounce	4	Clams
	Pork, cooked	28	1 ounce	4	Crab
	Veal, cooked	28	1 ounce	3	Lunch meat or cold cuts with milk solids added
	Bacon, fried crisp	8	1 strip	1	
	Bologna, no milk solids added	30	1 slice	2	Oysters
					Scallops
	Frankfurter, all beef, no milk solids added	50	1	3	Shrimp
					All other meats not listed
	Ham	28	1 ounce	3	
	Liver, cooked	28	1 ounce	3	
	Chicken, cooked	28	1 ounce	4	
	Turkey, cooked	28	1 ounce	2	
	Cod, cooked	28	1 ounce	9	
	Haddock, cooked	28	1 ounce	11	
	Halibut, cooked	28	1 ounce	5	
	Tuna, oil packed	40	¼ cup	3	
Egg	Egg	50	1 medium	28	
Nuts	Cashews	35	¼ cup	13	Almonds
	Peanuts	36	¼ cup	27	Brazil nuts
	Walnuts, black			—	All other nuts
	Peruvian or English, halves	25	¼ cup	25	
	Peanut butter	32	2 tablespoons	19	
Fruit	Apple	150	1 medium	9	Blackberries
	Apple juice	120	½ cup	7	Boysenberries
	Applesauce	150	½ cup	6	Raw or dried figs
	Apricots, canned halves	100	3 medium	11	Kumquats
	Avocado	100	½	10	Loganberries
	Banana	100	1 small	8	Dried peaches or pears
	Blueberries	80	½ cup	12	
	Cantaloupe	100	¼, 5 in. diameter	14	Raspberries
					Rhubarb
	Cherries, sweet	100	15 large	22	Ripe olives
	Cranberries, raw	100	1 cup	14	Pumpkin
	Cranberry sauce, canned	60	½ cup	4	

Table 35-2. Calcium-Restricted Food Exchange Group [*Continued*]

Food Group	Foods Allowed/ Description	Serving Sizes: Weight (g)	Serving Sizes: Household Measure	Calcium (mg)	Foods to Avoid
	Cranberry juice	120	½ cup	6	All other fruits not listed
	Fruit cocktail	100	½ cup	9	
	Grapefruit	100	½	16	
	Grapefruit sections	100	½ cup	8	
	Grapefruit juice	120	½ cup	12	
	Grapes				
	American	100	22 medium	16	
	European	100	24 medium	12	
	Thompson seedless, canned	100	½ cup	8	
	Honeydew melon	100	¼ small, 5 in. diameter	14	
	Lemon	100	1 medium	26	
	Lemon juice, fresh	61	¼ cup	4	
	Mangos	200	1 medium	20	
	Nectarines	50	1 medium	2	
	Orange, peeled	75	½ medium	31	
	Orange juice	120	½ cup	13	
	Olives, green, pickled	13	2 medium	8	
	Peaches	100	1 medium	9	
	Peaches, canned	100	2 halves	6	
	Peach nectar	120	½ cup	5	
	Pears	200	1 medium	16	
	Pear nectar	120	½ cup	4	
	Pineapple, raw diced	67	½ cup	11	
	Pineapple, canned slice	100	1 large	11	
	Pineapple, frozen chunks	131	½ cup	12	
	Plums, raw	50	1 medium	9	
	Plums, canned	100	3 medium	9	
	Prunes, dried and cooked	100	5 medium	19	
	Raisins, dried seedless	10	1 tablespoon	6	
	Strawberries	100	10 large	21	
	Tangerines	58	½ small	23	
	Watermelon, diced	100	½ cup	7	
Vegetable	Asparagus	75	½ cup	16	Artichokes
	Bean sprouts, Mung, raw	60	1 cup	11	Broccoli
	Beans, snap, green, cooked	66	½ cup	30	Cabbage
					Dry beans and peas
	Beets, canned	83	½ cup	16	Lima beans
	Carrots, raw	81	1 medium	27	Okra
	Carrots, cooked	78	½ cup	25	Parsley
	Cauliflower, raw	100	1 cup	25	Parsnips
	Cauliflower, cooked	57	½ cup	25	Rutabaga
	Celery, raw outer stalk	50	1	20	Sauerkraut
	Corn, fresh ear	100	1 medium	3	Spinach and other greens
	Corn, canned	100	½ cup	5	
	Cucumber, raw, pared	50	½ medium	9	Sweet potato

TABLE 35-2. Calcium-Restricted Food Exchange Group [*Continued*]

Food Group	Foods Allowed/ Description	Serving Sizes		Calcium (mg)	Foods to Avoid
		Weight (g)	Household Measure		
	Eggplant, cooked, diced	100	½ cup	11	All other vegetables not listed
	Lettuce, iceberg	55	1 cup	11	
	Mushrooms, fresh	100	10 small	6	
	Mushrooms, canned	136	½ cup	8	
	Onion, raw	100	1 (2¼ in. diameter)	27	
	Peas, frozen	67	½ cup	13	
	Peas, canned	67	½ cup	17	
	Pepper, green, raw	100	1 large	9	
	Pickles, dill	100	1 large	26	
	Pickles, sour	105	1 large	18	
	Pickles, sweet	100	1 large	12	
	Potato, white, baked	100	1 medium	9	
	Potato, pared, boiled	100	1 medium	7	
	Potato, fried	170	1 cup	26	
	Potato chips	20	10 pieces	8	
	Radishes	50	5 small	15	
	Squash, summer, boiled	100	½ cup	25	
	Squash, winter, baked	100	½ cup	28	
	Tomato, canned[1]	100	½ cup	6	
	Tomato, raw	100	1 small	13	
	Tomato juice	120	½ cup	8	
	Tomato catsup	17	1 tablespoon	4	
	Tomato paste	114	½ cup	31	
Grain	Bread, milk free	23	1 slice	4	Instant cereals Commercial corn bread Pancakes Pizza Waffles Wheat bran All other items not listed
	Bread, white, enriched with 1–2% nonfat dry milk	23	1 slice	16	
	Bread, whole wheat, enriched with 2% nonfat dry milk	23	1 slice	23	
	Crackers, soda or saltines	12	4 squares	3	
	Crackers, graham	14	2 squares	6	
	Rusk	12	1	2	
	40% Bran Flakes	37	1 cup	26	
	Cornflakes	25	1 cup	4	
	Rice Krispies	28	1 cup	5	
	Puffed Rice	13	1 cup	3	
	Shredded wheat	22	1 biscuit	9	
	Farina, enriched, cooked	123		5	
	Cornmeal, enriched, cooked	120	½ cup	10	
	Macaroni, enriched, cooked	140	1 cup	11	
	Noodles, egg, enriched, cooked	160	1 cup	16	
	Rice, milled, white, cooked	150	1 cup	15	

Table 35-2. Calcium-Restricted Food Exchange Group [*Continued*]

Food Group	Foods Allowed/ Description	Serving Sizes Weight (g)	Household Measure	Calcium (mg)	Foods to Avoid
	Rice, brown, cooked	150	1 cup	18	
	Spaghetti, enriched, cooked	146	1 cup	12	
	Flour, wheat all purpose, enriched	110	1 cup	18	
Other Beverage[2]	Coffee	240	1 cup	5	All milk beverages
	Tea	240	1 cup	—	Diet pop sweetened with calcium
					Saccharine[3]
Fat	Butter or margarine	5	1 teaspoon	1	Cream
	Coffee whitener,				Cream cheese
	nondairy, liquid, frozen	15	1 tablespoon	1	Sour cream
	Coffee whitener, powdered	3	1 teaspoon	1	Creamy salad dressing
	Mayonnaise	14	1 tablespoon	3	Other items not listed
	Salad or cooking oil	5	1 teaspoon	0	
	Salad dressings				
	French	14	1 tablespoon	2	
	Italian	14	1 tablespoon	1	
	Thousand Island	14	1 tablespoon	2	
	Russian	14	1 tablespoon	3	
	Tartar sauce	20	1 tablespoon	4	
Sweet	Assorted jams, jellies, and preserves	20	1 tablespoon	4	Caramels
					Chocolate bars
	Honey	21	1 tablespoon	1	Cream pies
	Sugar, white	12	1 tablespoon	0	Fudge
	Corn syrup	20	1 tablespoon	3	Pecan pie
	Chocolate syrup, thin type	20	1 tablespoon	4	Brown sugar
					Maple syrup
	Cake, home recipe				Molasses
	Angel food	45	1 slice	4	
	Pound	30	1 slice	6	
	Sponge	50	1 slice	15	
	Cookies, assorted	20	1 cookie (2 in. diameter)	7	
	Lady finger	14	1 large	6	
	Macaroons	14	1 medium	4	
	Vanilla wafers	11	3	5	
	Shortbread cookie	8	1 piece	6	
	Pie				
	Apple	160	$\frac{1}{6}$ of 9 in.	13	
	Blueberry	160	$\frac{1}{6}$ of 9 in.	30	
	Cherry	160	$\frac{1}{6}$ of 9 in.	22	
Miscellaneous	Hard candies	As desired			Soups unless made from allowed ingredients
	Cornstarch				
	Pepper, salt, spices				
	Vegetable oil				

TABLE 35-2. Calcium-Restricted Food Exchange Group [*Concluded*]

Food Group	Foods Allowed/ Description	Serving Sizes		Calcium (mg)	Foods to Avoid
		Weight (g)	Household Measure		
	Shortening, lard, salt pork				
	Vinegar				

[1] Federal standards provide for addition of certain calcium salts as firming agents; if used, these salts may add calcium not to exceed 26 mg/100 g of finished product.
[2] The calcium content of beverages will vary according to the type of water used in their preparation. The use of distilled water is recommended.
[3] The calcium content of carbonated beverages depends on the calcium content of the water supply. Avoid them unless the manufacturer has provided information on the calcium content of the beverage distributed in your area.

REFERENCES CITED

1. DeLuca, H. F. 1980. The vitamins. B. Vitamin D. In *Modern nutrition in health and disease,* eds., R. S. Goodhart and M. E. Shils, pp. 160–170. 6th ed. Philadelphia: Lea & Febiger.
2. Williams, H. E. 1974. Nephrolithiasis. *N. Eng. J. Med.* 290:33.
3. Gallagher, J. C., and Riggs, B. L. 1978. Nutrition and bone disease. *N. Eng. J. Med.* 298:193.
4. Personal communication with Yuk-Kai Lau, M.D., Assistant Professor of Internal Medicine, Nephrology, University Hospital, University of Michigan; Ann Arbor, Mich., March 1980.
5. Bell, N. H.; Gill, J. R., Jr.; and Barter, F. C. 1964. On the abnormal calcium absorption in sarcoidosis. *Am. J. Med.* 36:500.
6. Bell, N. H.; Stern, P. H.; Pantzer, E.; Sinha, T. K.; and DeLuca, H. F. 1979. Evidence that increased circulating 1α,25-dihydroxy-vitamin D is the probable cause for abnormal calcium metabolism in sarcoidosis. *J. Clin. Invest.* 64:218.
7. Papapoulos, S. E.; Fraher, L. J.; Sandler, L. M.; Clemens, T. L.; Lewin, I. G.; and O'Riordan, J. L. H. 1979. 1,25-Dihydroxycholecalciferol in the pathogenesis of the hypercalcemia of sarcoidosis. *Lancet* 1:627.
8. Heaney, R. P.; Saville, P. D.; and Recker, R. R. 1975. Calcium absorption as a function of calcium intake. *J. Lab. Clin. Med.* 85:881.
9. Avioli, L. V. 1980. Major minerals: A. Calcium and phosphorus. In *Modern nutrition in health and disease,* eds., R. S. Goodhart and M. E. Shils, pp. 294–309. 6th ed. Philadelphia: Lea & Febiger.
10. Prien, E. L. 1975. Calcium oxalate renal stones. *Ann. Rev. Med.* 26:173.
11. Gordan, G. S.; Lichtenstein, L.; and Roof, B. S. 1971. Metabolic bone diseases associated with malignancy. *Israel J. Med. Sci.* 7:499.
12. Smith, L. H.; Van Den Berg, C. J.; and Wilson, D. M. 1978. Nutrition and urolithiasis. *N. Eng. J. Med.* 298:87.
13. Gill, W. B.; Silvert, M. A.; and Roma, M. J. 1974. Supersaturation levels and crystallization rates of calcium oxalate from urines of normal humans and stone formers determined by a ^{14}C-oxalate technique. *Invest. Urol.* 12:203.
14. Kark, R. M., and Oyama, J. H. 1980. Nutrition, hypertension and kidney diseases. In *Modern nutrition in health and disease,* eds., R. S. Goodhart and M. E. Shils, pp. 998–1044. 6th ed. Philadelphia: Lea & Febiger.

Oxalate Restricted

INDICATIONS FOR USE

A low-oxalate diet may be indicated for individuals with the following conditions:

Calcium oxalate renal stones. There is evidence that increased oxalate excretion is due mainly to increased oxalate absorption. (1–3)

Enteric hyperoxaluria. This condition may occur secondary to a variety of chronic gastrointestinal disorders including chronic inflammatory bowel disease, chronic pancreatic and biliary tract disease, bacterial overgrowth syndrome, blind loop syndrome, after small bowel resections, and after jejunoileal bypass procedures. (4–16)

CONTRAINDICATIONS FOR USE

A low-oxalate diet is not beneficial for hyperoxaluria resulting from the following:

Primary hyperoxaluria. Primary hyperoxaluria is a familial disorder characterized by calcium oxalate renal stones, nephrocalcinosis, recurrent urinary tract infections, and death at an early age. Dietary treatment is not effective. (17)

Vitamin B_6 (pyridoxine) deficiency. A deficiency of vitamin B_6 induces hyperoxaluria in animals and humans. Adequate replacement of the vitamin quickly reverses the hyperoxaluria. (18, 19)

Ascorbic acid (vitamin C) in very large doses. Intakes of ascorbic acid greater than 3 g/day have been reported to increase urinary oxalate excretion. Ingestion of large amounts of vitamin C may be hazardous to some individuals and may lead to nephrolithiasis. (19, 20)

DESCRIPTION

Calcium oxalate renal stones. In the long-term treatment of patients with renal stones, it may become necessary to restrict dietary oxalate as well as calcium. Calcium binds oxalate in the gut, making oxalate unavailable for absorption. The restriction of dietary calcium reduces the intraluminal concentrations of calcium and results in increased absorption of oxalate. (1–3)

Of major importance in the treatment of stone disease, regardless of type, is the maintenance of an adequate fluid intake. (21, 22) Stone formation has been controlled, in many cases, with diet adjustment and adequate fluid intake to maintain the urine volume above 2500 ml/24 hr. (2)

Enteric hyperoxaluria. The most common hyperoxaluric syndrome is that associated with chronic gastrointestinal disorders and is termed enteric hyperoxaluria. Hyperoxaluria results from increased intestinal oxalate absorption; the mechanism of hyperabsorption is controversial. (4) It has been hypothesized that nonabsorbed fatty acids and bile salts in the intestine bind calcium, preventing the formation of insoluble calcium oxalate and thus increasing the concentration of oxalate in the aqueous phase of intestinal fluid. (9, 23) This increase in oxalate concentration results in an increase in oxalate absorption. The colon appears to be the major site of the increased oxalate absorption. (6, 23) Nutrition therapy, including restriction of dietary fat (Chapter 29), use of medium-chain triglycerides, reduction of dietary oxalate, and oral calcium supplements, is recommended to bring urinary oxalate excretion toward normal levels. (8, 9, 11, 12, 21, 23, 24)

GUIDELINES FOR NUTRITIONAL MANAGEMENT

Restrict dietary oxalate. It is impractical to calculate an accurate level of oxalate in the diet since analytical data reported on the oxalic acid content of food are variable, probably due to seasonal variation in oxalate content of vegetables and inaccuracies in analytical methods. (24 29) A low-oxalate diet is achieved by avoidance of foods that are known to be high in oxalic acid. Table 36-1 lists foods known to be high in oxalic acid. A 24 hour urine oxalate measured periodically is recommended to detect hyperoxaluria and evaluate the effect of dietary management.

In addition to dietary oxalate restriction, nutritional management for stone disease should include a liberal intake of fluid. The individual is encouraged to take 250–300 ml of fluid hourly while awake and to drink 250–300 ml of fluid upon rising to void during the night. At least 50% of this fluid intake should be water. (21)

NUTRIENT ADEQUACY

Actual nutrient intake depends upon the individual's appetite, preferences, and ability to eat. Provided that the individual consumes a wide variety of foods in adequate amounts, the diet will meet the recommended daily allowances, 1980. When individuals are under stressful conditions, the recommended dietary allowances may not be adequate to meet nutrient needs.

TABLES

TABLE 36-1. Foods High in Oxalic Acid

Food Group	Foods to Avoid
Milk and calcium equivalents	Chocolate-flavored products
Meat and protein equivalents	Kidney Liver
Fruit	Grapefruit peel Lemon peel Lime peel Orange peel Rhubarb
Vegetable	Beans, snap, green and wax Beets Carrots Celery Greens: beet leaves, chard, dandelion leaves, endive, kale, lamb's quarters, poke, purslane, spinach, turnip tops Parsley
Grain	None
Other	
Beverage	Cocoa Cola beverages Tea
Fats	None
Sweet	Citrus fruit marmalade, chocolate products
Miscellaneous	Chocolate

REFERENCES CITED

1. Hodgkinson, A. 1978. Evidence of increased oxalate absorption in patients with calcium-containing renal stones. *Clin. Sci. & Mol. Med.* 54:291.
2. Marshall, R. W.; Cochran, M.; and Hodgkinson, A. 1972. Relationships between calcium and oxalic acid intake in the diet and their excretion in the urine of normal and renal-stone-forming subjects. *Clin. Sci.* 43:91.
3. Zarembski, P. M., and Hodgkinson, A. 1969. Some factors influencing the urinary excretion of oxalic acid in man. *Clin. Chim. Acta* 25:1.
4. Andersson, H., and Gillberg, R. 1977. Urinary oxalate on a high-oxalate diet as a clinical test of malabsorption. *Lancet* 2:677.
5. McDonald, G. B.; Earnest, D. L.; and Admirand, W. H. 1977. Hyperoxaluria correlates with fat malabsorption in patients with sprue. *Gut* 18:561.
6. Dobbins, J. W., and Binder, H. J. 1977. Importance of the colon in enteric hyperoxaluria. *N. Eng. J. Med.* 296:298.
7. Smith, L. H.; Fromm, H.; and Hofmann, A. F. 1972. Acquired hyperoxaluria, nephrolithiasis, and intestinal disease. *N. Eng. J. Med.* 286:1371.
8. Chadwick, V. S.; Modha, K.; and Dowling, R. H. 1973. Mechanism for hyperoxaluria in patients with ileal dysfunction. *N. Eng. J. Med.* 289:172.
9. Earnest, D. L.; Johnson, G.; Williams, H. E.; and Admirand, W. H. 1974. Hyperoxaluria in patients with ileal resection: An abnormality in dietary oxalate absorption. *Gastroenterology* 66:1114.
10. Stauffer, J. Q.; Humphreys, M. H.; and Weir, G. J. 1973. Acquired hyperoxaluria with regional enteritis after ileal resection. *Ann. Intern. Med.* 79:383.
11. Thomas, M. H., and Madura, J. A. 1977. Urolithiasis after intestinal bypass for morbid obesity. *Urology* 9:170.
12. Stauffer, J. Q. 1977. Hyperoxaluria and calcium oxalate nephrolithiasis after jejunoileal bypass. *Am. J. Clin. Nutr.* 30:64.
13. Bray, G. A., and Benfield, J. R. 1977. Intestinal bypass for obesity: A summary and perspective. *Am. J. Clin. Nutr.* 30:121.
14. Drenick, E. J.; Stanley, T. M.; Border, W. A.; Zawada, E. T.; Dornfeld, L. P.; Upham, T.; and Llach, F. 1978. Renal damage with intestinal bypass. *Ann. Intern. Med.* 89:594.
15. Barry, R. E.; Barisch, J.; Bray, G. A.; Sperling, M. A.; Morin, R. J.; and Benfield, J. 1977. Intestinal adaptation after jejunoileal bypass in man. *Am. J. Clin. Nutr.* 30:32.
16. Gelbart, D. R.; Brewer, L. L.; Fajardo, L. F.; and Weinstein, A. B. 1977. Oxalosis and chronic renal failure after intestinal bypass. *Arch. Intern. Med.* 137:239.
17. Williams, H. E., and Smith, L. H., Jr. 1972. Primary hyperoxaluria. In *The metabolic basis of inherited disease,* eds., J. B. Stanbury, J. B. Wyngaarden, and D. Fredrickson, pp. 196–219. 3rd ed. New York: McGraw-Hill.
18. Faber, S. R.; Feitler, W. W.; Bleiler, R. E.; Ohlson, M. A.; and Hodges, R. E. 1963. The effects of an induced pyridoxine and pantothenic acid deficiency on excretions of oxalic and xanthurenic acids in the urine. *Am. J. Clin. Nutr.* 12:406.
19. Hagler, L., and Herman, R. H. 1973. Oxalate metabolism. II. *Am. J. Clin. Nutr.* 26:882.
20. Briggs, M. H.; Garcia-Webb, P.; and Davies, P. 1973. Urinary oxalate and vitamin-C supplements. *Lancet* 2:201.
21. Smith, L. H.; Van Den Berg, C. J.; and Wilson, D. M. 1978. Nutrition and urolithiasis. *N. Eng. J. Med.* 298:87.
22. Williams, H. E. 1974. Nephrolithiasis. *N. Eng. J. Med.* 290:33.
23. Dobbins, J. W., and Binder, H. J. 1976. Effect of bile salts and fatty acids on the colonic absorption of oxalate. *Gastroenterology* 70:1096.
24. Williams, H. E. 1978. Oxalic acid and the hyperoxaluric syndromes. *Kidney Int.* 13:410.
25. Hodgkinson, A., and Zarembski, P. M. 1968. Oxalic acid metabolism in man: A review. *Calc. Tiss. Res.* 2:115.

26. Franco, V., and Krinitz, B. 1973. Determination of oxalic acid in foods. *J. Assoc. Off. Anal. Chem.* 56:164.
27. Andrews, J. C., and Viser, E. T. 1951. The oxalic acid content of some common foods. *Food Res.* 16:306.
28. Kohman, E. F. 1939. Oxalic acid in foods and its behavior and fate in the diet. *J. Nutr.* 18:233.
29. Sinclair, W. B., and Eny, D. M. 1947. Ether-soluble organic acids and buffer properties of citrus peels. *Botan. Gaz.* 108:398.

Copper Restricted

INDICATIONS FOR USE

A copper-restricted diet is indicated in the treatment of Wilson's disease. Wilson's disease is a permanent, inherited defect of copper metabolism involving abnormal copper metabolism in the liver and results in excessive amounts of copper deposited in soft tissue. (1–3)

The manifestations of Wilson's disease are low serum copper and ceruloplasmin concentrations, elevated urinary copper excretion, neurologic abnormalities, hepatic cirrhosis, renal damage, and deposition of copper in the liver, basal ganglia, cerebral cortex, kidney, and cornea (Kayser–Fleischer rings). (3)

Asymptomatic, aceruloplasminemic siblings of individuals with Wilson's disease, in whom the condition would develop, may be treated and kept clinically free of the disease. The copper-restricted diet may be started as early as one year of age and may be used in conjunction with an oral chelating agent, carbacrylamine resin. In individuals over the age of two, D-penicillamine may be added to the treatment. Since this regimen prevents excessive copper absorption and promotes copper excretion, symptoms may not develop or may be delayed. (1, 2)

DESCRIPTION

The accumulation of copper in individuals with Wilson's disease is thought to be due to a decrease in biliary copper excretion. The cause is either a defect in ceruloplasmin synthesis or in the incorporation of copper into ceruloplasmin. (4–6) Treatment is directed at achieving a negative copper balance by decreasing dietary copper and increasing copper excretion by drugs. (1–3, 7, 8)

The usual dietary copper intake in the United States is less than 1–5 mg/day; 25–50% is absorbed. (3, 4, 9, 10) Absorption is facilitated by amino acids (especially as derived from animal protein) and interfered with by cadmium, silver, zinc, molybdenum, ascorbic acid, soy–protein, phytic acid, and sulfide compounds. (4, 11) To achieve a negative copper balance on dietary copper restriction alone, an intake of less than 1.1 mg/day is required. Because this level of copper intake may be incompatible with a nutritionally adequate diet, a moderate intake of 1.5 mg/day is instituted. (2) There is some evidence that the use of a strict vegetarian diet can decrease the positive copper balance in untreated Wilson's disease. (11)

D-Penicillamine, a cupriuric agent, acts to reduce the tissue stores of copper. (1, 2, 5, 7) Oral chelators may be used to increase the fecal excretion of dietary copper. (1, 2, 7) Because the effectiveness of D-penicillamine is reduced on long-term usage and toxic reactions to it may occur, D-penicillamine therapy may be interrupted or discontinued, further increasing the importance of the copper-restricted diet. The combination of a low-copper diet and carbacrylamine resin is used in the periods when D-penicillamine is not used. (1, 2)

BASIC GUIDELINES FOR NUTRITIONAL MANAGEMENT

Dietary copper is restricted to 1.5 mg/day. This level can be achieved by avoiding the high-copper foods listed in Table 37-1, discarding cooking water since copper is leached into the water during the cooking process, and avoiding use of copper or bronze cooking utensils.

Drinking water can make a significant contribution to the daily copper intake. The copper level in water varies depending on the hardness of the water and the type of household piping. The local public health department should be contacted for the copper content of the local water supply. If the local water supply contains more than 1 ppm or 1 mg/l of copper, it is advisable for the patient to drink demineralized or distilled water. (1) For example, Ann Arbor city water does not contain copper before it enters copper pipes. (12)

NUTRIENT ADEQUACY

Actual nutrient intake depends upon the individual's appetite, preferences, and ability to eat. Provided that the individual consumes a wide variety of foods in adequate amounts, the diet will meet the recommended dietary allowances, 1980. When individuals are under stressful conditions, the recommended dietary allowances may not be adequate to meet nutrient needs. If vitamin or mineral supplements are used, their copper content should be evaluated.

TABLES

TABLE 37-1. Foods to Avoid for a Copper-Restricted Diet (13–20)

Food Group	Foods to Avoid
Milk and calcium equivalents	Malted milk, chocolate milk, cocoa, chocolate ice cream
Meat and protein equivalents	Organ meats: brains, heart, kidney, liver Shellfish: crab, lobster, oysters, shrimp Nuts, all except peanut butter[1] Seeds, all Split peas, soybeans, any other beans cooked from dry state except limas and lentils[2]
Fruit and vegetable	Applesauce, avocado, dried fruits except raisins Mushrooms, parsley, pimientos Any sprouted vegetable
Grain	Whole grain breads and cereals; bran, corn or wheat germ; high-protein dry baby cereal; Pablum; any cereal products made with ingredients not allowed such as chocolate or nuts Brown rice
Other	
Beverage	Bouillon, chocolate drinks, instant breakfast mixes, Ovaltine, tea, malted beverages
Fat	Olives in brine
Sweet	Chocolate, cocoa, molasses
Miscellaneous	Dry onion soup mix Dried yeast

[1] Limit to 2 tablespoons per day.
[2] Limit to $\frac{1}{2}$ cup cooked per day.

REFERENCES CITED

1. Scheinberg, I. H., and Sternlieb, I. 1960. The long-term management of hepatolenticular degeneration (Wilson's disease). *Am. J. Med.* 29:316.
2. Strickland, G. T.; Blackwell, R. Q.; and Watten, R. H. 1971. Metabolic studies in Wilson's disease. *Am. J. Med.* 51:31.
3. Dekaban, A. S. 1976. Inborn errors of copper metabolism: Kinky hair disease and hepatolenticular degeneration. Therapeutic approaches. *Mater. Med. Pol.* 8:167.
4. Evans, G. W. 1973. Copper homeostasis in the mammalian system. *Physiolog. Rev.* 53:535.
5. Rupp, H., and Weser, U. 1976. Reactions of D-penicillamine with copper in Wilson's disease. *Biochem. Biophys. Res. Commun.* 72:223.
6. Walshe, J. M., and Potter, G. 1977. The pattern of the whole body distribution of radioactive copper (^{67}Cu, ^{64}Cu) in Wilson's disease and various control groups. *Quart. J. Med. (N.S.)* 184:445.
7. Walshe, J. M. 1956. Penicillamine, a new oral therapy for Wilson's disease. *Am. J. Med.* 21:487.
8. Ohlson, M. A. 1972. *Experimental and therapeutic dietetics,* pp. 94–96. 2nd ed. Minneapolis, Minn.: Burgess Publishing.
9. Ting-Kai, Li, and Vallee, B. L. 1980. The biochemical and nutritional roles of other trace elements. In *Modern nutrition in health and disease,* eds., R. S. Goodhart and M. E. Shils, p. 413. 6th ed. Philadelphia: Lea & Febiger.
10. Food and Nutrition Board. 1980. *Recommended dietary allowances,* pp. 151–154. 9th rev. ed. Washington, D.C.: National Academy of Sciences.
11. Canelas, H. M.; DeJorge, F. B.; and Tognola, W. A. 1967. Metabolic balances of copper in patients with hepatolenticular degeneration submitted to vegetarian and mixed diets. *J. Neurol. Neurosurg. Psychiat.* 30:371.
12. Communication with City of Ann Arbor Utilities Department, March 1979.
13. Mattice, M. R., ed. 1950. *Bridges' food and beverage analyses.* 3rd ed. Philadelphia: Lea & Febiger.
14. Pennington, J. T., and Calloway, D. H. 1973. Copper content of foods. *J. Am. Dietet. A.* 63:143.
15. Gormican, A. 1970. Inorganic elements in foods used in hospital menus. *J. Am. Dietet. A.* 56:397.
16. Hodges, M. A., and Peterson, W. H. 1931. Manganese, copper, and iron content of serving portions of common foods. *J. Am. Dietet. A.* 7:6.
17. Hook, L., and Brandt, T. K. 1966. Copper content of some low-copper foods. *J. Am. Dietet. A.* 49:202.
18. Wong, N. P.; LaCroix, D. E.; and Alford, J. A. 1973. Mineral content of dairy products. *J. Am. Dietet. A.* 72:288.
19. Zook, E. G., and Lehmann, J. 1968. Mineral composition of fruits. *J. Am. Dietet. A.* 52:225.
20. Yale–New Haven Hospital. 1970. *Low copper diet.* New Haven, Conn.: Yale–New Haven Hospital.

Iron Supplemented

INDICATIONS FOR USE

An iron-supplemented diet is indicated for individuals at risk for developing iron deficiency anemia. Iron deficiency is one of the most commonly recognized nutrient deficiencies in developing and developed countries. (1)

Iron deficiency anemia results from increased demand for iron and/or inadequate iron intake and occurs most frequently in the following cases (2):

Infancy. Iron stores at birth are only sufficient for approximately six months and the iron content of milk is low.

Childhood and adolescence. Rapid growth is occurring demanding increased iron.

Female reproductive period. Iron is lost during menstruation.

Pregnancy. Iron requirement is increased due to expanded blood volume, provision of iron for the placenta and fetus, and blood loss at childbirth.

Prolonged low intake of iron may also occur among the very young, the elderly, chronic alcoholics, and individuals with pica. These individuals should be assessed for iron status.

Diet alone is not adequate therapy for iron deficiency anemia (3) but is used to supplement the intake of prescribed iron salts. Following discontinuation of the pharmaceutical supplement, the diet aids in maintaining adequate iron stores.

DESCRIPTION

The recommended dietary allowances for iron have been set at 10 mg/day for men and postmenopausal women and 18 mg/day for women of child-bearing age. (2) The RDAs for iron were established at levels to provide replacement of iron lost from the body and to take into account the low average rate of absorption of ingested iron, approximately 10%. (2, 4–8) The American diet provides approximately 6 mg iron/1000 kcal. (9) Women require careful guidance in food selection to meet their increased iron requirements at weight maintenance levels of energy intake.

The goals of nutritional management are to increase iron intake and increase iron absorption. Iron absorption is influenced by the individual's state of iron nutriture (iron deficiency increases iron absorption), the form of iron ingested, and the composition of the foods ingested with the iron. (2, 10)

The two principal forms of dietary iron are heme iron and nonheme iron. Although the percentage varies with the source, approximately 40% of the iron in animal tissue is heme iron. (10) The remaining iron in animal tissue and all the iron in eggs and vegetable products is nonheme iron. (10) Approximately 15–35% of ingested heme iron is absorbed; this percentage is not altered by other components of the meal. (10) The percentage of nonheme iron absorbed is generally less than 5% but can be altered markedly by other components of the meal ingested simultaneously. (6, 10)

The presence of animal tissue (e.g., beef, lamb, pork, liver, fish, and chicken) has been shown to increase nonheme iron absorption. (11, 12) Milk, cheese, and eggs are not effective in increasing iron absorption and may have an inhibitory effect. (11–13) The presence of ascorbic acid may increase nonheme iron absorption up to fivefold. (12, 14) EDTA, calcium phosphate salts, phytate, and the tannic acid in tea inhibit nonheme iron absorption. (15–18)

The iron content of acidic foods can be increased by cooking in iron utensils. (19, 20) The amount of iron released from the utensil is increased with increased acidity of the cooked food. (19)

Iron supplements may be necessary to meet increased physiologic demands, to supply adequate iron for individuals on low-calorie, low-protein, or vegetarian diets, or to treat iron deficiency anemia. The primary form of iron used in supplements is the ferrous (Fe^{+2}) salt, which is well absorbed. Ferrous sulfate, containing 65 mg elemental iron per 325 mg tablet, is the most popular and least expensive form used. The daily dose (Table 38-1) is generally divided among three meals. (21)

GUIDELINES FOR NUTRITIONAL MANAGEMENT

Nutritional management is planned after assessment of the individual's present eating habits and iron requirements as identified from the recommended dietary allowances. (2)

The two factors involved in nutritional management are to

- Provide foods high in iron in the daily diet. Table 38-2 lists foods containing approximately 2.5 mg iron per serving. Table 38-3 lists foods containing approximately 1.5 mg iron per serving. The food lists are based on the iron content of the foods and not on the actual availability of the iron.
- Utilize food combinations and preparation methods to increase iron intake and absorption.

  Include a source of ascorbic acid in the same meal containing nonheme iron sources.

  Use infant iron-fortified cereals mixed with vitamin C-fortified juice for infants and young children.

  Include meat in the same meal containing nonheme iron sources.

  Use foods that are iron fortified or enriched with iron. Read labels, particularly of breads, cereals, and pastas.

  Substitute iron-fortified dry cereal for flour where appropriate in meatloaf, casseroles, or baked products.

  Cook foods high in iron in small amounts of liquids to retain iron content.

  Avoid large amounts of tea with meals containing nonheme iron sources.

NUTRIENT ADEQUACY

Actual nutrient intake depends upon the individual's appetite, preferences, and ability to eat. Provided that the individual consumes a wide variety of foods in adequate amounts, the diet will meet the recommended dietary allowances, 1980. When individuals are under stressful conditions, the recommended dietary allowances may not be adequate to meet nutrient needs.

TABLES

TABLE 38-1. Elemental Iron Prescribed Prophylactically or for Treatment of Iron Deficiency Anemia

	Daily Dose Elemental Iron	
Age Group	Prophylactic	For Treatment of Iron Deficiency Anemia
Children	1–2 mg/kg	6 mg/kg
Adults	65–180 mg	180–240 mg

TABLE 38-2. Foods Containing 2.5 mg Iron Per Serving

Food Group	Food Item	Serving Size: Weight (g)	Serving Size: Household Measure
Meat and protein equivalents	Beef, cooked	70	2½ ounces
	Beef, dried	56	2 ounces
	Clams, canned	56	2 ounces
	Ham, canned	84	3 ounces
	Heart		
	Beef, lean, cooked	42	1½ ounces
	Calf, cooked	56	2 ounces
	Chicken, cooked	70	2½ ounces
	Kidney, beef, cooked	21	¾ ounce
	Liver		
	Beef, cooked	28	1 ounce
	Calf, cooked	21	¾ ounce
	Chicken, cooked	28	1 ounce
	Liverwurst	42	1½ ounces
	Oysters, canned or raw	42	1½ ounces
	Pork, cooked	70	2½ ounces
	Salami	84	3 ounces
	Sardines	84	3 ounces
	Scallops	23	2
	Shrimp	70	2½ ounces
	Veal, cooked	64	2⅓ ounces
	Beans, dry, cooked		
	Navy or northern	90	½ cup
	Kidney	105	⅔ cup
	Lima	80	½ cup
	Cowpeas, including blackeye peas	190	¾ cup
	Tofu (soybean curd)	130	2½ in. × 3 in. × 1 in.
Fruit and vegetable	Greens, cooked		
	Mustard	140	1 cup
	Spinach	112	⅔ cup
	Peaches, dried	44	3 large halves
	Prunes, cooked, fruit and liquid	186	⅔ cup
	Prune juice	60	¼ cup
	Raisins	72	½ cup
Grain	Baby cereals, precooked, dry	3	1⅓ tablespoon
	Ready-to-eat cereals, iron fortified	Variable[1]	

[1] The amount of iron in iron-fortified cereals will vary with brand and type. Refer to product labeling to determine the amount of iron provided. Cereals are often fortified with 25–100% of the RDA for iron.

TABLE 38-3. Foods Containing 1.5 mg Iron Per Serving

Food Group	Food Item	Serving Size: Weight (g)	Serving Size: Household Measure
Meat and protein equivalents	Chicken, cooked		
	Dark meat	84	3 ounces
	Light meat	112	4 ounces
	Knockwurst	68	1 link
	Mackerel, Pacific, canned	63	2¼ ounces
	Tongue, cooked	70	2½ ounces
	Tuna, solid and liquids		
	Packed in oil	126	4½ ounces
	Packed in water	84	3 ounces
	Turkey, without skin		
	Dark meat	56	2 ounces
	Light meat	112	4 ounces
	Brazil nuts	45	9–12
	Cashew nuts	40	¼ cup
	Egg	100	2 medium
	Peanuts	75	½ cup
	Peanut butter	79	⅓ cup
Fruit and vegetable	Apple juice	240	1 cup
	Greens		
	Beet, cooked	78	½ cup
	Dandelion, cooked	83	¾ cup
	Kale, leaves only, cooked	110	1 cup
	Spinach, raw, chopped	55	1 cup
	Swiss chard, cooked		
	Leaves and stalks	80	⅔ cup
	Leaves only	83	½ cup
	Turnip, cooked	145	1 cup
	Peas		
	Cooked	88	½ cup
	Dried, cooked	88	½ cup
	Strawberries, whole	150	1 cup
	Tomato juice	180	¾ cup
	Watermelon, diced	240	1½ cups
Grain	Bread, white or wheat, enriched	69	3 slices
	Farina, cooked, instant	183	¾ cup
	Oatmeal, cooked	245	1 cup
	Noodles, enriched, cooked	160	1 cup
	Tortilla, corn	45	1½

TABLE 38-3. Foods Containing 1.5 mg Iron Per Serving [*Concluded*]

Food Group	Food Item	Serving Size: Weight (g)	Serving Size: Household Measure
Other			
Sweets	Corn syrup, light and dark	40	2 tablespoons
	Molasses, cane		
	Light	34	1⅔ tablespoons
	Medium	25	1⅓ tablespoons
	Dark	10	½ tablespoon
Miscellaneous	Wheat germ, without salt and sugar toasted	18	3 tablespoons

REFERENCES CITED

1. Dallman, P. R.; Siimes, M. A.; and Stekel, A. 1980. Iron deficiency in infancy and childhood. *Am. J. Clin. Nutr.* 33:86.
2. Food and Nutrition Board. 1980. *Recommended dietary allowances,* pp. 137–144. 9th rev. ed. Washington, D.C.: National Academy of Sciences.
3. Hickman, S. G. 1977. Anemia. In *Manual of medical therapeutics,* eds., N. V.. Costrini and W. M. Thomson, pp. 244–245. 22nd ed. Boston: Little, Brown.
4. Hallberg, L.; Hogdahl, A. M.; Nilsson, L.; and Rybo, G. 1966. Menstrual blood loss–A population study. *Acta Obst. et Gynec. Scandinav.* 45:320.
5. Finch, C. A. 1952. Body iron exchange in man. *J. Clin. Invest.* 38:392.
6. Bjorn-Rasmussen, E.; Hallberg, L.; Isaksson, B.; and Arvidsson, B. 1974. Food iron absorption in man. *J. Clin. Invest.* 53:247.
7. Layrisse, M.; Cook, J. D.; Martinez, C.; Roche, M.; Kuhn, I. N.; Walker, R. B.; and Finch, C. A. 1969. Food iron absorption: A comparison of vegetable and animal foods. *Blood* 33:430.
8. Green, R.; Charlton, R.; Seftel, H.; Bothwell, T.; Mayet, F.; Adams, B.; Finch, C.; and Layrisse, M. 1968. Body iron excretion in man. *Am. J. Med.* 45:336.
9. *Ten state nutrition survey 1968–1970. IV. Biochemical.* DHEW Pub. No. (HSM) 72–8132, 1972.
10. Monsen, E. R.; Hallberg, L.; Layrisse, M.; Hegsted, D. M.; Cook, J. D.; Mertz, W.; and Finch, C. A. 1978. Estimation of available dietary iron. *Am. J. Clin. Nutr.* 31:134.
11. Cook, J. D., and Monsen, E. R. 1976. Food iron absorption in human subjects. III. Comparison of the effect of animal proteins on nonheme iron absorption. *Am. J. Clin. Nutr.* 29:859.
12. Layrisse, M.; Martinez-Torres, C.; and Gonzalez, M. 1974. Measurement of the total daily dietary iron absorption by the extrinsic tag model. *Am. J. Clin. Nutr.* 27:152.
13. Monsen, E. R., and Cook, J. D. 1979. Food iron absorption in human subjects. V. Effects of the major dietary constituents of a semisynthetic meal. *Am. J. Clin. Nutr.* 32:804.
14. Cook, J. D. 1977. Absorption of food iron. *Fed. Proc.* 36:2028.
15. Monsen, E. R., and Cook, J. D. 1976. Food iron absorption in human subjects. IV. The effect of calcium and phosphate salts on the absorption of nonheme iron. *Am. J. Clin. Nutr.* 29:1142.
16. Cook, J. D., and Monsen, F. R. 1976. Food iron absorption in man. II. The effect of EDTA on absorption of dietary nonheme iron. *Am. J. Clin. Nutr.* 29:614.
17. Disler, P. B.; Lynch, S. R.; Charlton, R. W.; Torrance, J. D.; Bothwell, T. H.; Walker, R. B.; and Mayet, F. 1975. The effect of tea on iron absorption. *Gut* 16:193.
18. Finch, C. A. 1977. Iron nutrition. *Ann. N.Y. Acad. Sci.* 300:221.
19. Burroughs, A. L., and Chan, J. J. 1972. Iron content of some Mexican–American foods. *J. Am. Dietet. A.* 60:123.
20. Walker, A. R. P., and Arvidsson, U. B. 1953. Iron "overload" in the South African Bantu. *Trans. R. Soc. Trop. Med. Hyg.* 47:536.
21. Communication, January 1980, with C. E. Johnson, Pharm. D., Clinical Pharmacist, University Hospital, University of Michigan, Ann Arbor, Mich.

Phosphorus Restricted

INDICATIONS FOR USE

This diet, indicated for individuals with chronic renal failure, is designed to prevent hyperphosphatemia.

DESCRIPTION

In chronic renal failure the serum phosphate concentration shows recurrent transient increases as the glomerular filtration rate (GFR) decreases. The exact mechanism for increased phosphorus is not known. (1) However, this hyperphosphatemia will reduce serum calcium and lead to secondary hyperparathyroidism resulting in bone disease. (2–4) A diet restricted to 600–700 mg/day phosphorus and supplemented with calcium has been effective in preventing secondary hyperparathyroidism when instituted at a creatinine level of 3 mg/100 ml. (2) The incidence of osteoclastic bone disease has been observed to be significantly higher when the phosphorus restriction is started later, after plasma creatinine is greater than 4 mg/100 ml. (2)

Phosphorus intake in the average American diet is approximately 1500 mg/day. A diet can be planned to progressively reduce phosphorus intake as renal failure progresses.

Agents that bind phosphorus in the gastrointestinal tract and interfere with its absorption are used as necessary to further lower serum phosphorus (5) to the desired 4–6 mg/100 ml range. If binding agents are not tolerated, the diet is of greater importance.

GUIDELINES FOR NUTRITIONAL MANAGEMENT

In the early stages of renal failure, reduce phosphorus by avoiding foods very high in phosphorus and limiting foods high in phosphorus. Use the guidelines in Table 39-1.

As renal failure progresses and the diet is restricted in protein, phosphorus is further reduced. Phosphorus is found in a wide variety of foods but is found in greater concentration in foods high in protein. Phosphorus-restricted food systems, listed in Tables 39-2 and 39-3, are used in meal planning. The average phosphorus content for each food group listed in Table 39-2 may be used for calculation of the diet. The specific phosphorus values for each food item listed in Table 39-3 may be used when a more exact determination of phosphorus intake is indicated.

To make phosphate binders more acceptable, a cookie recipe has been developed incorporating the powdered form of aluminum hydroxide gel (Amphojel). Each cookie contains 1.8 g aluminum hydroxide gel, which is equivalent to 3 Amphojel tablets or 1 ounce of liquid Amphojel. (6) Table 39-4 contains the recipe for an Amphojel cookie.

NUTRIENT ADEQUACY

A diet restricted in phosphorus will generally restrict calcium. Calcium supplementation may be indicated.

TABLES

TABLE 39-1. Guidelines for Decreasing Dietary Phosphorus Intake Early in Chronic Renal Failure

Avoid	Limit (per day)
Baking powder	Cheese to 1 ounce
Chocolate	Meats, poultry, fish to 5 ounces
Dates	Milk to ½ cup
Dried beans	
Lima beans and peas	
Liver	
Whole grain breads and cereals	

TABLE 39-2. Average Phosphorus Content of One Serving (Exchange), Phosphorus-Restricted Food System

	Phosphorus	
Food Group	Average Per Serving (mg)	Range (mg)
Milk	115	114–123
Meat and protein equivalents		
Meat, poultry, cheese	60	36–112
Fish and shellfish	75	49–94
Egg whites	10	
Fruit	20	5–33
Vegetable	20	4–35
Grain		
Bread	20	15–34
Cereal	15	2–33
Potato or substitute	45	21–65
Other		
Beverage	Varies[1]	4–70
Fat	2	1–4
Sweet	Varies[1]	0–36
Miscellaneous	Varies[1]	0–60

[1] Refer to Table 39-3 for specific values.

TABLE 39-3. Phosphorus-Restricted Food Exchange Group

Food Group	Foods Allowed	Serving Size: Weight (g)	Serving Size: Household Measure	Phosphorus (mg)	Foods to Avoid
Milk and calcium equivalents	Whole milk	120	½ cup	114	Yogurt
	Low-fat milk	120	½ cup	116	
	Skim milk	120	½ cup	123	
	Half and half	120	½ cup	115	
Meat and protein equivalents	Beef, cooked	28	1 ounce	58	Beef or calves liver
	Lamb, cooked	28	1 ounce	51	
	Pork, cooked	28	1 ounce	54	Sweetbreads
	Veal, cooked	28	1 ounce	54	
	Bacon, cooked	21	3 strips	47	
	Canadian bacon, cooked	28	1 ounce	61	Peanut butter
	Chicken livers, cooked	28	1 ounce	45	Dried beans,
	Chicken, cooked	28	1 ounce	69	Dried peas, nuts
	Turkey, cooked	28	1 ounce	112	
	Cream cheese	28	1 ounce	30	
	Cottage cheese	56	¼ cup	75	Other cheeses
	Fish, cooked				
	Crab	28	1 ounce	49	Other fish
	Scallops	28	1 ounce	95	
	Shrimp	28	1 ounce	74	
	Lobster	28	1 ounce	54	
	Cod	28	1 ounce	77	
	Haddock	28	1 ounce	69	
	Halibut	28	1 ounce	69	
	Tuna, oil packed	40	¼ cup	94	
	Egg white	60	2	9	Egg yolks
					Nuts
					Poppy, mustard, and sesame seeds
Fruit	Apple	150	1 medium	15	Avocado
	Applesauce	150	½ cup	8	Banana
	Apricots, fresh	100	2–3 medium	23	Dates
	Apricots, canned	200	6 halves	30	Prunes
	Blackberries or boysenberries	150	½ cup	29	Dried fruits
	Blueberries	75	½ cup	10	
	Cherries, fresh	100	15 large	19	
	Cherries, canned	100	½ cup	13	
	Cranberries, fresh	50	½ cup	5	
	Figs, canned	130	4 medium	17	
	Fruit cocktail	100	½ cup	12	
	Grapefruit, fresh	100	½ medium	16	
	Grapefruit, canned	100	½ cup	14	
	Grapes, American	100	22 medium	12	
	Grapes, European	100	24 medium	20	
	Cantaloupe and honeydew	100	½ cup or ¼ of 5 in. diameter	16	

TABLE 39-3. Phosphorus-Restricted Food Exchange Group [*Continued*]

Food Group	Foods Allowed	Serving Size		Phosphorus (mg)	Foods to Avoid
		Weight (g)	Household Measure		
	Orange	150	1 medium	30	
	Peach, fresh	100	1 medium	13	
	Peach, canned	100	½ cup	16	
	Pear, fresh	200	1 large	22	
	Pear, canned	100	½ cup	7	
	Pineapple, fresh	100	¾ cup	8	
	Pineapple, canned	200	2 large slices	14	
	Plums, fresh	100	2 medium or 3 prune type	18	
	Plums, canned	100	2 medium	10	
	Raisins	10	1 tablespoon	10	
	Raspberries, fresh	67	½ cup	15	
	Rhubarb, cooked	130	½ cup	20	
	Strawberries, fresh	100	10 large	21	
	Strawberries, frozen	125	½ cup	21	
	Tangerine	100	1 large	18	
	Juices				
	Apple	180	¾ cup	17	Prune juice
	Apricot nectar	180	¾ cup	22	
	Cranberry juice cocktail	180	¾ cup	24	
	Grapefruit	180	¾ cup	28	
	Grape juice, bottled	180	¾ cup	22	
	Grape juice, frozen	180	¾ cup	6	
	Orange	180	¾ cup	33	
	Pineapple, canned	180	¾ cup	17	
Vegetable	Beans, green or yellow	50	½ cup	20	Asparagus
	Beets	83	½ cup	19	Broccoli
	Beet greens	100	½ cup	25	Brussels sprouts
	Cabbage, raw	50	½ cup	15	Collards
	Cabbage, cooked	83	½ cup	35	
	Carrots, raw	50	1 small	18	Corn, popcorn
	Carrots, cooked	75	½ cup	23	Dandelion greens
	Cauliflower	55	½ cup	23	Dried beans
	Celery, raw	50	½ cup	14	Dried peas
	Celery, cooked	60	½ cup	13	
	Swiss chard	83	½ cup	20	Mushrooms
	Cucumber	50	½ medium	7	Okra
	Eggplant	100	½ cup	21	Parsnips
	Lettuce	55	1 cup	14	Peas
	Onions, raw	10	1 tablespoon	4	Winter squash
	Onions, cooked	100	½ cup	29	Turnip greens
	Green sweet peppers	50	½ large	11	
	Radishes	50	5 small	16	
	Spinach, raw	50	2 ounces	26	
	Spinach, cooked	90	½ cup	34	
	Squash, summer, diced, cooked	105	½ cup	26	
	Tomato, raw	100	1 small	27	
	Tomato, cooked	100	½ cup	32	
	Turnips	75	½ cup	18	

TABLE 39-3. Phosphorus-Restricted Food Exchange Group [*Continued*]

Food Group	Foods Allowed	Serving Size		Phosphorus (mg)	Foods to Avoid
		Weight (g)	Household Measure		
Grain	Breads				
	French or Vienna	20	1 slice	17	Whole grain breads
	Italian	23	1 slice	18	
	White	23	1 slice	23	
	Rolls				
	Hard	35	1	32	Muffins
	Panroll	38	1	32	Biscuits
	Brown and serve	35	1	31	
	Roll mix	35	1	34	
	Graham crackers, plain	14	2–2½ in. square	21	Honey graham crackers
	Saltine crackers	16	5	14	Cheese crackers
	Soda crackers	28	4	25	Wheat crackers
					Pancakes, waffles
	Cereal				
	Cornflakes	25	1 cup	11	Bran cereals
	Puffed Rice	13	1 cup	12	Puffed Wheat
	Crisped rice	28	1 cup	33	Oatmeal
	Farina, cooked regular	123	½ cup	15	
	Macaroni, cooked	70	½ cup	41	
	Noodles, cooked	80	½ cup	47	
	Potato or substitute				
	White				
	Baked	100	1 medium	65	
	Boiled	100	1 medium	53	
	Fries	50	10	43	
	Mashed with milk	100	½ cup	49	
	Sweet				
	Baked	100	1 small	58	
	Boiled	100	½ cup	47	
	Spaghetti, cooked	75	½ cup	44	
	Rice, white, cooked	75	½ cup	21	Wild or brown rice
Other					
Beverage	Alcohol				
	Beer	240	8 ounces	72	
	Wine (table)	100	3½ ounces	10	
	Coffee	240	1 cup	10	
	Tea	240	1 cup	4	
	Lemonade	480	2 cups	5	
	Carbonated		As desired		Dr Pepper
Fat	Butter	15	1 tablespoon	3	
	Margarine	15	1 tablespoon	2	
	Oil		As desired		
	Salad dressings				
	French	14	1 tablespoon	2	Blue cheese
	Italian	14	1 tablespoon	1	
	Mayonnaise	14	1 tablespoon	4	
	Thousand Island	14	1 tablespoon	2	

TABLE 39-3. Phosphorus-Restricted Food Exchange Group [*Concluded*]

Food Group	Foods Allowed	Serving Size		Phosphorus (mg)	Foods to Avoid
		Weight (g)	Household Measure		
Sweets	Sugar, granulated or powdered	—	As desired	0	
	Gum drops	—	As desired	0	Caramels
	Hard candy	15	3	1	Chocolate
	Jellies	20	1 tablespoon	2	
	Jelly beans	28	10	1	
	Marshmallows	33	3	2	Molasses
	Maple syrup	40	2 tablespoons	3	
	Sugar, brown	14	1 tablespoon	3	
	Cake, angel food	45	$\frac{1}{10}$ average	10	
	White cake, white icing	60	2 in. × 3 in. × 2 in.	21	
	Cookies				
	Butter cookies	22	2–2½ in.	21	
	Fig bars	32	2	19	
	Shortbread cookies	14	2	22	
	Sugar wafers	22	4	18	
	Vanilla wafers	22	6	14	
	Pie				
	Apple	120	⅛ of 9 in.	26	
	Blackberry	120	⅛ of 9 in.	31	
	Blueberry	120	⅛ of 9 in.	28	
	Cherry	120	⅛ of 9 in.	30	
	Peach	120	⅛ of 9 in.	35	
	Pineapple	120	⅛ of 9 in.	25	
	Raisin	90	⅛ of 9 in.	36	
	Rhubarb	120	⅛ of 9 in.	31	
	Strawberry	85	⅛ of 9 in.	21	
	Sherbet	150	¾ cup	20	
Soups[1]	Beef broth, bouillon or consomme	200	⅓ can	26	Cream soups
	Beef noodle	200	⅓ can	40	
	Chicken consomme	200	⅓ can	60	
	Chicken gumbo	200	⅓ can	20	
	Chicken noodle	200	⅓ can	30	
	Chicken rice	200	⅓ can	21	
	Chicken vegetable	200	⅓ can	32	
	Onion	200	⅓ can	22	
	Turkey noodle	200	⅓ can	36	
	Vegetable beef	200	⅓ can	40	
	Vegetable, beef broth	200	⅓ can	32	
	Vegetarian vegetable	200	⅓ can	32	
Miscellaneous	Barbeque sauce	68	¼ cup	14	All nuts; poppy, mustard, and sesame seeds
	Catsup	34	1 tablespoon	17	
	Cranberry sauce	20	1 tablespoon	1	
	Mustard				
	Yellow	5	1 tablespoon	4	
	Brown	5	1 tablespoon	7	
	Seasonings	—	As desired		

[1] Prepared with water.

TABLE 39-4. Recipe: Amphojel Cookies (32 Cookies)[1]

Directions	Ingredients	Amounts
Mix thoroughly	Margarine	½ cup
	Sugar	¾ cup
	Egg	1
	Lemon juice	3 tablespoons
	Lemon rind, grated	4 tablespoons
Sift together and stir in	Flour–Amphojel mix[2]	1¾ cup
	Baking powder	1½ teaspoons
	Salt	¼ teaspoon
Chill dough and divide into 32 walnut-sized balls. Bake on greased cookie sheets at 400°F for 12 to 15 minutes.		

[1] One cookie has the following nutrients: kcal, 63; carbohydrate, 8 g; protein, 1 g; fat, 3 g; phosphorus, 9 mg; sodium, 36 mg; potassium, 8 mg; calcium, 10 mg.

[2] Ninety-six Amphojel tablets, powdered, and add enough sifted flour to make 1¾ cups.

REFERENCES CITED

1. Fiaschi, E.; Maschio, G.; D'Angelo, A.; Bonucci, E.; Tessitore, N.; and Messa, P. 1978. Low-protein diets and bone disease in chronic renal failure. *Kidney Int.* 13 (Suppl.) :79.
2. Bricker, N. S.; Slatopolsky, E.; Reiss, E.; and Avioli, L. V. 1969. Calcium, phosphorus, and bone in renal disease and transplantation. *Arch. Intern. Med.* 123:543.
3. Slatopolsky, E.; Caglar, S.; Gradowska, L.; Canterbury, J.; Reiss, E.; and Bricker, N. S. 1972. On the prevention of secondary hyperparathyroidism in experimental chronic renal disease using "proportional reduction" of dietary phosphorus intake. *Kidney Int.* 2:147.
4. Massry, S. G.; Ritz, E.; and Verberckmoes, R. 1977. Role of phosphate in the genesis of secondary hyperparathyroidism of renal failure. *Nephron* 18:77.
5. Schoolwerth, A. C., and Engle, J. E. 1975. Calcium and phosphorus in diet therapy or uremia. *J. Am. Dietet. A.* 66:460.
6. Johnson, K. 1979. Review of Amphojel cookies and Kayexalate candy. *Dialysis and Transplant.* 8:145.

40

Potassium Supplemented

INDICATIONS FOR USE

The potassium-supplemented diet is indicated for individuals at risk of developing hypokalemia. Potassium depletion may result from the long-term use of potassium-losing diuretics such as thiazides and furosemide, corticosteroid therapy, and primary aldosteronism and in edematous states associated with cardiac or hepatic disorders. (1–6) Diuretic therapy is the most common cause of potassium depletion and hypokalemia. (1–3)

The potassium-supplemented diet is generally used in conjunction with pharmaceutical potassium supplements. (1, 4) Diet alone may be used by individuals who are on short-term diuretic therapy, by individuals who have a mild potassium depletion, or by those who are not able to tolerate pharmaceutical potassium supplements.

CONTRAINDICATIONS FOR USE

Dietary potassium supplementation is not indicated when potassium-retaining diuretics such as amiloride, triameterene, and spironolactone are used due to the danger of inducing hyperkalemia. (1, 2, 7)

DESCRIPTION

Potassium is the principal intracellular cation. In a delicate balance with sodium, it influences cellular osmotic pressure and acid–base balance. The ratio between extra- and intracellular potassium plays an important role in the maintenance of neuromuscular activity. (1)

Individuals with mild potassium depletion may experience no symptoms. Those with mild to moderate depletion may experience lassitude, depression, weakness, and muscle cramps. More severe depletion may result in drowsiness, confusion, anorexia, nausea, hypotension, polyuria, polydipsia, changes in the electrocardiogram, and potentially fatal arrythmias. Hypokalemia predisposes the individual to digitalis-induced arrhythmias. (1)

The normal daily intake of potassium is approximately 2400–4000 mg (60–100 mEq) per day (8) but may vary widely due to diverse dietary habits (refer to Table A.6-4 for milligram–milliequivalent conversions). Potassium chloride in the form of a salt substitute may add a considerable amount of potassium to the diet. Refer to Table 41-3 for the sodium and potassium content of salt substitutes.

The common daily dosage of potassium supplements prescribed for the correction of hypokalemia ranges from 600–3200 mg (or 15–30 mEq). (1–4, 7, 9, 10) The most common form of potassium supplement used is potassium chloride. (1, 2, 4, 7) The chloride is important in correcting the diuretic-induced hypochloremic alkalosis that may be present. Unless the existing chloride deficit is corrected, supplementary potassium may not be effectively retained. (1, 4, 11) The most severe potential side effect of potassium supplementation is hyperkalemia, which may cause fatal arrythmias. (7, 12)

GUIDELINES FOR NUTRITIONAL MANAGEMENT

A high-potassium diet is provided in conjunction with any pharmaceutical potassium supplement prescribed to meet the desired level of potassium intake.

The procedure for calculating a potassium-supplemented diet is as follows:

1. Obtain a diet history and establish a reasonable average daily intake of potassium. Use Table 40-1 and the level of dietary potassium supplementation that will be practical for the individual to achieve.
2. Consult the physician to determine the level of dietary potassium intake desired for the individual.
3. Calculate the number of additional servings of foods from the high-potassium food groups listed in Tables 40-2 and 40-3 necessary to achieve the recommended potassium intake.
4. Record in the medical record the estimated past daily dietary intake of potassium and the estimated level of dietary potassium supplementation achievable.
5. Instruct the individual to include the recommended number of high-potassium foods in the diet. Emphasize the use of fresh fruits and vegetables that have a higher potassium content than those that are processed. Discourage cooking vegetables in water for prolonged periods or cooking in large quantities of water, which causes leaching of potassium. (13) If desired, add potassium chloride salt substitutes to the diet.

NUTRIENT ADEQUACY

Actual nutrient intake depends upon the individual's appetite, preferences, and ability to eat. Provided that the individual consumes a wide variety of foods in adequate amounts, the diet will meet the recommended dietary allowances, 1980. When individuals are under stressful conditions, the recommended dietary allowances may not be adequate to meet nutrient needs.

TABLES

TABLE 40-1. Potassium Content of One Serving of Foods from the Basic Food Groups

Food Group	Serving Size	Potassium Average (mg)	Potassium Range (mg)
Milk and calcium equivalents	8 ounces	345	335–420
Meat and protein equivalents (fish, poultry)	1 ounce	100	80–175
Cheese	1 ounce	30	25–45
Egg	1	60	65–75
Fruit and vegetable[1]	½ cup	180	75–205
Grain	1 slice or ½ cup	50	15–70
Other			
Beverage			
Coffee, brewed	6 ounces	105	
Coffee, instant	1 teaspoon	35	
Tea	6 ounces	40	
Fat	1 teaspoon	0	

[1] Do not count high-potassium fruits and vegetables. Refer to Tables 40-2 and 40-3.

TABLE 40-2. High-Potassium Foods, 500 mg Potassium Per Serving

		Serving Size	
Food Group	Food Item	Weight (g)	Household Measure
Fruit	Avocado	100	½
	Banana	150	1 medium
	Dates	80	½ cup or 8 medium
	Figs, dried	80	4 medium
	Orange juice	240	1 cup
	Prunes	80	8 large
	Prune juice	240	1 cup
	Raisins	70	½ cup
	Tomato juice	240	1 cup
	Watermelon	500	1 medium slice or 2½ cups diced
Vegetable	Dried beans and dried lima beans, cooked	135	⅔ cup
	Dried peas, cooked	200	1 cup
	Parsnips, raw	100	½ large
	Potato, white, boiled	125	1 medium with skin
	Potato, sweet, baked	180	1 large with skin
	Soybeans, cooked	100	½ cup
	Squash, winter, baked	100	½ cup
	Tomato, fresh	200	1 large
	Tomato paste	55	2 ounces
	Tomato puree	125	½ cup
Miscellaneous	Milk	360	1½ cups
	Salt substitute (potassium chloride)	1	¼ teaspoon

TABLE 40-3. High-Potassium Foods, 250 mg Per Serving

Food Group	Food Item	Serving Size: Weight (g)	Serving Size: Household Measure
Fruit	Apricots, canned	135	4 medium halves
	Apricots, dried, cooked	100	4 halves
	Apricot nectar	180	¾ cup
	Cantaloupe	100	¼ melon
	Grapefruit, raw	200	1 medium
	Grapefruit juice	180	¾ cup
	Honeydew melon	100	¼ small
	Nectarines	100	2 medium
	Orange, fresh	150	1 medium
	Peach, fresh	150	1 large
	Pear, fresh	200	1 medium
	Pineapple juice	180	¾ cup
	Plums, fresh	100	2 medium
	Strawberries	150	1 cup
Vegetable	Artichoke, cooked	100	½ cup
	Beet greens, cooked	100	½ cup
	Broccoli, cooked	100	⅔ cup
	Carrots, raw	100	1 large
	Chard, cooked	80	½ cup
	Mushrooms, fresh	70	7 small
	Potatoes, white, mashed or boiled	100	½ cup
	Pumpkin, canned	125	½ cup
	Spinach, cooked	90	½ cup
Miscellaneous	Milk	180	¾ cup
	Molasses, second extraction	30	1½ tablespoon
	Nuts	50	½ cup
	Peanut butter	45	3 tablespoons

REFERENCES CITED

1. Jellett, L. B. 1978. Potassium therapy: When is it indicated? *Drugs* 16:88.
2. Morgan, T. O. 1973. Clinical use of potassium supplements and potassium sparing diuretics. *Drugs* 6:222.
3. Edmonds, C. J., and Jasani, B. 1972. Total-body potassium in hypertensive patients during prolonged diuretic therapy. *Lancet* 2:8.
4. Cooper, I. 1975. Potassium supplementation during diuretic therapy. *Curr. Ther. Res.* 17:555.
5. Manner, R. J.; Brechbill, D. O.; and DeWitt, K. 1972. Prevalence of hypokalemia in diuretic therapy. *Clin. Med.* 79:15.
6. Shenfield, G. M.; Knowles, G. K.; Thomas, N.; and Paterson, J. W. 1975. Potassium supplements in patients treated with corticosteroids. *Br. J. Dis. Chest* 69:171.
7. Lawson, D. H. 1977. The clinical use of potassium supplements. *Drug Ther. Rev.* 1:137.
8. Randall, H. T. 1980. Water, electrolytes, and acid–base balance. In *Modern nutrition in health and disease,* eds., R. S. Goodhart and M. E. Shils, p. 377. 6th ed. Philadelphia: Lea & Febiger.
9. Ramsay, L. E., and Ramsay, M. H. 1977. Rational potassium prescribing. *Pract.* 219:529.
10. Schwartz, A. B., and Swartz, C. D. 1974. Dosage of potassium chloride elixir to correct thiazide-induced hypokalemia. *JAMA* 230:702.
11. Kassirer, J. P.; Berkman, P. M.; Lawrenz, D. R.; and Schwartz, W. B. 1965. The critical role of chloride in the correction of hypokalemic alkalosis in man. *Amer. J. Med.* 38:172.
12. Lawson, D. H. 1974. Adverse reactions to potassium chloride. *Quart. J. Med. (N.S.)* 43:433.
13. Tsaltas, T. T. 1969. Dietetic management of uremic patients. I. Extraction of potassium from foods for uremic patients. *Am. J. Clin. Nutr.* 22:490.

41

Sodium Restricted

INDICATIONS FOR USE

A sodium-restricted diet may be indicated for individuals with hypertension or fluid retention often resulting from cardiovascular or liver disease. Refer to Chapters 26, 27, and 28. (1–8)

CONTRAINDICATIONS FOR USE

A sodium-restricted diet is contraindicated for the following conditions:

Lithium carbonate therapy Lithium carbonate is used in the treatment of manic episodes in manic depressive illness. The kidney does not always discriminate between sodium and lithium; consequently, a state of sodium depletion results in increased reabsorption of both lithium and sodium. With a low-sodium intake, sodium and lithium are conserved, serum lithium rises more rapidly, and lithium toxicity may result. (9, 10)

Pregnancy. The edema of normal pregnancy is a physiological response to normal processes. There is no current evidence supporting routine sodium restriction in pregnancy. (11, 12)

Nephrotic syndrome treated with ACTH. Intensive sodium supplementation may be necessary for a brief period to prevent severe sodium depletion. (13)

DESCRIPTION

Sodium is the predominant cation of the extracellular fluid. The important functions of sodium are the regulation of the osmotic pressure of body fluid, preservation of normal muscle function, and preservation of the permeability of the cells. (14)

Retention of abnormal amounts of sodium and water is associated with hypertension and edema. These are generally treated with a combination of dietary sodium restriction, diuretics, and/or fluid restriction. (1, 3, 5, 6)

Excess sodium intake resulting in expanded extracellular fluid volume has been implicated as an important factor in the development of essential hypertension, hypertension of unknown origin. (8, 15) Reviews of epidemiologic studies support this hypothesis, indicating that, in populations with low-sodium intakes, essential hypertension is rare. When these people increase sodium intake, the incidence of hypertension increases. (8, 15) The habitual intake of sodium, 2000–4600 mg (90–200 mEq) per day for adults in Western industrialized countries often exceeds body need by tenfold or more and may be a major contributor to the 9–20% incidence of hypertension in the United States. (15) Dietary recommendations for controlling hypertension include a sodium restriction of 1400–1600 mg (60–70 mEq) per day and achievement and maintenance of ideal body weight. (6, 7, 15, 16)

Edema in congestive heart failure may result from increased renal conservation of sodium, an increased level of circulating aldosterone, and possibly an increased level of antidiuretic hormone. (3) Edema in liver disease results from portal hypertension, hypoalbuminemia, and overproduction of lymph. Fluid diffuses into the abdominal cavity and ascites results. (4)

The level of dietary sodium restriction required will depend upon the individual condition, drug therapy, and the individual response to sodium restriction. Sodium restriction may start as low as 250 mg (11 mEq) per day.

GUIDELINES FOR NUTRITIONAL MANAGEMENT

Provide a sodium-restricted diet. The majority of sodium in the diet is from sodium chloride salt used in processed foods and added to foods as a seasoning agent by the consumer. Unprocessed meat, fruits, vegetables, grains, and fats are very low in sodium.

The procedure for calculating the diet is as follows:

1. Obtain a diet history and establish the average daily intake of sodium using Tables 41-1 and 41-2 and food composition tables that include sodium values.
2. Consult the physician to determine the level of dietary sodium intake desired for the individual. The diet prescription should designate level of sodium desired, not level of salt. Sodium restriction may start as low as 250 mg (11 mEq) of sodium per day. The prescription is generally done in increments of approximately 250 mg (11 mEq) of sodium. A diet of 1000 mg sodium or less per day requires use of specially processed and prepared food items.
3. Use the diet history to adjust the diet with the individual to meet the dietary prescription. Tables 41-1 and 41-2 are used to calculate the sodium content of the diet. If additional high-sodium foods are desired, the dietitian may be able to calculate them into the diet using sodium values from food composition tables or information from manufacturers.
4. Evaluate the individual's drug therapy and renal status to determine if potassium-containing salt substitutes are appropriate. (17) The use of potassium-retaining diuretics or presence of impaired renal function may contraindicate their use. Table 41-3 lists the potassium and sodium contents of various salt substitutes compared with sodium chloride, table salt.
5. The sodium content of water may need to be evaluated and distilled water used depending on the level of sodium restriction and sodium content of the water supply. Information regarding sodium content of the water supply can be obtained from the local public health department. For example, the sodium content of Ann Arbor water is 36 mg/l. (18) Commercially softened water replaces calcium and magnesium ions with sodium ions. The amount of sodium in softened water will depend on the original hardness of the water.

NUTRIENT ADEQUACY

Actual nutrient intake depends upon the individual's appetite, preferences, and ability to eat. Provided that the individual consumes a wide variety of foods in adequate amounts, the diet will meet the recommended dietary allowances, 1980. When individuals are under stressful conditions, the recommended dietary allowances may not be adequate to meet nutrient needs.

TABLES

TABLE 41-1. Average Sodium Content of One Serving (Exchange), Sodium-Restricted Food Exchange System

Food Group	Food Item	Sodium Per Serving (mg)
Milk	Regular	120
	Low sodium	10
Meat and protein equivalents	Unsalted beef, pork, fish, poultry	30
	Egg	60
Fruit	Regular	Trace
Vegetable	Regular	200
	Unsalted	Trace
Grain	Breads, regular	120
	Breads, unsalted	2
	Cereals, regular	300
	Cereals, unsalted	2
Fat	Regular	50
	Unsalted	Trace
Sweet	Regular	300
	Unsalted	15
	Ice cream or gelatin dessert	50
Soup	Unsalted, commercial	40
High-sodium foods	Group A	550
	Group B	200

TABLE 41-2. Sodium-Restricted Food Exchange Group

Food Group	Foods Allowed	Serving Size (household measure)	Foods to Avoid[1]
Milk			
Regular	Milk: whole, 2%, skim	1 cup	Buttermilk; malted milk
	Yogurt	1 cup	Processed cocoa
Low sodium	Milk, low sodium	1 cup	
Meat and protein equivalents (unsalted)	Beef; cheese (specially processed without sodium); fish; pork; poultry; veal; wild game	1 ounce	Canned, salted, or smoked meat or fish, such as bacon, cold cuts, chipped, corned or dried beef, frankfurters, ham, kidney, salt pork, sardines, and sausages
	Cottage cheese	¼ cup	TV dinners Canned or frozen mixed dishes
	Peanuts, peanut butter; cooked soybeans	2 tablespoons	Meat extracts; regular cheese and cottage cheese; regular peanut butter
	Cooked kidney, lima, or navy beans; split peas	½ cup	
Fruit	Fresh, frozen, canned; juice	Unlimited	
Vegetable			
Regular	Canned vegetables	½ cup	Canned tomato paste, puree, and sauce; olives; pickles; sauerkraut
Unsalted	Fresh, frozen, canned	Unlimited	
Grain			
Breads, regular	Bread	1 slice	Corn bread; pancakes; waffle mixes
Regular	Cooked noodles, rice, macaroni	½ cup	Saltines and other salted crackers Regular potato chips; pretzels; other processed or salted snack-type products
Breads, unsalted	Bread Crackers; noodles, rice; and macaroni prepared without salt	Unlimited	
Cereal			
Regular	Ready-to-eat cereals	¾ cup	Quick-cooking and instant cereals
Unsalted	Puffed Wheat or Rice, Shredded Wheat, other commercial unsalted cereals; cooked cereals prepared without salt	Unlimited	
Fat			
Regular	Butter, margarine	1 teaspoon	Regular commercial salad dressings; regular gravies or sauces; salted nuts

TABLE 41-2. Sodium-Restricted Food Exchange Group [*Continued*]

Food Group	Foods Allowed	Serving Size (household measure)	Foods to Avoid[1]
Unsalted	Butter, margarine; cream sauces, gravies; nuts; salad dressings, oil, vegetable shortening	Unlimited	
Sweet			
Regular	Cake	3 in. × 3 in. × 2 in.	Mince-meat pie; molasses
	Cookies	2 medium	
	Pie	$\frac{1}{6}$ of 9 in.	
	Pudding	$\frac{1}{2}$ cup	
Unsalted	Cakes and cookies made with sodium-free baking powder; fruit and fruit whip; dietetic gelatin dessert; unsalted custards and puddings; unsalted fruit pie	Unlimited	
	Honey; jam, jelly; sugar; syrup		
	Sweets including hard candies, gum drops, marshmallows, and jelly beans		
Ice cream or gelatin dessert	Regular ice cream, ice milk, and gelatin dessert	$\frac{1}{2}$ cup	
Soup			
Unsalted	Commercial or homemade soups made with unsalted broth and no salt added in preparation	1 cup	Regular canned, dried, or packaged soup; bouillon cubes or powder; regular homemade salted soups
High-sodium food			
Group A (550 mg-Na/serving)	Bologna or other luncheon meats	1 ounce	
	Buttermilk	1 cup	
	Canadian bacon, cooked	$\frac{1}{2}$ ounce	
	Corned beef, cooked	1 ounce	
	Cottage cheese	$\frac{1}{2}$ cup	
	Fish, canned	$\frac{1}{4}$ cup	
	Ham, cooked	$1\frac{1}{2}$ ounces	
	Hot dog	1	
	Natural cheese	2 ounces	
	Processed cheeses (e.g., American)	1 ounce	
	Salt	$\frac{1}{4}$ teaspoon	
	Sausage links	2 average	
	Soup (regular) canned, dried, or frozen	$\frac{1}{2}$ cup	
	Tomato juice, regular, V-8 or vegetable juice, regular	1 cup	
	Morton's Lite salt	$\frac{1}{2}$ teaspoon	

TABLE 41-2. Sodium-Restricted Food Exchange Group [*Concluded*]

Food Group	Foods Allowed	Serving Size (household measure)	Foods to Avoid[1]
Group B (200 mg Na/serving)	Bacon	2 slices	
	Barbecue sauce	1 tablespoon	
	Buttermilk	½ cup	
	Catsup	1 tablespoon	
	Chili sauce	1 tablespoon	
	Malted milk	1 cup	
	Mayonnaise	1 tablespoon	
	Mustard	1 tablespoon	
	Peanut butter	2 tablespoons	
	Salad dressings	1 tablespoon	
	Tartar sauce	1 tablespoon	
	Tomato paste	1 tablespoon	
	Tomato sauce	2 tablespoons	

[1] Foods listed under foods to avoid may be used provided that the sodium content has been calculated into the diet.

TABLE 41-3. Potassium and Sodium Content of Various Salt Substitutes and Table Salt

Product Name	Potassium		Sodium	
	mg/g	mg/tsp	mg/g	mg/tsp
Co-Salt	481	2285	<1	<1
Adolph's Salt Substitute	480	2352	<1	<1
Morton's Salt Substitute	493	2662	1	<1
Morton's Lite-Salt	195	1131	240	1392
Table salt (sodium chloride)	0	0	393	2358

From product manufacturers and Oexmann-Wannamaker, M.J. 1976. Salt substitutes, *Am. J. Clin. Nutr.* 29:599.

REFERENCES CITED

1. Abelmann, W. H. 1978. Treatment of congestive cardiomyopathy. *Postgrad. Med. J.* 54:477.
2. Tobin, J. R. 1978. The treatment of congestive heart failure. *Arch. Intern. Med.* 138:453.
3. Sidd, J. J. 1978. Congestive heart failure. *Orthopedic Clin. N. Am.* 9:745.
4. Arroyo, V., and Rodés, J. 1975. A rational approach to the treatment of ascites. *Postgrad. Med. J.* 51:558.
5. Editorial. 1978. Management of hepatic ascites. *Lancet* 1:311.
6. Carney, S.; Morgan, T.; Wilson, M.; Matthews, G.; and Roberts, R. 1975. Sodium restriction and thiazide diuretics in the treatment of hypertension. *Med. J. Aust.* 1:803.
7. Morgan, T.; Gillies, A.; Morgan, G.; Adam, W.; Wilson, M.; and Carney, S. 1978. Hypertension treated by salt restriction. *Lancet* 1:227.
8. Freis, E. D. 1976. Salt, volume and the prevention of hypertension. *Circulation* 53:589.
9. Varda, V. A.; Bartak, B. R.; and Slowie, L. A. 1979. Nutritional therapy of patients receiving lithium carbonate. *J. Am. Dietet. A.* 74:149.
10. Platman, S. R., and Fieve, R. R. 1969. Lithium retention and excretion. The effect of sodium and fluid intake. *Arch. Gen. Psych.* 20:285.
11. Kaminetzky, H. 1978. Sodium in pregnancy. Part II. *Ariz. Med.* 35:401.
12. Oakes, G. K.; Chez, R. A.; and Morelli, I. C. 1975. Diet in pregnancy. Meddling with the normal or preventing toxemia. *Am. J. Nurs.* 75:1134.
13. Kinsell, L. W.; Partridge, J. W.; Boling, L.; and Margen, S. 1952. Dietary modification of the metabolic and clinical effects of ACTH and cortisone. *Ann. Intern. Med.* 37:921.
14. Harper, H. A.; Rodwell, V. W.; and Mayes, P. A. 1977. *Review of physiological chemistry,* pp. 526–527. 16th ed. Los Altos, Calif.: Lange Medical Publications.
15. Tobian, L. 1979. The relationship of salt to hypertension. *Am. J. Clin. Nutr.* 32:2739.
16. Reisin, E.; Abel, R.; Modan, M.; Silverberg, D. S.; Eliahou, H. E.; and Modan, B. 1978. Effect of weight loss without salt restriction on the reduction of blood pressure in overweight hypertensive patients. *N. Eng. J. Med.* 298:1.
17. Lakhanpal, R. K. 1978. When salt substitutes are required in low-sodium diets. *J. Nat. Med. Assoc.* 70:255.
18. Communication with Ann Arbor Water Works, October 1979.

REFERENCES FOR THE LAY PUBLIC

Dosti, R.; Kidushim, D.; and Wolke, M. 1979. *Light style. The new American cuisine.* New York: Harper & Row.

Krause, B. 1974. *The dictionary of sodium, fats and cholesterol.* New York: Grosset and Dunlap.

Margie, J. D., and Hunt, J. C. 1978. *Living with high blood pressure: The hypertension diet cookbook.* Bloomfield, N.J.: HLS Press.

Trice-Sanders, E. 1977. *Recipes for sodium-restricted diets.* Pacoima, Calif.: Community Education System for High Blood Pressure Control.

PART X
Food Sensitivity

Food Allergies

INTRODUCTION

Allergy is defined as an exaggerated response to a specific substance, resulting from prior experience with that substance or with a closely chemically related compound. (1) Food allergies are associated with a large spectrum of symptoms. Definitive diagnosis is by an elimination diet (Chapter 60). Skin tests and blood tests as yet have limited value in identifying specific food allergies unless confirmed by elimination diet. (2, 3)

Individuals vary in their tolerance to specific allergens, and sensitivity to allergens may decrease over time. It is important to retest individuals periodically to determine tolerance levels and adjust the diet accordingly. (2, 3)

Egg

INDICATIONS FOR USE

The egg-restricted diet is indicated for individuals with a demonstrated allergic reaction to eggs.

DESCRIPTION

The egg-restricted diet eliminates egg in all forms. Egg white or albumin is an extremely potent allergen and is a more common cause of egg allergy than the egg yolk. (4) Coagulation of the egg white by heating will change the protein character to such an extent that some individuals may be able to tolerate a cooked egg. (4) Individuals allergic to egg may also be allergic to poultry or the odor of an egg cooking. (4)

GUIDELINES FOR NUTRITIONAL MANAGEMENT

Avoid eggs in any form including fresh, dried, or powdered whole eggs or egg white and low-cholesterol egg substitutes. Table 42-1 lists foods to use and foods to avoid. To be assured that a product does not contain egg, read the label or recipe carefully. The following ingredients indicate the presence of egg: egg albumin, yolk, globulin, ovomucoid, ovomucin, livetin, vitellin, ovovitellin. (5)

Thoroughly wash and rinse utensils used for cooking to avoid contamination of foods with egg previously in contact with the utensil.

The following suggestions can be used to alter recipes of baked products using eggs:

Substitute for one egg:

½ teaspoon baking powder, or

2 tablespoons flour, or

½ tablespoon shortening, or

2 tablespoons liquid

Try the recipe without eggs if the recipe calls for 2 or more teaspoons baking powder or 1½ or more teaspoons baking soda. Increase flavoring ingredients when omitting eggs to cover flavor changes.

Beat eggless cakes thoroughly between each addition of ingredients. When all ingredients have been added, handle the batter as little as possible and bake immediately.

NUTRIENT ADEQUACY

Actual nutrient intake depends upon the individual's appetite, preferences, and ability to eat. Provided that the individual consumes a wide variety of foods in adequate amounts, the diet will meet the recommended dietary allowances, 1980. When individuals are under stressful conditions, the recommended dietary allowances may not be adequate to meet nutrient needs.

Milk

INDICATIONS FOR USE

The milk-restricted diet is indicated for individuals with a demonstrated allergic reaction to milk protein. This diet is not indicated for a lactose-restricted diet (Chapter 43).

DESCRIPTION

This diet eliminates milk and products containing milk proteins. The two main groups of milk proteins are casein, which coagulates with natural souring or rennet, and whey, which remains after removal of the casein. (6) Individuals sensitive to casein are generally not able to tolerate goat's milk or heat-treated cow's milk and must avoid hard cheeses as casein forms the cheese curd. (5) The whey is composed primarily of lactoglobulin and lactalbumin. The whey proteins are denatured by heating and may thereby be rendered less allergenic. The heat treatment of pasteurization does not cause significant denaturation; boiling does. (6) Individuals sensitive to whey proteins may tolerate boiled, evaporated, or dried cow's milk. (4, 5) Goat's milk may also be tolerated as the whey fraction differs from that of cow's milk. (5)

The degree of avoidance necessary to prevent symptoms will vary with each individual. Often the small amount of milk protein found in butter, margarine, and many bread products can be tolerated.

GUIDELINES FOR NUTRITIONAL MANAGEMENT

Avoid milk and products containing milk proteins. Table 42-2 lists foods to use and foods to avoid. To be certain that a product is milk free, read the label or recipe carefully. The following ingredients may indicate the presence of milk protein:

butter	lactalbumin
casein	lactoglobulin
caseinate	lactose
cheese	milk solids
cream	whey
curds	

Some individuals may be able to tolerate boiled, evaporated, or dried milk or milk heated for 20 minutes in a double boiler. (4, 5, 7) The skin or film that forms on the surface of heated milk should be removed. (5)

Individuals sensitive to whey may tolerate the following cheeses high in casein but low in whey (5):

American (not processed)
Cheddar
Edam
Gruyere
Parmesan
Romano
Swiss

The following cheeses contain larger amounts of whey and may not be tolerated by whey-sensitive individuals (5):

cottage cheese
cream cheese
Gervais
Neufchatel
ricotta

NUTRIENT ADEQUACY

The milk-restricted diet can be planned to meet the recommended dietary allowances, 1980, provided that a milk substitute fortified with vitamins and minerals is used. If an appropriate milk substitute is not used, the diet may be deficient in calcium, riboflavin, and vitamin D. When individuals are under stressful conditions, the recommended dietary allowances may not be adequate to meet nutrient needs.

Fungus or Mold

INDICATIONS FOR USE

The fungus- or mold-restricted diet is indicated for individuals with a demonstrated allergic reaction to fungus or mold.

DESCRIPTION

The fungus family includes ergot, Iceland moss, Jew's ear, mushrooms, truffels, yeast, and antibiotics derived from mold cultures. (8) Dietary elimination of fungus includes avoidance of foods that are not freshly prepared or opened. Fungus may grow readily in vegetable containers, refrigerator drip trays, garbage pails, house plants, planters, and sink and laundry areas. It is important that these areas be kept clean and, if possible, separated from food storage and preparation areas.

GUIDELINES FOR NUTRITIONAL MANAGEMENT

Avoid all foods that are known to contain fungus. Avoid foods that are aged, cured, pickled, or fermented. Avoid foods prepared with vinegar as vinegar may be produced with the use of yeast. (9) Table 42-3 lists foods to use and foods to avoid.

Serve foods as fresh as possible. Check for any evidence of mold. Store food in tightly covered containers or wrap securely to prevent air-borne spores from reaching the food.

Use canned foods, juices, and frozen juices when freshly opened or within 48 hours after opening or preparation. Clean the tops of all cans prior to opening.

Use honey, jams, jellies, and preserves within two weeks of opening.

Use meat and fish within 72 hours of purchase. Hamburger must be from freshly ground meat. When large portions of meat are being used, serve the inside portions that will be freer of possible contamination to the allergenic individual.

Avoid foods that contain yeast (often called leavening on the label) or vitamins derived from yeast. (8) Contact individual companies to determine content of products and type of vitamins when in doubt.

NUTRIENT ADEQUACY

Actual nutrient intake depends upon the individual's appetite, preferences, and ability to eat. Provided that the individual consumes a wide variety of foods in adequate amounts, the diet will meet the recommended dietary allowances, 1980. When individuals are under stressful conditions, the recommended dietary allowances may not be adequate to meet nutrient needs.

Wheat

INDICATIONS FOR USE

The wheat-restricted diet is indicated for individuals with a demonstrated allergic reaction to wheat gluten or wheat starch.

This diet is not indicated for a gluten-free diet, which eliminates the glutens of wheat, rye, oats, and barley from the diet (Chapter 44).

DESCRIPTION

The wheat-restricted diet eliminates wheat and products made with wheat. The two allergenic fractions of wheat are the wheat protein gluten and wheat starch. (5) Gluten is a vegetable protein that differs in its characteristics depending upon the grain in which it occurs.

Malt is avoided in the wheat-restricted diet because it may be derived from wheat. Malt derived from barley and corn is acceptable. (9) Because wheat-sensitive individuals are often sensitive to buckwheat flour, this flour should be introduced into the diet with caution. (5, 8)

GUIDELINES FOR NUTRITIONAL MANAGEMENT

Avoid wheat and wheat products in any form. Table 42-4 lists foods to use and foods to avoid. Individual manufacturers must be contacted to determine the specific content of products in question.

The following ingredients indicate the presence of wheat:

Flours:	*Others:*
all-purpose	bran
bread	bread crumbs
cake	cracked meal
cracked wheat	farina
durum	food starch
graham	malt
pastry	modified food starch
phosphated	semolina
self-rising	wheat germ
wheat	
white	

The following flours are acceptable alternatives in recipes for baked products using wheat flour. A combination of these flours often results in more acceptable products. Substitutes for 1 cup wheat flour are (5)

$\frac{1}{2}$ cup barley flour
$\frac{7}{8}$ cup rice flour
$1\frac{1}{4}$ cups rye flour
$1\frac{1}{3}$ cups rolled oats
$\frac{5}{8}$ cup potato starch
1 cup rye meal
$\frac{3}{4}$ cup soya flour
$\frac{3}{4}$ cup cornmeal (coarse)
1 cup corn flour

When preparing gravies, sauces, and puddings the following can be substituted for 1 tablespoon of wheat flour (5):

$\frac{1}{2}$ tablespoon potato starch
$\frac{1}{2}$ tablespoon arrowroot starch
$\frac{1}{2}$ tablespoon rice flour
2 teaspoons quick-cooking tapioca
$\frac{1}{2}$ tablespoon corn starch

NUTRIENT ADEQUACY

Actual nutrient intake depends upon the individual's appetite, preferences, and ability to eat. Provided that the individual consumes a wide variety of foods in adequate amounts, the diet will meet the recommended dietary allowances, 1980. When individuals are under stressful conditions, the recommended dietary allowances may not be adequate to meet nutrient needs.

TABLES

Table 42-1. Foods Allowed and Foods to Avoid for an Egg-Protein-Restricted Diet[1]

Food Group	Foods Allowed	Foods to Avoid
Milk and calcium equivalents	Milk; cheese; yogurt; cocoa beverage	Eggnog; custard; cream pies; puddings; most ice cream
Meat and protein equivalents	Meat; poultry; fish; shellfish; organ meats; cold cuts; frankfurters; peanut butter; legumes	Eggs; meat, fish, or poultry prepared with eggs in any form, such as casseroles, croquettes, loaves, soufflés, omelets
Fruit and vegetable	All fresh, frozen, or canned	Any prepared with eggs
Grain	Cereal or grain products not processed or prepared with eggs; ready-to-eat and cooked cereals	Any cereal or grain product containing egg or albumin as an ingredient or glazed with eggs; including doughnuts, French toast, muffins, pancakes, waffles, rolls, prepared baking mixes, egg noodles
Other		
Beverage	Beverages not containing foods to avoid	Malted drinks such as Ovaltine and Ovomalt; coffee, tea, and wine if cleared with egg; foaming-type root beer, Orange Julius, or similar beverages
Fat	Butter; cream; margarine; vegetable oil; shortening	Boiled salad dressing; sauces made with eggs; mayonnaise; mayonnaise-type dressings; some commercial oil–vinegar salad dressings; tartar sauce
Sweet	Gelatin desserts; fruit pie filling; hard candy; desserts made from recipes without egg or modified to contain no egg	Cakes; cookies; meringue; cream pies; pies glazed with egg; icings and frostings unless egg free; marshmallows; all candies except hard candies without soft centers
Miscellaneous	Nuts; seasonings; corn syrup; honey; jam, jelly; molasses; sugar; cornstarch; flour; vinegar; Royal and Cellu baking powder	Broth-based soups; beef bouillon or consomme if cleared with egg; soups with egg noodles; egg drop soup and mock turtle soup; some baking powders

[1] This food list is not comprehensive. Product labels must be read to determine whether individual products contain eggs or are egg free.

TABLE 42-2. Foods Allowed and Foods to Avoid for a Milk-Protein-Restricted Diet[1]

Food Group	Foods Allowed	Foods to Avoid[2]
Milk and calcium equivalents	Soy milk substitutes; Isomil (Ross); Prosobee (Mead Johnson)	Milk; buttermilk; cream; milk drinks; cocoa drink mixes made with milk; ice cream; cheeses; yogurt; cream cheese; "nondairy" products containing caseinate
Meat and protein equivalents	Eggs; meat; poultry; fish; shellfish; organ meats; peanut butter; legumes prepared without milk or meat products	Eggs or meats prepared with milk, butter, or margarine; cold cuts; hot dogs; packaged mixed dishes containing milk or milk products
Fruit and vegetable	All fresh, frozen, or canned, prepared without milk products	Any prepared or served with milk, butter, margarine or other milk products such as creamed or escalloped vegetables
Grain	Cereal or grain products made without milk or milk products; graham crackers; rice wafers; Ry-Krisp; cereals not fortified with milk solids or with milk protein; macaroni, noodles, rice	Baked products made with milk, milk solids, whey, butter, or margarine; French toast, pancakes, waffles; cereals processed or prepared with milk or milk products
Other		
Beverage	Carbonated beverages; black coffee and tea; alcoholic beverages	Any containing milk or milk products
Fat	Milk-free margarine, mayonnaise, shortening, oil, vinegar–oil salad dressings	Butter, margarine except milk free; salad dressings made with milk products; gravy made with milk
Sweet	Gelatin dessert, cookies, pies, and cakes prepared without milk products; hard candy; fruit ices; sugars; syrups; jelly, jams; honey	Puddings, cream pies, cakes, and cookies made with milk or milk products; candy unless hard sugar candy; some sherbets; whipped cream
Miscellaneous	Nuts; seasonings; bouillon; soups made from allowed ingredients; catsup; mustard	Cream soups, sauces, or chowders made with milk or milk products

[1] This list is not comprehensive. Product labels must be read to determine whether individual products contain milk proteins or are milk protein free.
[2] Individual tolerances will vary; some individuals may be able to tolerate foods listed under foods to avoid.

TABLE 42-3. Foods Allowed and Foods to Avoid for Fungus- and Mold-Restricted Diet[1]

Food Group	Foods Allowed	Foods to Avoid
Milk and calcium equivalents	Milk or milk products fortified with synthetic vitamins; yogurt; eggnog; custards; puddings made from allowed foods	Milk or milk products fortified with vitamins derived from yeast; milk drinks containing malt; cheeses ripened with mold such as Brie, Camembert, Blue, and Roquefort; other cheeses, cottage cheese, buttermilk, and sour cream that may contain yeast or mold (contact manufacturer)
Meat and protein equivalents	Eggs; meat; poultry; fish; shellfish; organ meats; peanut butter; legumes	Cold cuts; hamburger unless 100% beef and freshly ground; pickled or smoked meat, fish, and eggs (including delicatessen foods); corned beef; frankfurters; sausage; pickled tongue; foods made from leftovers such as meatloaf, hash, or croquettes
Fruit and vegetable	All fresh, frozen, or canned except those with mushrooms and those listed as containing fungus	Dried fruits including apricots, dates, figs, prunes, and raisins; vegetables served with cheese or cured with mold; chili peppers, pickled vegetables; truffles; sauerkraut; canned tomatoes and canned tomato products such as sauce, paste, or puree unless homemade; all pickles, any prepared with mushrooms
Grain	Breads, cereals, pasta, and rice not containing yeast or yeast-derived vitamins; products leavened with baking powder Cornstarch; flour with allowed vitamins	Breads leavened with yeast and those containing vitamins that are yeast derived; flour enriched with yeast-derived vitamins; crackers, noodles, and similar products enriched with yeast-derived vitamins; cereals containing malt; canned refrigerator biscuits (Borden, Pillsbury, and General Mills); Gerber's oatmeal and barley cereal
Other		
Beverage	Carbonated beverages, coffee, and tea (except those to avoid)	Cider; black tea, the leaves of which are yeast fermented; brandy, gin, fermented beverages; gingerale, homemade root beer; rum, vodka, whiskey, and wine; dried beverage powders containing yeast-derived vitamins
Fat	Margarine; butter; vegetable oil; shortening	Green or black olives; mayonnaise and salad dressings containing vinegar
Sweet	Fruit ice, gelatin, cakes, cookies, and pies made with allowed ingredients	Candy with malt or malted chocolate; any dessert containing large amounts of yeast or vinegar (e.g., mince pie)
Miscellaneous	Nuts; seasonings; broth; corn syrup; honey; molasses; hard candy	Mushrooms; homemade or canned soups made with any of the foods to avoid; canned foods that have been opened for over 48 hrs; vinegar or products that contain vinegar such as pickles, catsup, chili sauce, relishes, and horseradish; brewer's yeast or flavored yeast

[1] The food list is not comprehensive. Product labels must be read to determine whether individual products contain fungus, mold, or yeast or are fungus, mold, and yeast free.

Table 42-4. Foods Allowed and Foods to Avoid for a Wheat-Protein-Restricted Diet[1]

Food Group	Foods Allowed	Foods to Avoid
Milk and calcium equivalents	Milk, cheese, yogurt, all cottage cheese, cream cheese, sour cream, and yogurt not containing wheat; custard and puddings made with cornstarch, rice or tapioca; some ice cream	Some commercial chocolate milk, malted milk; some commercial ice cream; custard and puddings made with wheat flour
Meat and protein equivalents	Eggs; meat; poultry; fish; shellfish; organ meats; peanut butter not processed or prepared with wheat or wheat products; legumes	Meat, fish, or poultry patties or loaves made with bread or bread crumbs; croquettes, canned meat, cold cuts, hot dogs or sausages unless certified as pure meat; chili con carne; soufflés or omelets (unless all ingredients are known to be wheat free); stews with noodles, dumplings, or sauces
Fruit and vegetable	Fresh, frozen, or canned not processed or prepared with wheat or wheat products	Any prepared with wheat products including au gratin, creamed, escalloped vegetables, vegetables dipped in wheat flour batter for frying
Grain	Arrowroot; barley; cornmeal; cornstarch; oats; potato flour; rice; rice flour; soya flour; tapioca; rice bread; rice wafers; Ry-Krisp; 100% rye bread; products made from allowed flours; Cream of Rice cereal; oatmeal; Puffed Rice; rice	Wheat; wheat flours; any baked product made with wheat flour including baking powder biscuits, white, whole wheat, or rye breads; crackers made with wheat flours; doughnuts; muffins; matzos; pancakes; waffles; pretzels; rolls; rusk; zweiback; graham crackers; gluten breads; pita bread; popovers; sweet rolls; taco shells and corn chips commercially made; any cereal listing wheat or malt; bran cereals; farina; macaroni, noodles, ravioli, spaghetti, vermicelli; dumplings; bulgar
Other		
Beverage	Carbonated beverages; noninstant coffee or tea; cider; wine; pure cocoa	Beer; distilled liquors; cereal beverages (Postum); Ovaltine; instant coffee or tea containing wheat products
Fat	Butter, margarine; pure mayonnaise; oil–vinegar dressings; shortening; vegetable oil	Salad dressings containing wheat products
Sweet	Sugar; honey; corn syrup; maple syrup; molasses; jelly, jam; custard and puddings made with cornstarch, rice, or tapioca; chocolate, cocoa, fruit ice, fruit whip, gelatin, junket, meringue, homemade ice cream, commercial ice cream and sherbet if made without a wheat source; candies made without a gluten source	Commercial puddings or puddings thickened with flour; bread puddings, cakes, cookies, unless made with allowed ingredients; ice cream cones, ice cream, and sherbet if a wheat source is present; candies containing a wheat source including most fillings for chocolate or candy bars
Miscellaneous	Seasonings, except those that contain a gluten source; clear meat and vegetable soups; some canned and frozen soups; sauces and gravies if prepared with allowed thickeners and ingredients; vinegar; olives; nuts without flour coating; coconut; popcorn; potato and corn chips	Seasonings containing fillers, stabilizers, or hydrogenated vegetable protein; all soups containing ingredients not allowed; all commercial thickened soups, sauces, and gravies made with gluten sources; nuts with flour coating; chips made with a gluten source

[1] This food list is not comprehensive. Product labels must be read to determine whether individual products contain wheat or are wheat free.

REFERENCES CITED

1. Bleumink, E. 1970. Food allergy. The chemical nature of the substances eliciting symptoms. *World Rev. Nutr. Dietet.* 12:507.
2. May, C. D. 1974. Food allergy. In *Infant nutrition,* ed., S. J. Fomon, pp. 435–458. 2nd ed. Philadelphia: W. B. Saunders.
3. Personal communication with J. A. McLean, M.D., M.S., Prof. of Internal Medicine, Allergy Division, University Hospital, University of Michigan, Ann Arbor, Mich.
4. Tuft, L., and Mueller, H. L. 1970. *Allergy in children.* Philadelphia: W. B. Saunders.
5. Frazier, C. A. 1974. *Coping with food allergy.* New York: Quadrangle/New York Times Book Company.
6. Palumbo, M. 1972. Milk and milk products. In *Food theory and applications,* eds., P. C. Paul and H. H. Palmer, pp. 563–611. New York: John Wiley.
7. Fontana, V. J. 1969. *Practical management of the allergic child.* New York: Appleton-Century-Crofts Educational Division, Meredith Corporation.
8. Breneman, J. C. 1978. *Basics of food allergy.* Springfield, Ill.: Charles C Thomas.
9. Miller, J. B. 1978. Hidden food ingredients, chemical food additives and incomplete food labels. *Ann. Allerg.* 41:93.

REFERENCES AND SOURCES OF PRODUCTS AND RECIPES FOR THE LAY PUBLIC

American Dietetic Association. *Allergy diet recipes.* 430 N. Michigan Ave., Chicago, Ill. 60611.

Chicago Dietetic Supply House, Inc., *Cellu Foods.* 405 East Shawmut Ave., La Grange, Ill. 60525.

Energy Foods, Inc., P.O. Box 24723, 6901 Fox Ave., South Seattle, Washington 98124.

Good Housekeeping. *125 great recipes for allergy diets.* Good Housekeeping Bulletin Service, P.O. Box 2317, FDR Station, New York, New York 10022.

Public Health Service, National Institutes of Health. *Food allergy.* DHEW Pub. No. (NIH) 75-533.

Quaker Oats Company. *Wheat, milk, and egg free recipes.* Consumer Services, Merchandise Mart Plaza, Chicago, Ill. 60654.

Smoekh, E. 1974. *Allergy and your child.* New York: Harper & Row.

43

Disaccharidase Deficiencies

INTRODUCTION

A disaccharide is a carbohydrate or sugar composed of two simple sugars (monosaccharides). For utilization within the body, disaccharides must be hydrolized by the disaccharidases and absorbed from the gastrointestinal tract by monosaccharide transport mechanisms. (1) The hydrolysis of disaccharides to monosaccharides occurs in the brush border membrane of the intestinal villus. (1, 2) Figure 43-1 illustrates the disaccharidase enzymes required and the end products of intestinal hydrolysis. When a disaccharidase is deficient, the disaccharide cannot be absorbed. The unabsorbed disaccharides exert a hyperosmolar effect on the intraluminal contents, causing large volumes of water to be drawn into the intestinal lumen resulting in diarrhea. (2) Abdominal bloating occurs and is due to the osmotic load and the bacterial fermentation of the unabsorbed carbohydrate that produces volatile acids and carbon dioxide. Production of the acids results in stools with an acidic pH. (2) Severity of the symptoms may depend upon the age of the individual when sugars were introduced into the diet, the amount of sugars ingested, and the extent of disaccharidase activity impairment. (2)

Disaccharidase deficiencies may be primary or may occur secondary to another disease process. Two primary disaccharidase deficiencies are lactase deficiency and sucrase–isomaltase deficiency. Secondary disaccharidase deficiencies occur when there are gastrointestinal disorders affecting the small intestinal mucosa. Such disorders include gluten-sensitive enteropathy, cystic fibrosis, kwashiorkor, tropical sprue, intractable diarrhea, gastroenteritis, short bowel syndrome, gastric surgery, and malnutrition of infancy. (3–8)

Lactase

INDICATIONS FOR USE

A lactose-restricted diet is indicated for individuals who have a clinical diagnosis of lactase deficiency. Lactase sensitivity varies among individuals due to varying amounts of lactase present and the condition of the intestinal mucosa. (8, 9) Duration of the need of the diet may be short or long.

DESCRIPTION

Lactase deficiency may occur as a congenital disorder, as secondary to intestinal disorders, or at an age where lactase activity is normally low. (8) Congenital lactase deficiency is rare and becomes apparent shortly after lactose is introduced into the infant's diet. (8) A temporary intestinal lactase deficiency may exist in light-treated jaundiced infants due to increased amounts of unconjugated bilirubin. (10) Lactase activity returns when the jaundice is resolved. Lactase appears to be the disaccharidase most depressed by disease states or disorders affecting the small intestine mucosa; the lactase deficiency may persist after clinical remission of the disorder. (2, 4) For many ethnic groups, lactase activity is low after the age of three to five years. (8)

GUIDELINES FOR NUTRITIONAL MANAGEMENT

Avoid lactose. Milk and milk products are the natural sources of lactose in the diet. Table 43-1 lists foods to use and foods to avoid. The degree of avoidance necessary will depend upon the individual's sensitivity and occurrence of symptoms.

Read food labels carefully. The following ingredients may indicate the presence of lactose:

butter	lactose
cheese	milk
cream	milk solids
curds	whey

Milk may be used after treatment with a commercial product containing the enzyme lactase such as Lact-Aid.[1] These products hydrolyze lactose.

Substitute water, fruit juice, water from cooked vegetables, or milk substitutes in recipes containing milk.

Refer to Chapter 49 for lactose-free infant formulas and Chapter 4 for lactose-free tube feedings.

NUTRIENT ADEQUACY

The lactose restricted diet can be planned to meet the recommended dietary allowances, 1980, provided that a milk substitute fortified with vitamins and minerals is used. If an appropriate milk substitute is not used, the diet may be deficient in calcium, riboflavin, and vitamin D. When individuals are under stressful conditions, the recommended dietary allowances may not be adequate to meet nutrient needs.

Sucrase–Isomaltase

INDICATIONS FOR USE

A low-sucrose diet is indicated for those individuals with a clinical diagnosis of sucrase–isomaltase deficiency. Failure to follow a sucrose-restricted diet results in immediate diarrhea. An increase of small amounts of sucrose may be tolerated as the child grows older. (11)

DESCRIPTION

Sucrase–isomaltase deficiency is an inherited disease of the autosomal recessive type. (12) Congenital deficiency of sucrase is always combined with a deficiency of isomaltase. (3) Symptoms of a disaccharidase deficiency begin when sucrose is introduced into the diet, usually in infant formulas or strained fruits. (2, 3) Infants with a congenital deficiency of sucrase who have been fed a sucrose-containing formula from birth will show impaired growth and dehydration. (13, 14) Breast-fed infants or infants receiving formula with lactose, dextrose, or invert sugar as the carbohydrate remain well until sucrose is introduced. Sucrose intolerance is a lifelong abnormality. (2) Occasionally it is necessary to reduce starches in the diet as sucrase and isomaltase are responsible for some maltase activity and maltose and small oligosaccharides from starch digestion may not be adequately hydrolyzed. (3)

[1] Lact-Aid lactase enzyme is available from Sugarlo Co., P.O. Box 1017, Atlantic City, N.J. 08404.

GUIDELINES FOR NUTRITIONAL MANAGEMENT

Avoid foods containing sucrose including sugar in all forms, honey, molasses, and syrups. Table 43-2 lists foods to use and foods to avoid.

Read ingredient lists on all food labels. Sugar and other sweeteners are common ingredients in processed foods.

Use artificial sweeteners in recipes calling for sucrose-containing sweeteners or try the recipe without any form of sweetener.

For infant feeding, use breast milk or sucrose-free formulas, for example, Enfamil (Mead Johnson), Similac (Ross) or Similac 24 LBW (Ross). Refer to Chapter 49 for more details about sugars contained within infant formulas and to Chapter 4 for details about sugars contained within tube feedings.

Many vitamin and pharmaceutical preparations contain sucrose. A pharmacist should be consulted for this information.

NUTRIENT ADEQUACY

Vitamin C will be deficient and daily supplementation is recommended. Adequacy of other nutrients will be dependent on how well the individual tolerates fruits and vegetables and on the food choices made. A vitamin–mineral supplement may be indicated. Evaluation of nutrition status should be completed periodically.

TABLES AND FIGURES

TABLE 43-1. Foods Allowed and Foods to Avoid for a Lactose-Restricted Diet[1]

Food Group	Foods Allowed	Foods to Avoid[2]
Milk and calcium equivalents	Lactose-free formulas and lactose-free milk substitutes; milk treated with lactose-hydrolyzing products such as Lact-Aid	Whole, skim, fresh, dried, evaporated, or condensed milk; buttermilk; cream; malted, chocolate, or cocoa made with milk; eggnot; milkshakes; yogurt; nondairy creamers; whipped cream; ice cream; sherbet
		Cottage cheese, ricotta cheese, and American cheese spread containing greater than 2 g lactose per 1 ounce serving; all other cheeses contain less than 2 g lactose per 1 ounce serving (may be tolerated)
Meat and protein equivalents	Eggs; meat; poultry; fish; shellfish; organ meats; kosher meats; peanut butter; legumes	Any eggs, fish, or meat prepared with butter, margarine, milk, cream, or cheese; cold cuts, frankfurters, and packaged mixed dishes
Fruit and vegetable	All fresh, frozen, or canned prepared without milk products	Any prepared or served with milk, butter, margarine, or other milk products, such as creamed or escalloped vegetables
Grain	Cereal or grain products made without milk or milk products; graham crackers, rice wafers, Ry-Krisp, cereals not fortified with milk solids or with milk protein; macaroni; noodles; rice	Baked products made with milk, milk solids, whey, butter, or margarine; French toast, pancakes, waffles; cereals processed or prepared with milk or milk products
Other		
Beverage	Carbonated beverages; black coffee and tea; alcoholic beverages	Any containing milk or milk products
Fat	Lactose-free margarine, mayonnaise, shortening, oil; vinegar–oil salad dressings	Butter, margarine (except those not containing lactose); boiled salad dressings, salad dressings with cheese; gravy made with milk
Sweet	Gelatin dessert, cookies, pies, and cakes prepared without milk products; hard candy; fruit ices; sugars; syrups; jelly, jam; honey	Puddings, cream pies, cakes, and cookies made with milk or milk products; candy unless hard sugar candy; some sherbet; whipped cream
Miscellaneous	Nuts; seasonings; bouillon; soups made from allowed ingredients; catsup; mustard	Cream soups, sauces and chowders made with milk or milk products

[1] This food list is not comprehensive. Product labels must be read to determine whether individual products contain lactose or are lactose free.

[2] Individual tolerance will vary; some individuals may be able to tolerate foods listed under foods to avoid.

TABLE 43-2. Foods Allowed and Foods to Avoid for a Sucrose-Restricted Diet (15)[1]

Food Group	Foods Allowed	Foods to Avoid[2]
Milk and calcium equivalents	Milk and milk products not processed with sugar including plain cottage cheese, plain yogurt, cream cheese, and natural cheeses	Chocolate milk; flavored yogurt; ice cream; some processed cheese spreads; sweetened condensed milk
Meat and protein equivalents	Eggs; meat; poultry; fish, organ meats	Cold cuts, frankfurters; almonds, chestnuts, macadamia nuts; peanuts, peanut butter, lentils, chick peas; field or garden peas; soybeans; nuts, beans, and peas containing less than 2 g sucrose/100 g portion may be tolerated and include black or green mung beans, cow peas, pigeon peas, pecans
Fruit and vegetable	None	Sweetened fruits and fruit juices; sweetened vegetables and vegetable juices; all other fruits and vegetables not listed Fruits containing less than 2 g sucrose/100 g portion may be tolerated and include blackberries, bing cherries, boysenberries, cranberries, currants (red or black), figs, grapes (Concord or Malaga), guava, lemons and lemon juice, loganberries, pears, plums (Damson and sour), raspberries, strawberries Vegetables containing less than 2 g sucrose/100 g portion may be tolerated and include bamboo shoots, beans (snap), cabbage (raw), carrots (raw), cauliflower, celery, corn, cucumbers, eggplant, lettuce, white potatoes, pumpkin, radishes, squash (butternut, crookneck, Hubbard)
Grain	Oats; cornmeal; rye flour; wheat flour; brown rice; white rice; Puffed Rice; Shredded Wheat cereal; Puffed Wheat; Triscuits; saltines; macaroni; spaghetti	Barley flour; soybean flour and meal; wheat germ; sweet rolls; sweetened baked products including breads, cereals, crackers, and muffins containing sugar
Other Beverage	Coffee, tea; artificially sweetened beverages; distilled liquor	Fruit punches; regular carbonated beverages; beer; wine
Fat	Butter, margarine; vegetable oil and shortening; some salad dressings	Salad dressings containing sucrose
Sweet	Artificial sweeteners; corn syrup	Any foods containing sugar, honey, molasses; golden, maple, or sorghum syrup Gelatin desserts; jellies, jams; sherbet
Miscellaneous	Pure spices and herbs	Allspice; catsup; sweet pickles

[1] This food list is not comprehensive. Product labels must be read to determine whether individual products contain sucrose or are sucrose free.
[2] Individual tolerance may vary; some individuals may be able to tolerate foods listed under foods to avoid; others may also need to avoid starches.

$$\text{Lactose} \xrightarrow{\text{Lactase}} \text{Glucose} + \text{galactose}$$

$$\text{Sucrose} \xrightarrow[\text{}]{\text{Sucrase–isomaltase}} \text{Fructose} + \text{glucose}$$

$$\text{Maltose} \xrightarrow{\text{Maltase}} \text{Glucose} + \text{glucose}$$

FIGURE 43-1. *Intestinal hydrolysis of disaccharides.*

REFERENCES CITED

1. Barnes, G. L. 1976. Management of sugar intolerance in children. *N. Zealand Med. J.* 83:149.
2. Lebenthal, E. 1975. Small intestinal disaccharidase deficiencies. *Pediatr. Clin. N. Amer.* 20:757.
3. Anderson, T. A.; Meeuwisse, G. W.; and Fomon, S. J. 1974. Carbohydrate, In *Infant nutrition.* ed., S. J. Fomon, pp. 193–208. 2nd ed. Philadelphia: W. B. Saunders.
4. Gray, G. M.; Walter, W. M.; and Colver, E. H. 1968. Persistent deficiency of intestinal lactase in apparently cured tropical sprue. *Gastroenterology* 54:552.
5. Sunshine, P.; and Kretchmer, N. 1964. Studies of small intestine during development. III. Infantile diarrhea associated with intolerance to disaccharides. *Pediatrics* 34:38.
6. Weijers, H. A., and Van De Kamer, J. H. 1962. Diarrhoea caused by deficiency of sugar-splitting enzymes. II. *Acta Paediatr.* 51:371.
7. Welsh, J. D.; Shaw, R. W.; and Walker, A. 1966. Isolated lactase deficiency producing postgastrectomy milk intolerance. *Ann. Intern. Med.* 64:1252.
8. Johnson, J. D.; Kretchmer, N.; and Simoons, F. J. 1974. Lactose malabsorption: Its biology and history. *Adv. in Pediatrics* 21:197.
9. Gudmand-Hoyer, E., and Simony, K. 1977. Individual sensitivity to lactose in lactose malabsorption. *Digestive Diseases* 22:177.
10. Bakken, A. F. 1977. Temporary intestinal lactase deficiency in light-treated jaundiced infants. *Acta Paediatr. Scand.* 66:91.
11. Burgess, E. A.; Levin, B.; Mahalanabis, D.; and Tonge, R. E. 1964. Hereditary sucrose intolerance: Levels of sucrase activity in jejunal mucosa. *Arch. Dis. Child.* 39:431.
12. Burke, V., and Anderson, C. M. 1966. Sugar intolerance as a cause of protracted diarrhoea following surgery of the gastrointestinal tract in neonates. *Aust. Paediatr. J.* 2:219.
13. Ament, M. E.; Perera, D. R.; and Esther, L. J. 1973. Sucrase–isomaltase deficiency—A frequently misdiagnosed disease. *J. Pediatr.* 83:721.
14. Gudmand-Hoyer, E., and Krasilnikoff, P. A. 1977. The effect of sucrose malabsorption on the growth pattern in children. *Scand. J. Gastroent.* 12:103.
15. Hardinge, M. G.; Swarner, J. B.; and Crooks, H. 1965. Carbohydrates in foods. *J. Am. Dietet. A.* 46:197.

OTHER REFERENCES

Bayless, T. M., Rothfeld, B.; Massa, C.; Wise, L.; Paige, D.; and Bedine, M. S. 1975. Lactose and milk intolerance: Clinical implications. *N. Eng. J. Med.* 292:1156.

Harrison, M., and Walker-Smith, J. A. 1977. Reinvestigation of lactose intolerant children: Lack of correlation between continuing lactose intolerance and small intestinal morphology, disaccharidase activity, and lactose tolerance tests. *Gut* 18:48.

Read, N. W.; Davies, R. J.; Holdworth, C. D.; and Levin, R. J. 1977. Electrical assessment of functional lactase activity in conscious man. *Gut* 18:640.

Welsh, J. D. 1978. Diet therapy in adult lactose malabsorption: Present practices. *Amer. J. Clin. Nutr.* 31:592.

U.S. Department of Agriculture. 1979. USDA analyzes cereals for five food sugars. *CNI Weekly Report* 9:7.

Gluten-Sensitive Enteropathy

INDICATIONS FOR USE

A gluten-free diet is defined as a diet free of the glutens of wheat, rye, oats, and barley. The gluten-free diet is indicated for individuals with gluten-sensitive enteropathy, also referred to as celiac disease. Forms of the disorder include celiac disease of children, adult celiac disease, non-tropical sprue, idiopathic steatorrhea, and Gee–Herter syndrome. (1–3) Celiac disease may appear at any age, is the same entity for all age groups, and shows a definite familial incidence. (4–6)

Symptoms of untreated celiac disease may include diarrhea, steatorrhea, abdominal cramps and distension, flatulence, anorexia, osteomalacia, anemia, amenorrhea, weight loss, muscle wasting, growth failure, and dermatitis herpetiformis. (1, 5, 7–10) Untreated celiac disease is also associated with increased risk of malignancy of the gastrointestinal tract. Treatment with a gluten-free diet may reduce the risk of malignancy. (11–13)

The diet is implemented as soon as celiac disease is diagnosed and is recommended for the entire life of the individual. (1, 2, 7, 10)

A gluten-free diet may also be indicated for some individuals with dermatitis herpetiformis. (14, 15) Most individuals with dermatitis herpetiformis have the same intestinal mucosal lesion seen in celiac disease. Treatment with a gluten-free diet improves the mucosa and the skin, decreases the deposition of subepidermal IgA, and lowers the daily requirement of medication (dapsone). Complete remission often occurs. (14, 15)

DESCRIPTION

Gluten-sensitive enteropathy or celiac disease is defined as a gluten-induced abnormal jejunal mucosa resulting in malabsorption of most nutrients. (1, 7, 9, 12, 16–20) The mucosal damage may be associated with an immunologic reaction to gliaden, a polypeptide component of the cereal grain protein, gluten. (7, 21–25) Only the glutens of wheat, rye, oats, and barley contain this component. (1, 8)

When celiac disease is diagnosed, the initial diet is gluten free, high in carbohydrate and protein, and may be cereal starch free. (4) Depending on the severity of the malabsorption, milk and fat may also need to be restricted. (1) Refer to Chapters 42, 43, and 29. The diet is gradually liberalized to include all foods except those that contain the glutens of wheat, rye, oats, and barley. (4) The degree of recovery is dependent on the degree of gluten sensitivity and the level of adherence to the diet. (1, 26)

Individuals who do not recover in spite of strict dietary adherence may need to have corticosteroids added to their treatment. (7, 21, 27, 28)

GUIDELINES FOR NUTRITIONAL MANAGEMENT

The gluten-free diet avoids all foods containing glutens from wheat, rye, oats, and barley. Malt is also avoided as it may be made from these grains. Malt flavoring used in cereals is acceptable. Table 44-1 lists foods to allow and foods to avoid.

Labels must be read carefully. The following ingredients may contain glutens:

cake meal	matzo meal
cereals	millet
emulsifiers	modified food starch
fillers	stabilizers
graham	starch
hydrolyzed vegetable or plant protein	wheat germ
	wheat starch

Products containing these ingredients should not be used unless the contents of the ingredient is known to be acceptable (without glutens of wheat, rye, oats and barley). Some manufacturers are not required to list their ingredients. Avoid any product if there is a question about the ingredients. MSG (monosodium glutamate) is not a gluten-containing item and may be used.

Catalogs and order forms for gluten-free baked products are available from the following companies:

SUPPLIER	SUGGESTED PRODUCTS
Cellu Foods Chicago Dietetic Supply, Inc. P. O. Box 40 LaGrange, Ill. 60525	Corn, grainless, potato, rice, soybean, and tapioca flours; rice cakes and wafers
General Mills, Special Foods 4620 West 77th Street Minneapolis, Minn. 55435	A-Proten line of imitation macaroni, spaghetti, pasta
Jolly Joan Products Ener-G Foods, Inc. P. O. Box 24723 6901 Fox Ave. South Seattle, Wash. 98124	Rice bread, potato bread, cornbread mixes
Vita Grain Giusta Specialty Foods, Inc. South San Francisco, Calif. 94080	Lima potato bread
Vita Wheat Baking Products, Inc. 1839 Hilton Rd. Ferndale, Mich. 48220	Low-protein cookies (gluten free), rice bread

Low-gluten baked products and wheat starch are distributed by Cellu Foods and General Mills. These products are made with wheat starch (0.2% gluten) from wheat flour specially processed to reduce its gluten content. However, wheat starch is not sufficiently low in gluten, and the use of these products is not recommended. The physician may feel this level is safe for some individuals. Individual tolerance to these products varies.

Intolerance to other foods such as milk, fat, and gas-forming vegetables may occur; individualization of the diet is required.

NUTRIENT ADEQUACY

Although the diet may be planned to meet the recommended dietary allowances, nutrient supplementation may be necessary when intestinal malabsorption is present. Supplementation of potassium, folic acid, vitamin B_{12}, and other water-soluble vitamins; vitamin D and other fat-soluble vitamins; and calcium, iron, and magnesium may be indicated. Parenteral vitamin–mineral preparations are used when absorption by the oral route is insufficient. Supplementation is discontinued as the diet becomes effective. (1, 10) Evaluation of nutritional status should be completed periodically.

TABLES

Table 44-1. Foods Allowed and Foods to Avoid for a Gluten-Free or Low-Gluten Diet[1]

Food Group	Foods Allowed	Foods to Avoid[2]
Milk and calcium equivalents	All milk, cream, sour cream, yogurt, cottage cheese, cream cheese, natural cheese, and processed cheese not containing a gluten source; custard and puddings made with cornstarch, rice, or tapioca	Malted milk; some commercial chocolate milk; some commercial ice cream Processed cheese, cheese foods, and cheese spreads that contain a gluten source
Meat and protein equivalents	All eggs, meat, poultry, fish, shellfish, organ meats not processed or prepared with a gluten source	Meat, fish, or poultry patties or loaves made with bread or bread crumbs; croquettes; canned meat; cold cuts, hot dogs, or sausages unless certified as pure meat; chili con carne; soufflés or omelets (unless all ingredients are known to be gluten free); stews with noodles, dumplings, or sauces
Fruit and vegetable	All fresh, frozen, and canned prepared without a gluten source	Any prepared with a gluten source such as au gratin, creamed, escalloped vegetables and vegetables dipped in wheat flour batter for frying
Grain	Breads or other baked products made with cornmeal, cornstarch, rice, soy, or potato starch flour and without a gluten source	Baked products made with wheat, rye, oats, barley, malt, kasha, or wheat germ including biscuits, cakes, cookies, crackers, pancakes, pastries, pretzels, rolls, waffles, or commercial mixes for baked products
	Cream of Rice cereal; rice, hominy, or grits; corn or rice cereals such as cornflakes, Puffed Rice	Cereals, flours, and pastas containing wheat, rye, oats, barley, or malt; malt flavoring in cereals acceptable
	Corn, potato, rice, tapioca, soy, chick pea, or other bean flours	Wheat, rye, oat, or barley flour
	Gluten-free pasta or homemade pasta made with allowed flours	All regular pasta made from wheat flour
	Sprouted alfalfa or other allowed grains	Sprouted wheat or other grains not allowed
Other		
Beverage	Cider; fruit-flavored drinks without a gluten source; pure cocoa; noninstant coffee and tea; carbonated beverages	Cereal beverages such as Postum and Ovaltine; instant coffee and tea if containing a gluten source; cocoa mixes
	Distilled liquor; wine	Beer and ale
Fat	Butter, margarine; vegetable oils, and other fats; pure mayonnaise; commercial salad dressings not containing a gluten source	Commercial salad dressings if ingredients are not allowed or unknown
Sweet	Sugar; honey; corn syrup; molasses; jelly, jam	

TABLE 44-1. Foods Allowed and Foods to Avoid for a Gluten-Free or Low-Gluten Diet[1] [*Concluded*]

Food Group	Foods Allowed	Foods to Avoid[2]
	Puddings made with cornstarch, rice, or tapioca; chocolate, cocoa, custard; fruit ice, fruit whip; gelatin; junket; meringue	Commercial puddings or puddings thickened with flour; bread puddings; cakes, cookies, chocolate or candy bars made with gluten sources
	Homemade ice cream; commercial ice cream and sherbet if made without a gluten source	Ice cream cones; ice cream and sherbet if a gluten source is present
	Candies made without a gluten source	Candies containing a gluten source including most fillings for chocolate or candy bars
Miscellaneous	Seasonings, except those that contain a gluten source	Seasonings containing fillers, stabilizers, or hydrogenated vegetable protein
	Clear meat and vegetable soups; some canned and frozen soups	All soups containing ingredients not allowed; all commercial thickened soups
	Sauces and gravies if prepared with allowed thickeners and ingredients	Sauces and gravies made with gluten sources
	Vinegar; olives; nuts without flour coating; peanut butter; coconut; popcorn; potato and corn chips	Nuts with flour coating; chips made with a gluten source

[1] This food list is not comprehensive. Product labels must be read or manufacturers contacted to ensure that individual products are gluten free.
[2] Individual tolerance will vary; some individuals may be able to tolerate foods listed under foods to avoid.

REFERENCES CITED

1. BROITMAN, S. A., and ZAMCHECK, N. 1980. Nutrition in diseases of the gastrointestinal tract. B. Nutrition in diseases of the intestines. In *Modern nutrition in health and disease,* eds., R. S. Goodhart and M. E. Shils, pp. 912–952. 6th ed. Philadelphia: Lea & Febiger.
2. KOWLESSAR, O. D. 1972. Dietary gluten sensitivity updated. *J. Am. Dietet. A.* 60:475.
3. TRIER, J. S. 1978. Celiac sprue disease. In *Gastrointestinal disease,* eds., M. H. Sleisenger and J. S. Fordtran, pp. 1029–1051. 2nd ed. Philadelphia: W. B. Saunders.
4. DI SANT'AGNESE, P. A., and JONES, W. O. 1962. The celiac syndrome (malabsorption) in pediatrics. *JAMA* 180:308.
5. ANDERSON, D. M. 1959. History of celiac disease. *J. Am. Dietet. A.* 35:1158.
6. MACDONALD, W. C.; DOBBINS, W. O.; and RUBIN, C. E. 1965. Studies of the familial nature of celiac sprue using biopsy of the small intestine. *N. Eng. J. Med.* 272:448.
7. BOOTH, C. C. 1977. Coeliac disease. *Nutr. Metab.* 21:65.
8. LORENZ, K., and LEE, V. A. 1977. The nutritional and physiological impact of cereal products in human nutrition. *CRC Critical Rev. in Food Sci. and Nutr.* 8:383.
9. HAJJAR, E. T.; VINCENTI, F.; and SALTI, I. S. 1974. Gluten-induced enteropathy: Osteomalacia as its principal manifestation. *Arch. Intern. Med.* 134:565.
10. YOUNG, W. F., and PRINGLE, E. M. 1971. 110 children with coeliac disease, 1950–1969. *Arch. Dis. Child* 46:421.
11. AUSTAD, W. I.; CORNES, J. S.; GOUGH, K. R.; MCCARTHY, C. F.; and READ, A. E. 1967. Steatorrhea and malignant lymphoma. *Am. J. Digest. Dis. (N.S.)* 12:475.
12. MCCRAE, W. M.; EASTWOOD, M. A.; MARTIN, M. R.; and SIRCUS, W. 1975. Neglected coeliac disease. *Lancet* 1:187.
13. HARRIS, O. D.; COOKE, W. T.; THOMPSON, H.; and WATERHOUSE, J. A. H. 1967. Malignancy in adult coeliac disease and idiopathic steatorrhoea. *Am. J. Med.* 42:899.
14. REUNALA, T.; BLOMQVIST, K.; TARPILA, S.; HALME, H.; and KANGAS, K. 1977. Gluten-free diet in dermatitis herpetiformis. *Br. J. Derm.* 97:473.
15. HARRINGTON, C. I., and READ, N. W. 1977. Dermatitis herpetiformis: Effect of gluten-free diet on skin IgA and jejunal structure and function. *Br. Med. J.* 1:872.
16. STEWART, J. S.; POLLOCK, D. J.; HOFFBRAND, A. V.; MOLLIN, D. L.; and BOOTH, C. C. 1967. A study of proximal and distal intestinal structure and absorptive function in idiopathic steatorrhoea. *Quart. J. Med. (N.S.)* 36:425.
17. READ, N. W.; LEVIN, R. J.; and HOLDSWORTH, C. D. 1976. Electrogenic glucose absorption in untreated and treated coeliac disease. *Gut* 17:444.
18. SCHEDL, H. P.; PIERCE, C. E.; RIDER, A.; and CLIFTON, J. A. 1968. Absorption of 1-methionine from the human small intestine. *J. Clin. Invest.* 47.417.
19. HALSTED, C. H.; REISENAUER, A. M.; ROMERO, J. J.; CANTOR, D. S.; and REUBNER, B. 1977. Jejunal perfusion of simple and conjugated folates in celiac sprue. *J. Clin. Invest.* 59:993.
20. SCHEDL, H. P., and CLIFTON, J. A. 1963. Solute and water absorption by the human small intestine. *Nature* 199:1264.
21. HAMILTON, J. D.; CHAMBERS, R. A.; and WYNN-WILLIAMS, A. 1976. Role of gluten, prednisone, and azathioprine in non-responsive coeliac disease. *Lancet* 1:1213.
22. DISSANAYAKE, A. S.; JERROME, D. W.; OFFORD, R. E.; TRUELOVE, S. C.; and WHITEHEAD, R. 1974. Identifying toxic fractions of wheat gluten and their effect on the jejunal mucosa in coeliac disease. *Gut* 15:931.
23. RATNAIKE, R. N., and WANGEL, A. G. 1977. Immunological abnormalities in coeliac disease and their response to dietary restriction. I. Serum immunoglobulins, antibodies and complement. *Aust. N. Zealand J. Med.* 7:349.

24. Lancaster-Smith, M.; Joyce, S.; and Kumar, P. 1977. Immunoglobulins in the jejunal mucosa in adult coeliac disease and dermatitis herpetiformis after the reintroduction of dietary gluten. *Gut* 18:887.
25. Falchuk, Z. M., and Strober, W. 1974. Gluten-sensitive enteropathy; Synthesis of antigliadin antibody *in vitro. Gut* 15:947.
26. Dissanayake, A. S.; Truelove, S. C.; and Whitehead, R. 1974. Jejunal mucosal recovery in coeliac disease in relation to the degree of adherence to a gluten-free diet. *Quart. J. Med. (N.S.)* 43:161.
27. Wall, A. J.; Douglas, A. P.; Booth, C. C.; and Pearse, A. G. E. 1970. Response of the jejunal mucosa in adult coeliac disease to oral prednisolone. *Gut* 11:7.
28. Holdstock, D. J., and Oleesky, S. 1973. Successful treatment of collagenous sprue with combination of prednisolone and gluten-free diet. *Postgrad. Med. J.* 49:664.

45

Salicylate and Tartrazine

INDICATIONS FOR USE

This diet is indicated for individuals sensitive to salicylates and tartrazine. Urticaria, rhinitis, asthma, or many other symptoms of allergy may be present. (1–4) If the diet succeeds in significantly reducing or eliminating symptoms, the diet is prescribed for an indefinite period of time. (4)

DESCRIPTION

Salicylates are found either naturally or as chemical additives in many drugs, foods, beverages, and flavorings. (4) Many individuals sensitive to salicylates are also sensitive to tartrazine. (1, 4) The sources of salicylates and tartrazine include a wide variety of nonfood items and drugs that must be eliminated to control symptoms. (1–4) An extensive listing of these sources is available elsewhere. (3)

GUIDELINES FOR NUTRITIONAL MANAGEMENT

Avoid foods containing salicylates or tartrazine. Table 45-1 lists foods to use and foods to avoid.

Read labels carefully. The words "flavor" and "color" are often used without specifying the agent used. Any products that are shades of yellow, orange, green, or red may contain tartrazine and should be suspect. Manufacturers must be contacted to determine specifically which commercially processed foods contain salicylates or tartrazine.

NUTRIENT ADEQUACY

Although this diet may be planned to meet the recommended dietary allowances, 1980, the restricted choices from the fruit and vegetable group may result in a diet low in vitamin C. A vitamin supplement devoid of tartrazine is recommended for daily use. (4)

TABLES

Table 45-1. Foods Allowed and Foods to Avoid for a Salicylate and Tartrazine-Restricted Diet (3, 4)[1]

Food Group	Foods Allowed	Foods to Avoid
Milk and calcium equivalents	Evaporated, condensed, dry, and fresh milk; buttermilk; cream	All instant breakfast drinks and quick-mix powdered drinks; chocolate milk; yogurt; ice cream and ice milk; colored cheese; commercially prepared mixes for puddings or custards; puddings
Meat and protein equivalents	Eggs; meat; poultry; fish; organ meats; peanut butter; legumes	Cold cuts including bologna and salami; frankfurters, sausage, meatloaf, ham, bacon; barbecued meats; "self-basting" turkeys; frozen fish fillets or fish sticks that are dyed or flavored
Fruit and vegetable	Bananas; blueberries; cranberries; dates; figs; grapefruit; loganberries; lemons; limes; mangos; mandarin oranges; papayas; pears; pineapples; tangarines; and rhubarb	Apples; apricots; blackberries; boysenberries; dewberries; gooseberries; raspberries; strawberries; cherries; currants; grapes and raisins or products made of grapes or raisins; nectarines; oranges; peaches; plums and prunes
	All vegetables except those listed to avoid	Cucumbers; pickles; green bell peppers, peppers; tomatoes; potatoes (white)
Grain	Bread; cereal; crackers; grains; flours without added salicylates or tartrazine	Cereals with artificial colors and flavors; instant breakfast preparations; all manufactured baked products such as cakes, cookies, pastries, sweet rolls, doughnuts, pie crusts, frozen baked goods, egg bread, and whole wheat bread; gingersnaps; prepackaged baking mixes
Other		
Beverage	Allowed fruit juices; coffee, decaffeinated coffee	Cider; wine; beer; diet and regular carbonated beverages; instant breakfast drinks; powdered drink mixes; tea
Fat	Bacon; oil; cream cheese; sour cream; nuts except almonds	Almonds; salad dressings; olives; mayonnaise; avocados; margarine; colored butter; cooking fats
Sweet	Sugar; honey; corn syrup; allowed fruits and fruit ices; homemade cakes, cookies, candies made from allowed ingredients	Ice cream, sherbets, ices, gelatins, junkets; dessert mixes; mint-flavored items; commercial chocolate syrups; manufactured candies, hard or soft; desserts made with raisins; jams, jelly
Miscellaneous		Mustard; mint or wintergreen-flavored items; soy sauce; cider vinegar; wine vinegar; barbeque-flavored potato chips; cloves; catsup; chili sauce; almond extract; all items prepared with cider or wine vinegar

[1] This food list is not comprehensive. Product labels must be read and manufacturers contacted to determine if a specific food contains salicylates or tartrazine or is salicylate and tartrazine free.

REFERENCES CITED

1. FISHERMAN, E. W., and COHEN, G. N. 1973. Aspirin and other cross-reacting small chemicals in known aspirin intolerant patients. *Ann. Allergy* 31:476.
2. LOCKEY, S. D. 1977. Hypersensitivity to tartrazine (FD&C Yellow No. 5) and other dyes and additives present in foods and pharmaceutical products. *Ann. Allergy* 38:206.
3. BRENEMAN, J. C. 1978. *Basics of food allergy.* Springfield, Ill.: Charles C Thomas.
4. NOID, H. E.; SCHULZE, T. W.; and WINKLEMANN, R. K. 1974. Diet plan for patients with salicylate-induced urticaria. *Arch. Dermatol.* 109:866.

OTHER REFERENCES

FISHERMAN, E. W., and COHEN, G. N. 1976. Recurring and chronic urticaria: Identification of etiologies. *Ann. Allergy* 36:400.

LEIST, E. R., and BANWELL, J. G. 1974. Products containing aspirin. *N. Eng. J. Med.* 291:710.

PART XI
Maternal

46

Pregnancy (Normal and High Risk)

INDICATIONS FOR USE

This diet is indicated throughout the course of pregnancy. Nutritional assessment and dietary counseling are an essential aspect of obstetric management. (1)

DESCRIPTION

Nutrient requirements for calories, protein, vitamins, and minerals are increased during pregnancy. (2) In general, an increased caloric intake of 300 kcal/day and an increased protein intake of 30 g/day are recommended. Hematological changes markedly increase iron and folate requirements; routine supplementation during pregnancy is recommended. Refer to the recommended dietary allowances (Appendix 1) for recommended intakes of other vitamins and minerals.

No scientific evidence exists for routine restriction of calories or limitation of weight gain during pregnancy, regardless of pre-pregnancy weight. Severe restriction of calories is harmful to the developing fetus and the mother. When maternal intake is reduced to a point at which maternal fat stores are utilized to provide energy, ketosis and acetonuria may result. (3) Maternal acetonuria has been associated with fetal neuropsychological deficits. (4) Adequate maternal weight gain is important and has been positively correlated to the infant's birth weight, an index of the quality of fetal development. (5–8) Because of these factors, weight reduction should be accomplished between, not during, pregnancies.

An average weight gain of 22.0–27.5 lb (10.0–12.5 kg) is currently recommended. No single figure for weight change can be considered normal, with the implication that different figures are abnormal. (3, 10, 11) A wide range is compatible with clinical normality and normal outcome. (11) Weight gain is often minimal during the first three months, with steady, progressive, and linear gains averaging 0.75–1.0 lb (0.35–0.40 kg) per week during the remainder of pregnancy (Figure 46-1). (3, 10, 11)

Routine restriction of dietary sodium is not advised. When indicated by a medical condition, intake should ordinarily not be restricted below 2000 mg (87 mEq) sodium per day to meet the physiologic needs for pregnancy. (12, 13) Use of iodized salt is recommended. (2)

Alcohol intake during pregnancy has been correlated with the incidence of birth defects. (14) A risk to the fetus exists when a pregnant woman consumes alcohol. (15)

A number of medical, social, economic, environmental, and other risk factors influence nutritional needs during pregnancy and must be considered in nutritional management.

GUIDELINES FOR NUTRITIONAL MANAGEMENT OF "NORMAL" PREGNANCY

Nutrient requirements of pregnant women vary greatly because of differences in body size, age, activity, and nutritional status at the onset of pregnancy. The diet for pregnancy is based on the general diet for healthy adults (Chapter 8) and should include foods from the four food groups in the minimum amounts listed in Table 46-1. These foods may be consumed in greater amounts or other foods added to supply sufficient calories to meet individual needs.

GUIDELINES FOR NUTRITIONAL MANAGEMENT OF THE "AT-RISK" PREGNANCY

Nutritional management of any "at-risk" patient should take into account both the nutritional factors of pregnancy and the additional factors related to the patient's specific at-risk condition. Guidelines for commonly encountered conditions are as follows:

Adolescence. During adolescent pregnancy, nutritional needs of pregnancy are superimposed on the nutritional needs associated with uncompleted physical growth and maturation. It is suggested that the total daily protein intake be 1.5 g/kg body weight for the adolescent aged 15 to 18 years, and 1.7 g/kg for younger girls. (1, 2, 10) Adequate caloric intake is essential for optimal protein utilization. Total caloric needs may be as high as 3500 kcal/day for the young pregnant adolescent.

Diabetes mellitus. General guidelines for the nutritional management of pregnant women with diabetes are as follows (16):

1. *Noninsulin-Dependent Diabetes Mellitus.* Women not requiring exogenous insulin are counseled to eliminate concentrated sweets, eat at least four evenly spaced meals daily, and distribute carbohydrate intake throughout the day. Total intake should support normal weight gain. A rigid diet pattern (food intake plan) is usually not necessary.
2. *Insulin-Dependent Diabetes Mellitus.* A diet pattern is constructed that is individualized to the patient's life-style, insulin action, activity, and nutrient needs. Three meals and a minimum of two snacks are generally necessary to prevent ketosis resulting from hypoglycemia. Energy intake for pregnancy is recommended as a minimum of 36 kcal/kg of body weight (2) with adjustments made for age, activity, weight, gestational period, and loss of glucose calories through the urine. The diet should supply sufficient calories to permit normal weight gain throughout the gestational period. The approximate proportion of caloric intake from carbohydrate, protein, and fat should be 50%, 20%, and 30%, respectively. The diet pattern should be evaluated and revised throughout the gestational period. Rising energy and nutrient needs are usually best met by gradual dietary increases over time.

Anemias. Iron deficiency anemia and folic acid deficiency anemia may occur because of increased requirements and defects in absorption and/or utilization. (10) These individuals generally require additional supplementation of iron and folate.

Women with sickle cell anemia appear to have higher folate requirements than do normal pregnant women; supplementation with 1 mg folic acid daily is recommended. Storage iron in these women is usually adequate or even increased, and routine iron supplementation may not be indicated.

Cardiac disease and hypertensive disorders. Moderate sodium restriction (2–4 g) may be indicated with careful medical monitoring.

Obesity. Restriction of weight gain in the obese pregnant woman should not be practiced. Regardless of the patient's pre-pregnancy weight, a nutritionally adequate intake should be encouraged to prevent ketosis and support normal weight gain.

NUTRIENT ADEQUACY

Provided that individual caloric requirements are met to promote adequate weight gain, a general diet with emphasis on dairy products can be expected to meet the recommended dietary allowances for all nutrients except iron and folic acid. Most women are unable to meet the increased requirement for iron by diet and iron stores. A daily supplement of 30–60 mg ferrous iron throughout pregnancy is recommended. (1, 2, 10) Dietary levels of folate may not be adequate to meet pregnancy needs. Routine supplementation of 0.4 mg/day of folate is recommended. (1, 2, 10) Most vitamins and minerals are required in increased amounts during pregnancy. However, the necessity of routine supplements other than iron and folate is controversial. (1)

TABLES AND FIGURES

TABLE 46-1. Recommended Minimum Daily Intake from the Four Basic Food Groups for Women During Pregnancy

Food Group	Minimum Daily Amount
Milk and calcium equivalents	4 cups milk or equivalent[1]
Meat and protein equivalents	6 to 8 ounces meat or equivalent[1]
Fruit and vegetable	4 servings, including a dark green or dark yellow vegetable daily and a citrus fruit or juice daily
Grain	4 servings of whole grain or enriched breads and cereals
Fluid	6 to 8 cups

[1] Refer to Chapters 8 and 9 for listings of calcium and protein equivalents.

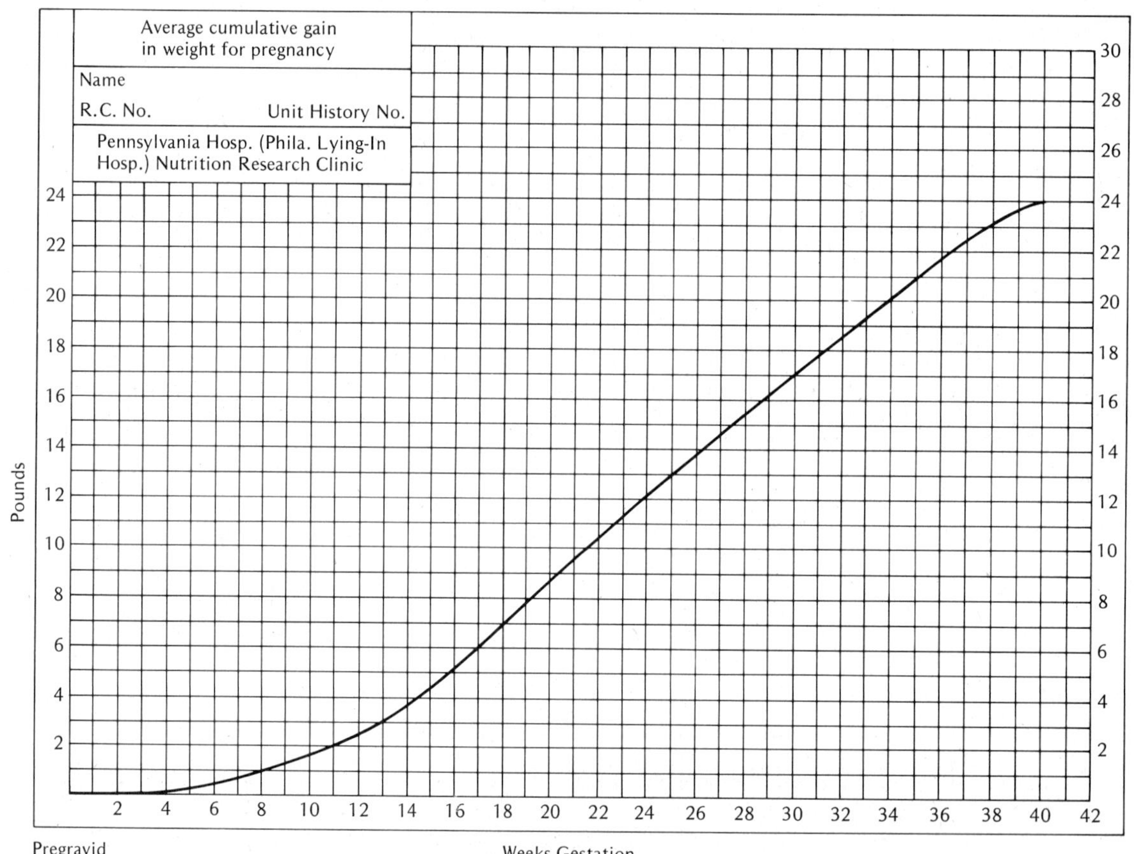

FIGURE 46-1. *Average cumulative gain in weight for pregnancy.*[1]

[1] Tompkins, W. 1953. Nutrition and nutritional deficiencies in pregnancy. *Clinical obstetrics*, eds., C. B. Lull and R. A. Kimbrough, p. 213. Philadelphia: J. B. Lippincott.

REFERENCES CITED

1. Pitkin, R. M.; Chesley, L. C.; Chez, R. A.; Kaminetzky, H. A.; Newton, M.; and Pritchard, J. A. 1974. *Nutrition in maternal health care.* Chicago: American College of Obstetrics and Gynecology.
2. Food and Nutrition Board. 1980. *Recommended dietary allowances.* 9th rev. ed. Washington, D.C.: National Academy of Sciences.
3. Pitkin, R. M.; Kaminetzky, H. A.; Newton, M.; and Pritchard, J. A. 1972. Maternal nutrition: A selective review of clinical topics. *Obstet. Gynecol.* 40:773.
4. Churchill, J. A.; Berendes, H. W.; and Nemore, J. 1969. Neuropsychological deficits in children of diabetic mothers. *Am. J. Obstet. Gynecol.* 105:257.
5. Jacobson, H. N. 1972. Nutrition and pregnancy. *J. Am. Dietet. A.* 60:26.
6. Jacobson, H. N. 1975. Weight and weight gain in pregnancy. *Clin. Perinatol.* 2:233.
7. Eastman, N. J., and Jackson, E. 1968. Weight relationships in pregnancy: The bearing of maternal weight gain and pre-pregnancy weight on birth weight in full term pregnancies. *Obstet. Gynecol. Surv.* 23:1003.
8. Simpson, J. W.; Lawless, R. W.; and Mitchell, A. C. 1975. Responsibility of the obstetrician to the fetus. II. Influence of prepregnancy weight and pregnancy weight gain on birth weight. *Obstet. Gynecol.* 45:481.
9. Niswander, K., and Jackson, E. C. 1974. Physical characteristics of the gravida and their association with birth weight and perinatal death. *Am. J. Obstet. Gynecol.* 119:306.
10. Food and Nutrition Board. 1970. *Maternal nutrition and the course of pregnancy.* Washington, D.C.: National Academy of Sciences.
11. Hytten, F. E., and Leitch, I. 1971. *The physiology of human pregnancy.* Oxford: Blackwell Scientific.
12. Pike, R. L., and Gursky, D. S. 1970. Further evidence of deleterious effects produced by sodium restriction during pregnancy. *Am. J. Clin. Nutr.* 23:883.
13. Lindheimer, M. D., and Katz, A. I. 1973. Sodium and diuretics in pregnancy. *N. Eng. J. Med.* 288:891.
14. Luke, B. 1979. *Maternal nutrition.* Boston: Little, Brown.
15. Witti, F. P. 1978. Alcohol and birth defects. In *FDA consumer.* DHEW Pub. No. (FDA) 78–1047.
16. Jouganatos, D. M., and Gabbe, S. G. 1978. Diabetes in pregnancy: Metabolic changes and current management. *J. Am. Dietet. A.* 73:168.

OTHER REFERENCES

Michigan State Medical Society, Michigan Dietetic Association, and Michigan Department of Public Health. 1979. *Suggested guidelines and standards for maternal and perinatal nutritional care.* Lansing: Michigan Department of Public Health, H-804.

Shank, R. E. 1970. A chink in our armor. *Nutr. Today* 5:2.

White, P. 1974. Diabetes mellitus in pregnancy. *Clin. Perinatol.* 1:331.

RECOMMENDED REFERENCES FOR THE LAY PUBLIC

Michigan Department of Public Health. 1979. *Food while you're pregnant.* Pamphlet H-731. Lansing: Michigan Department of Public Health.

National Foundation, March of Dimes. *Nutrition and pregnancy.* Pamphlet 9-0028. White Plains, N.Y.: National Foundation March of Dimes.

47 Lactation

INDICATIONS FOR USE

This diet is indicated throughout lactation.

DESCRIPTION

The lactating woman has increased requirements for calories, protein, vitamins, and minerals. Nutrient requirements during lactation are proportional to the quantity of milk produced and vary widely from one woman to another.

Approximately 90 kcal are required to produce 100 ml of human milk. Because average daily milk yield is estimated to be 850–1200 ml, daily energy requirements during lactation average 1000 kcal above the normal requirement. Women achieving a 22–27 lb (10–12 kg) weight gain during pregnancy will have stored 4.5–9.0 lb (2–4 kg) body fat that may be drawn upon to supply part of energy needs. (1)

During the first three months of lactation, it is recommended that daily intake be increased by 20 g protein and 500 kcal above normal requirements. (2) Additional calories will be required if lactation continues, maternal weight falls below ideal weight for height, or more than one infant is being nursed.

Environmental pollutants may enter breast milk and must be considered. For example, since 1973, Michigan residents have been exposed to polychlorinated biphenyls (PCB) and polybrominated biphenyls (PBB). Both pollutants are excreted in the breast milk of exposed mothers. However, the Michigan Department of Public Health does not recommend that women exposed to moderate levels of these chemicals make changes in nursing practices. (3)

GUIDELINES FOR NUTRITIONAL MANAGEMENT

The diet during lactation is based on the general diet for healthy adults (Chapter 8) and should include choices from the four food groups in the minimum amounts listed in Table 47-1. These foods may be taken in greater amounts or other food added to supply sufficient calories to meet individual needs.

Many food metabolites are excreted in breast milk and may cause gastrointestinal distress in the baby. Onions, garlic, spicy foods, chocolate, and cola should generally be consumed in moderation. Food metabolites usually appear in breast milk within four to six hours following ingestion. Alcoholic beverages may be permitted in moderate amounts. (4)

NUTRIENT ADEQUACY

Provided that individual caloric requirements are met, a general diet with emphasis on dairy products can meet nutrient needs for all essential nutrients except iron. Supplemental iron may be recommended.

Women who strictly exclude animal products from their diets should receive vitamin B_{12} supplementation. Infants exclusively breast fed by these vegetarian-diet mothers have been shown to exhibit striking dysfunction of the hematopoietic and central nervous systems unless the mother and/or child receives vitamin B_{12} supplementation. (5)

TABLES

TABLE 47-1. Recommended Minimum Daily Intake from the Four Food Groups for Lactating Women

Food Group	Minimum Daily Amount
Milk and calcium equivalents	4 cups milk or equivalent[1]
Meat and protein equivalents	6 to 8 ounces meat or equivalent[1]
Fruit and vegetable	4 servings, including a dark green or dark yellow vegetable daily and a citrus fruit or juice daily
Grain	4 servings of whole grain or enriched breads and cereals
Fluid	6 to 8 cups

[1] Refer to Chapters 8 and 9 for listings of calcium and protein equivalents.

REFERENCES CITED

1. Thomson, A. M.; Hytten, F. E.; and Billewicz, W. Z. 1970. The energy cost of human lactation. *Br. J. Nutr.* 24:565.
2. Food and Nutrition Board. 1980. *Recommended dietary allowances.* 9th rev. ed. Washington, D.C.: National Academy of Sciences.
3. Division of Environmental Epidemiology. 1979. *Breast feeding and PBB.* Pub. No. EE-Pl 30M 3/79. Lansing: Michigan Department of Public Health.
4. Smith, G. V.; Calvert, L. J.; and Kanto, W. P. 1978. Breast feeding and infant nutrition. *Am. Family Phys.* 17(4):92.
5. Higginbottom, M. C.; Sweetman, L.; and Nyhan, W. L. 1978. A syndrome of methylmalonic aciduria, homocystinuria, megaloblastic anemia, and neurologic abnormalities in a vitamin B_{12} deficient breast-fed infant of a strict vegetarian. *N. Engl. J. Med.* 299:317.

OTHER REFERENCES

Jelliffe, D. B., and Jelliffe, E. F. P. 1977. *Human milk in the modern world.* London: Oxford University Press.

Luke, B. 1979. *Maternal nutrition.* Boston: Little, Brown.

Nichols, M. G. 1978. Effective help for the nursing mother. J.O.G.N. 7(2):22.

Waletzky, L. R., ed. 1979. *Symposium on human lactation.* DHEW Pub. No. (HSA) 79-5107. Washington, D.C.: GPO.

RECOMMENDED REFERENCES FOR THE LAY PUBLIC

Eiger, M. S., and Olds, S. W. 1972. *The complete book of breastfeeding.* New York: Workman.

Pryor, K. 1973. *Nursing your baby.* New York: Pocket Books.

La Leche League. 1958. *The womanly art of breastfeeding.* Franklin Park, Ill.: La Leche League International, Inc.

PART XII
Infants and Children

48

Premature or Low-Birth-Weight Infants

INDICATIONS FOR USE

This diet is indicated for premature or low-birth-weight infants weighing less than 5.5 lb (2500 g) at birth.

DESCRIPTION

The goal for feeding low-birth-weight infants is a prompt postnatal resumption of growth to a rate approximating intrauterine growth. (1) This goal is rarely achieved, and failure to achieve such a rate of growth may not be deleterious to the infant. (2) In providing the special nutrient requirements of the low-birth-weight infant, care must be taken to avoid stress on the developing metabolic and excretory systems. (1) The very-low-birth-weight infants (less than 1250 g) often have special needs requiring adjustments in management. At University Hospital, refer to the *Holden House Staff Handbook* for further details. (3)

Nutritional management of the infant weighing less than 2500 g and more than 1250 g includes consideration of the following:

Calories. The basal metabolic rate of low-birth-weight infants is lower than that of full-term infants during the first week of life but reaches and exceeds that of full-term infants by the second week of life. There are considerable variations in caloric requirements depending on both physiological and environmental factors. However, caloric intakes of 110–150 kcal per kilogram body weight per day generally enable the low-birth-weight infant to achieve a satisfactory rate of growth. (1)

Protein. The essential amino acid requirements of the premature infant are greater in terms of body weight than at any other period in life and include the requirement for tyrosine and cystine, which are not required by the mature individual. (4)

The optimal protein intake for the low-birth-weight infant has not been precisely defined. The acceptable range is 2.25–5.00 g protein per kilogram body weight per day for cow's milk formulas. (1) Levels higher than 5 g protein per kilogram body weight per day have been associated with fever and lethargy (5) and increased blood urea nitrogen levels. (6–8) At University Hospital, formula protein levels do not exceed 3.5 g per kilogram body weight per day.

Although human milk has been considered inadequate in protein for preterm infants (9), recent research indicates that low-birth-weight infants receiving pooled human milk grow as well as infants receiving various formulas. (10) Other research has demonstrated that milk of mothers of pre-term infants averages approximately 20% more nitrogen than milk of mothers of full-term infants, providing the small premature infant with higher amounts of protein and other nitrogen-containing components utilizable for synthesis of body protein. (11, 12) Human milk also has an amino acid composition especially suited to the requirements of the pre-term infant. (13) Refer to Table 48-1 for nutrient composition of human milk, commercial infant formulas, and cow's milk and to Table 48-2 for nutrient content of special infant formulas.

Fat. The percentage of fat recommended is 40–50% of total calories. (1) Formulas of lower-fat content are not recommended as they may contain higher levels of protein that increase renal solute load. (1)

The normal infant's essential fatty acid requirement can be met by a feeding that supplies 300 mg of linoleic acid per 100 kcal (approximately 2.7% of total calories). (14) Human milk and commercial infant formulas both supply a generous allowance of linoleic acid. (1, 14)

Low-birth-weight infants have difficulty absorbing saturated fats such as butterfat. (15–18) Vegetable oils and human milk fat are absorbed well. (15, 16) Medium-chain triglycerides included as a fat source in the formula or with breast milk have been shown to improve fat absorption (19–22), increase weight gain (22), and enhance calcium absorption (21) and nitrogen retention. (20)

Carbohydrates. Most low-birth-weight infants can adequately digest disaccharides. (1) A slight delay of maturation of intestinal lactase may be of consequence in some low-birth-weight infants. (23)

Fluid. Increased caloric density of formula and limited capability of concentrating urine requires that special care be taken to meet minimum fluid requirements in low-birth-weight infants.

Iron. A low-birth-weight infant will have adequate iron stores for approximately two months postpartum. (24) It is not advisable to begin iron-fortified formula until the infant reaches 4.4 lb (2000 g) or two months of age, since iron oxidizes polyunsaturated fats and is thought to interfere with vitamin E absorption. (3)

Vitamin E. On admission, 75 mg vitamin E is given intramuscular to low-birth-weight infants of less than 3.8 lb (1750 g), since vitamin E stores in all infants are low and vitamin E is malabsorbed by pre-term infants. (3) The use of formulas high in polyunsaturated fat also increases the requirement for vitamin E. (1) If the infant is not receiving nutrition orally or by tube, the injection of vitamin E should be repeated weekly. When oral or tube feedings are being used, a daily oral dose of 25 IU vitamin E is recommended. (3) Daily vitamin E supplementation can be discontinued when the infant is feeding well and weight approaches 4.4 lb (2000 g). (3) An iron-containing formula may be used when vitamin E supplementation is discontinued. (3)

Other vitamins and minerals. Except for vitamin E, the minimum levels of vitamins recommended for infant formulas is probably adequate for the low-birth-weight infant. (1) However, the low-birth-weight infant may have low tissue stores and decreased absorption and may not be consuming sufficient formula in the early weeks to prevent a vitamin deficiency. (1) Therefore, an intramuscular injection of 0.5–1.0 mg vitamin K at birth and a daily oral multivitamin is recommended. (1, 3)

Some mineral requirements including those for calcium, sodium, and copper may be greater per 100 kcal for the low-birth-weight infant than for the full-term infant. (1)

GUIDELINES FOR NUTRITIONAL MANAGEMENT

Initial Feeding

Sterile water is generally recommended for the first feeding unless an oral–duodenal or oral–jejunal tube is in place, in which case formula may be given. (3) Expressed breast milk is also satisfactory for the first feeding. (3) Suggested initial feeding is 3–5 ml/kg. (3)

Subsequent Feedings

Human milk or commercial infant formula may be used for subsequent feedings. Refer to Table 48-1 for nutrient composition of human milk and to Table 48-2 for nutrient composition of special infant formulas.

Human milk. Advantages of using human milk include immunologic protection provided via secretory IgA, lactoferrin, lysozyme, and white plasma cells (25–27), decreased incidence of necrotizing enterocolitis due to passive transfer of milk phagocytes (28, 29), and an amino acid composition especially suited to the pre-term infant. (13) Infants fed with human milk should remain on multivitamins with iron as long as they are exclusively fed with breast milk. Supplementation with sodium may also be necessary. (1) When the infant is feeding well, MCT oil may be added to expressed breast milk at the rate of 0.5 ml MCT oil to 30 ml breast milk to increase calorie content to approximately 24 kcal/ounce. (3)

Infant formula. Special commercial infant formulas have been devel oped to help meet the needs of low-birth-weight and premature infants. The formulas may contain 24 kcal or more per ounce. Generally an infant can be switched to a 20 kcal/ounce formula if feeding well and weight is at least 4 lb (1800 g). All pre-term infants should remain on supplemental multivitamins until they are taking more than one l of formula per day.

Total Parenteral Nutrition

Total parenteral nutrition is indicated in infants unable or unlikely to tolerate adequate nutrition via the gastrointestinal tract before seven days of age. (3) Peripheral total parenteral nutrition is preferred. Constant monitoring of state of hydration and glucose status is necessary. (30) Interruption of infusion for greater than one-half hour is avoided because of the potential for reactive hypoglycemia. (3) Generally total parenteral nutrition is used only for short periods of time. At University Hospital, refer to the *Parenteral and Enteral Nutrition Manual* and the *Holden House Staff Handbook*.

NUTRIENT ADEQUACY

Nutrient adequacy of the diet is evaluated by ongoing assessment of the infant's rate of growth and development and presence of any signs of nutrient deficiencies.

TABLES

TABLE 48-1. Nutrient Composition of Human Milk, Commercial Infant Formulas, and Cow's Milk (per 30 ml)

Product (Manufacturer)	Indications	kcal	Protein (g)	Fat (g)	Carbohydrate (g)	Sodium (mg)	Potassium (mg)	Osmolality (mOsm/kg)
Human milk[1]	Routine	21	0.3	1.4	2.1	5.0	16.0	300
Enfamil, plain or with iron (Mead Johnson)	Routine	20	0.5	1.1	2.1	8.3	20.6	290
Similac, plain or with iron (Ross)	Routine	20	0.5	1.1	2.1	7.5	23.4	290
SMA (Wyeth)	Routine	20	0.5	1.1	2.2	4.5	16.8	300
Enfamil 24, with iron (Mead Johnson)	Increased calories	24	0.6	1.3	2.5	8.3	20.6	355
Similac 24, plain or with iron (Ross)	Increased calories	24	0.6	1.3	2.6	9.8	32.0	360
Evaporated whole milk formula	Routine when prepared formula unavailable	20	0.8	0.9	2.4	12.0	35.0	346
Cow's milk								
Whole	Not recommended for infants under 6 months of age	19	1.0	1.0	1.4	15.0	46.0	288
2%	Not recommended for children under 2 years of age	15	1.0	0.6	1.5	15.0	47.0	270
Skim	Not recommended for children under 2 years of age	11	1.0	—	1.5	16.0	51.0	270
Goat's milk		21	1.1	1.3	1.4	15.2	62.3	NA

[1] Composition varies with number of days postpartum, time of day, and duration of feeding.
[2] Protein includes casein, lactalbumin, and lactoglobulin.
[3] Powdered formula contains corn oil in place of soy oil.

Food Sources				
Protein	Fat	Carbohydrate	Other	Product (Manufacturer)
Human milk protein and 15% nonprotein nitrogen	50% saturated; 50% unsaturated	Lactose	Easily digested; protein forms soft curd in stomach; immunologic protection; infant controls intake; supplementation of fluoride, vitamin D recommended; iron supplementation optional	Human milk[1]
Nonfat cow's milk[2]	80% soy oil; 20% coconut oil	Lactose	Supplementation of iron recommended if plain formula used	Enfamil, plain or with iron (Mead Johnson)
Nonfat cow's milk[2]	60% coconut oil; 40% soy oil[3]	Lactose	Supplementation of iron recommended if plain formula used	Similac, plain or with iron (Ross)
Nonfat cow's milk[2]; demineralized whey	Safflower oil; coconut oil; soy oil	Lactose	Casein-to-lactalbumin ratio of 40:60	SMA (Wyeth)
Nonfat cow's milk[2]	80% soy oil; 20% coconut oil	Lactose		Enfamil 24, with iron (Mead Johnson)
Nonfat cow's milk[2]	60% coconut oil; 40% soy oil	Lactose	Supplementation of iron recommended if plain formula used	Similac 24, plain or with iron (Ross)
Cow's milk[2]	Butterfat	Lactose; corn syrup	Supplementation of iron and vitamin C required; less expensive than prepared formulas; parents will need instruction on preparation	Evaporated whole milk formula
				Cow's milk
Cow's milk[2]	Butterfat	Lactose	Protein forms hard curd in stomach; excessive protein content	Whole
Cow's milk[2]	Butterfat	Lactose	Inadequate caloric density may promote ingestion of large volume and formation of "full stomach" as signal of satiety	2%
Cow's milk[2]	Butterfat	Lactose	Inadequate caloric density as 2% milk; inadequate essential fatty acids	Skim
Goat's milk[2]	Higher percentage polyunsaturated and medium- and short-chain fatty acids than cow's milk	Lactose	Supplementation of 50 μg/day folacin required and iron, vitamin C and vitamin D supplements recommended if other food sources are not included in the diet	Goat's milk

TABLE 48-2. Nutrient Composition of Special Infant Formulas (per 30 ml)

Type	Product (Manufacturer)	Indications	kcal	Protein (g)	Fat (g)	Carbo-hydrate (g)	Sodium (mg)	Potas-sium (mg)	Osmol-ality (mOsm/kg)	Phenyl-alanine (mg)
Premature and Low Birth Weight	Enfamil Premature (Mead Johnson)	Low birth weight	24	0.7	1.2	2.7	9.4	33.0	407	32
	Similac 24 LBW (Ross)	Low birth weight	24	0.6	1.3	2.5	11.0	30.0	290	NA
	Similac PM 60/40 (Ross)	Need for low renal solute load or susceptibility to hypercalcemia	20	0.5	1.1	2.0	4.6	17.2	260	NA
Milk, Carbohydrate, or Protein Intolerance or Malabsorption	Isomil (Ross)	Intolerance to lactose, galactose, or milk protein	20	0.6	1.1	2.0	8.7	21.1	250	NA
	Prosobee (Mead Johnson)	Intolerance to lactose, galactose, sucrose, or milk protein	20	0.4	0.7	1.4	8.6	20.4	160	28
	Nutramigen (Mead Johnson)	Sensitivity to milk protein and lactose, or gastrointestinal disturbances; test or elimination diets	20	0.7	0.8	2.6	9.4	20.4	443	34
	CHO Free (Syntex)	Intolerance to certain carbohydrates	20	0.5	1.0	1.9	10.9	27.2	480/270[a]	31
	Meat-Base Formula (Gerber)	Galactosemia; milk allergy or glycogen storage disease	23	0.5	1.0	1.9	5.4	11.7	182	41
Fat Malabsorption	Pregestimil (Mead Johnson)	Disaccharidase deficiency; chronic diarrhea; detects indigestion or absorption	20	0.6	0.8	2.7	9.4	21.9	338	26
	Portagen (Mead Johnson)	Fat malabsorption (biliary obstruction, intestinal resection, lymphangiatasia)	20	0.7	1.0	2.3	9.4	25.0	236	32
Amino Acid Disorders	Lofenalac (Mead Johnson)	Phenylketonuria	20	0.7	0.8	2.6	9.4	20.2	454	4
	Phenyl Free (Mead Johnson)	Phenylketonurics who are also eating solid foods	25	1.2	0.4	4.1	15.6	43.7	NA	0

Food Sources			Nutrient Adequacy (per 960 ml)[1]	Other	Product (Manufacturer)
Protein	Fat	Carbohydrate			
Concentrated sweetened skim milk	MCT oil; corn oil; coconut oil	50% lactose; 50% sucrose	Inadequate	Does not meet RDAs for iron as iron would interfere with vitamin E absorption	Enfamil Premature (Mead Johnson)
Nonfat cow's milk[2]	50% MCT oil; 30% coconut oil; 20% soy oil	50% lactose; 50% glucose polymers	Inadequate	Does not meet RDAs for iron as iron would interfere with vitamin E absorption	Similac 24 LBW (Ross)
Purified casein salts; electrodialyzed whey	60% corn oil; 40% coconut oil	lactose	Inadequate	Does not meet RDAs for phosphorous or iron; calcium-to-phosphorous ratio, 2:1; not indicated for periods of rapid growth	Similac PM 60/40 (Ross)
Soy protein isolate	60% coconut oil; 40% soy oil	50% corn syrup; 50% sucrose	Adequate		Isomil (Ross)
Soy protein isolate supplemented with L-methionine	80% soy oil; 20% coconut oil	100% corn syrup solids (glucose polymers)	Adequate		Prosobee (Mead Johnson)
Hydrolyzed casein	Corn oil	70% sucrose; 30% modified tapioca starch	Adequate		Nutramigen (Mead Johnson)
Soy protein isolate	Soy oil	Dependent upon sugar/starch added	Inadequate	Dilute as directed; does not meet RDAs for iron	CHO Free (Syntex)
Beef	Tallow; sesame oil	Cane sugar; modified tapioca starch	Inadequate	Does not meet RDAs for folacin or iodine	Meat-Base Formula (Gerber)
Hydrolyzed casein	40% MCT oil; 60% corn oil	80% corn syrup solids (glucose polymers); 20% modified tapioca starch	Adequate	————	Pregestimil (Mead Johnson)
Hydrolyzed casein	87% MCT oil; 11% corn oil	75% corn syrup solids (glucose polymers); 25% sucrose; trace lactose	Adequate	Values are for powder prepared as directed	Portagen (Mead Johnson)
Hydrolyzed casein	Corn oil	83% corn syrup solids; (glucose polymers)	Adequate[5]	Casein is processed to remove most of the phenylalanine	Lofenalac (Mead Johnson)
Hydrolyzed casein	Corn oil	Corn syrup solids (glucose polymers); modified tapioca starch	Adequate[5]	An additional source of phenylalanine must be added	Phenyl Free (Mead Johnson)

(Continued)

TABLE 48-2. Nutrient Composition of Special Infant Formulas (per 30 ml) [*Concluded*]

Type	Product (Manufacturer)	Indications	kcal	Protein (g)	Fat (g)	Carbohydrate (g)	Sodium (mg)	Potassium (mg)	Osmolality (mOsm/kg)	Phenyalanin (mg)
	MSUD Powder (Mead Johnson)	Maple syrup urine disease	20	0.3	0.9	2.6	9.4	14.1	Varies with dilution	23
	Product 80056 (Mead Johnson)	Specific mixtures of amino acids required	4.5	—	0.2	0.7	0.7	1.1	Varies with dilution	0
Electrolyte Imbalances	Pedialyte (Ross)	Supplies fluid and electrolytes during diarrhea or in post-op states	6.0	—	—	1.5	20.7	17.5	290	—
	Lytren (Mead Johnson)	Supplies fluid and electrolytes during diarrhea or in post-op states	9.0	—	—	2.3	17.3	29.3	290	—

[1] Based on RDAs, 1980, for vitamin and minerals for 0–6 month infant.
[2] Protein includes casein, lactalbumin, and lactoglobulin.
[3] With monosaccharides added as directed.
[4] With disaccharides added as directed.
[5] Except for phenylalanine.
[6] Except for branched-chain amino acids.
[7] Except for protein.
NA = not available

Food Sources			Nutrient Adequacy (per 960 ml)[1]	Other	Product (Manufacturer)
Protein	Fat	Carbohydrate			
Free amino acids	Corn oil	Corn syrup solids (glucose polymers); modified tapioca starch	Adequate[6]	Values given for 134.5 g powder + 858 ml water; must supplement with formula or milk to provide adequate branched-chain amino acids	MSUD Powder (Mead Johnson)
Dependent upon amino acids added	Corn oil	Corn syrup solids (glucose polymers); modified tapioca starch	Adequate[7]	Dilute powder as directed	Product 80056 (Mead Johnson)
—	—	Dextrose	Inadequate		Pedialyte (Ross)
—	—	Corn syrup solids; dextrose	Inadequate		Lytren (Mead Johnson)

REFERENCES CITED

1. Committee on Nutrition, American Academy of Pediatrics. 1977. Nutritional needs of low-birth-weight infants. *Pediatrics* 60:519.
2. Heird, W. C. 1977. Feeding the premature infant: Human milk or an artificial formula? *Am. J. Dis. Child.* 131:468.
3. Sharp, M. J.; Donn, S. M.; and Roloff, D. W. 1979. *Holden House staff handbook: A guide to neonatal intensive care.* Ann Arbor: University Hospital, University of Michigan.
4. Snyderman, S. E. 1971. The protein and amino acid requirements of the premature infant. In *Metabolic processes in the foetus and newborn infant,* eds., J. H. P. Jonxis, H. K. A. Visser, and J. A. Troelstra, pp. 128–141. Baltimore, Md.: Williams & Wilkins.
5. Goldman, H. I.; Freudenthal, R.; Holland, B.; and Karelitz, S. 1969. Clinical effects of two different levels of protein intake on low-birth-weight infants. *J. Pediatr.* 74:881.
6. Davidson, M.; Levine, S. Z.; Bauer, C. H.; and Dann, M. 1967. Feeding studies in low-birth-weight infants. I. Relationships of dietary protein, fat, and electrolyte to rates of weight gain, clinical courses, and serum chemical concentrations. *J. Pediatr.* 70:695.
7. Omans, W. B.; Barness, L. A.; Rose, C. S.; and Gyorgy, P. 1961. Prolonged feeding studies in premature infants. *J. Pediatr.* 59:951.
8. Nichols, M. M., and Danford, B. H. 1966. Feeding premature infants: A comparison of effects on weight gain, blood and urine of two formulas with varying protein and ash composition. *South Med. J.* 59:1420.
9. Fomon, S. J.; Ziegler, E. E.; and Vazquez, H. D. 1977. Human milk and the small premature infant. *Am. J. Dis. Child.* 131:463.
10. Raiha, N. C. R.; Heinonen, K.; Rassin, D. K.; and Gaull, G. E. 1976. Milk protein quantity and quality in low-birth-weight infants: I. Metabolic responses and effects on growth. *Pediatrics* 57:659.
11. Atkinson, S. A.; Bryan, M. H.; and Anderson, G. H. 1978. Human milk: Difference in nitrogen concentration in milk from mothers of term and premature infants. *J. Pediatr.* 93:67.
12. Atkinson, S. A.; Anderson, G. H.; and Bryan, M. H. 1980. Human milk: Comparison of the nitrogen composition in milk from mothers of premature and full-term infants. *Am. J. Clin. Nutr.* 33:811.
13. Committee on Nutrition, American Academy of Pediatrics. 1978. Breast-feeding. *Pediatrics* 62:591.
14. Committee on Nutrition, American Academy of Pediatrics. 1976. Commentary on breast-feeding and infant formulas, including proposed standards for formulas. *Pediatrics* 57:278.
15. Tidwell, H. C.; Holt, L. E., Jr.; Farrow, H. L.; and Neale, S. 1935. Studies in fat metabolism. II. Fat absorption in premature infants and twins. *J. Pediatr.* 6:481.
16. Gordon, H. H.; Levine, S. Z.; Wheatley, M. A.; and Marples, E. 1937. Respiratory metabolism in infancy and in childhood. XX. The nitrogen metabolism in premature infants—Comparative studies of human milk and cow's milk. *Am. J. Dis. Child.* 54:1030.
17. Soderhjelm, L. 1952. Fat absorption studies in children. I. Influence of heat treatment of milk on fat retention by premature infants. *Acta Paediatr.* 41:207.
18. Davidson, M., and Bauer, C. H. 1960. Patterns of fat excretion in feces of premature infants fed various preparations of milk. *Pediatrics* 25:375.
19. Tantibhedhyangkul, P., and Hashim, S. A. 1971. Clinical and physiologic aspects of medium-chain triglycerides: Alleviation of steatorrhea in premature infants. *Bull. N.Y. Acad. Med.* 47:17.
20. Tantibhedhyangkul, P., and Hashim, S. A. 1975. Medium-chain triglyceride feeding in premature infants: Effects on fat and nitrogen absorption. *Pediatrics* 55:359.

21. ANDREWS, B. F., and LORCH, V. 1974. Improved fat and calcium absorption in LBW infants fed a medium-chain triglyceride containing formula. *Pediatr. Res.* 8:378.
22. ROY, C. C.; STE-MARIE, M.; CHARTRAND, L.; WEBER, A.; BARD, H.; and DORAY, B. 1975. Correction of the malabsorption of the preterm infant with a medium-chain triglyceride formula. *J. Pediatr.* 86:446.
23. BOELLNER, S. W.; BEARD, A. G.; and PANOS, T. C. 1965. Impairment of intestinal hydrolysis of lactose in newborn infants. *Pediatrics* 36:542.
24. DALLMAN, P. R. 1974. Iron, vitamin E, and folate in the preterm infant. *J. Pediatr.* 85:742.
25. GOLDMAN, A. S., and SMITH, C. W. 1973. Host resistance factors in human milk. *J. Pediatr.* 82:1082.
26. GOTHEFORS, L., and WINBERG, J. 1975. Host resistance factors. *Environ. Child Health* 21:260.
27. Editorial. 1976. Breast feeding: The immunological argument. *Br. Med. J.* 1:1167.
28. PITT, J. 1974. Passive transfer of milk phagocytes—Mechanism of protection in necrotizing enterocolitis. In *Necrotizing enterocolitis in the newborn infant,* ed., T. D. Moore. Columbus, Ohio, Ross Laboratories.
29. BARLOW, B.; SANTULLI, T. V.; HEIRD, W. C.; PITT, J.; BLANC, W. A.; and SCHULLINGER, J. N. 1974. An experimental study of acute neonatal enterocolitis. The importance of breast milk. *J. Pediatr. Surg.* 9:587.
30. DWECK, H. S. 1975. Feeding the prematurely born infant: Fluids, calories, and methods of feeding during the period of extrauterine growth retardation. *Clin. Perinatol.* 2:183.

OTHER REFERENCES

JELLIFFE, D. B., and JELLIFFE, E. F. P. 1977. "Breast is best": Modern meanings. *N. Eng. J. Med.* 297:912.

TOMARELLI, R. M. 1976. Osmolality, osmolarity, and renal solute load of infant formulas. *J. Pediatr.* 88:454.

Infants at Birth to 6 Months

INDICATIONS FOR USE

This diet is indicated for infants at birth to 6 months of age weighing greater than 5.5 lb (2500 g) at birth and requiring no dietary modifications.

DESCRIPTION

The general diet for infants at birth to 6 months is planned to provide the nutrients required for normal growth and maintenance of body tissues. Metabolic requirements of the full-term infant based on the recommended dietary allowances are 115 kcal per kilogram body weight per day and 2.2 g protein per kilogram body weight per day. (1) The energy requirement can vary considerably with age depending on the activity level of the child. (2) Consistent plotting of the infant's height and weight on a growth chart provides the most reliable determination of adequate nutrient intake. Refer to growth charts, Figures 49-1, 49-2, 49-3, and 49-4.

Human milk or infant formula provide the major source of nutrients for infants at birth to 6 months of age. Refer to Table 48-1 for nutrient composition of human milk, commercial infant formulas, and cow's milk.

Human milk. The Committee on Nutrition of the American Academy of Pediatrics and the Nutrition Committee of the Canadian Paediatric Society state that "Full term newborn infants should be breast-fed, except if there are specific contraindications or when breast-feeding is unsuccessful." (3) Human milk has special characteristics that meet the nutritional needs and physiological limitations of the infant. (4) The carbohydrate, protein, lipid, and vitamin and mineral components of human milk are in forms that are well absorbed and utilized and present the kidney with a low renal solute load. (3, 4) Human milk also provides nonnutritive advantages including:

- Immunologic protection via secretory IgA, lactoferrin, lysozyme and white plasma cells (notably macrophages and lymphocytes). (5–7)
- Presence of a growth factor specific for *Lactobacillus bifidus* and maintenance of a pH that promotes the growth of *L. bifidus* as the predominant microflora in the alimentary canal, preventing growth of gram negative anaerobes. (8, 9)
- Decreased risk of morbidity from a variety of illnesses, including both intestinal and respiratory disease, as compared with bottle-fed infants. (10, 11)

Supplementation of breast milk with vitamin D and iron remains a matter of controversy. Breast milk is low in lipid-soluble vitamin D (22 IU/L) (12) however it contains appreciable but variable amounts of water-soluble vitamin D sulfate whose biological activity has not yet been assessed. (13) The dietary requirement for vitamin D is dependent on the infant's exposure to sunlight; with adequate exposure to sunlight, there is no dietary requirement for vitamin D. (12) Supplements of 400 IU/day of vitamin D may be recommended for breast-fed infants. (14)

Conflicting evidence exists for the supplementation with iron of fully breast-fed infants. One study reports that the iron in human milk is sufficient to meet the iron requirements of the exclusively breast-fed, full-term infant until birth weight is tripled. (15) In addition, the low iron content of human milk may be extremely useful in maintaining the bacteriostatic properties of lactoferrin and transferrin. (16, 17) Others suggest that the possible interference with the lactoferrin system is a reasonable risk to take for the sake of ensuring iron nutritional status and therefore recommend supplementation of 7 mg/day of iron for the fully breast-fed infant. (14)

Since human milk contains little fluoride, fluoride supplementation of 0.25 mg daily is advised for infants who are exclusively breast fed. (18)

Infant formulas. Infant formulas are an acceptable substitution for human milk. Commercial infant formulas most closely approximate the nutritional characteristics of human milk, providing nutrients in easily digestible forms and presenting the kidney with a low renal solute load. (4) Iron-fortified commercial infant formulas are complete foods for infants and require no supplementation of vitamins or minerals. (14)

An acceptable infant formula can be made with evaporated whole milk, water, and corn syrup. Supplementation with vitamin C and iron is necessary. (2)

Other foods. Infants at birth to 6 months should not be fed skim milk since it provides neither adequate caloric intake nor essential fatty acid intake. (19) Whole cow's milk and 2% cow's milk are not recommended at this age due to their high protein content and their capacity to form a hard casein curd in the stomach and to increase gastric pH, which reduces pepsin activity. (20)

Introduction of beikost, foods other than human milk, or formulas is not recommended before 4 to 6 months of age. The digestive capacities of the infant less than 4 months of age are specifically well suited to the constituents of human milk. (20) An infant less than 5 months of age may not be physically able to signal satiety to beikost feeding. (14) Introducing solid foods before 4 months of age may interfere with establishment of sound eating habits and contribute to overfeeding. (14) There is no evidence to show that early introduction of beikost aids the infant in sleeping through the night.

GUIDELINES FOR NUTRITIONAL MANAGEMENT

Human milk or infant formula is used for feeding infants. Refer to Table 48-1 for the nutrient composition of human milk, commercial infant formulas, and cow's milk and to Table 49-1 for recommended intakes of human milk, commercial infant formulas, and vitamin–mineral supplements.

Human milk. Breast feeding on demand with supplementation of vitamin D and fluoride is the recommended feeding for infants at birth to 6 months.

Infant formulas. Infant formulas are an acceptable substitute for human milk. Commercial infant formulas, with or without iron fortification, are available in three forms: powdered, liquid concentrate, and ready to feed. Supplementation with vitamins and minerals is not necessary if an iron-fortified commercial formula is used. Provided that iron and vitamin C supplementation is supplied, an acceptable infant formula can be made with evaporated whole milk according to the recipe in Table 49-2. (14)

Other foods. The use of skim milk, 2% milk, whole milk, and beikost is not recommended for infants at birth to 6 months old. Refer to Chapter 50 for guidelines on introduction of cow's milk, goat's milk, and beikost.

NUTRIENT ADEQUACY

Nutritional adequacy of the diet is evaluated by ongoing assessment of the infant's rate of growth (height and weight plotted on a growth chart) and development. Refer to the growth charts for girls, birth to 36 months (Figures 49-1 and 49-2) and the growth charts for boys, birth to 36 months (Figures 49-3 and 49-4).

TABLES AND FIGURES

TABLE 49-1. Recommended Daily Intakes of Human Milk or Infant Formula and Vitamin–Mineral Supplements for the Infant at Birth to 6 Months

Feeding	Recommended Intake	Recommended Supplements			
		Vitamin D	Iron	Fluoride	Vitamin C
Human milk	On demand	Yes[1]	Optional	Yes	No
Commercial infant formula					
With iron	24–32 ounces	No	No	No[2]	No
Without iron	24–32 ounces	No	Yes	No[2]	No
Evaporated whole milk formula	24–32 ounces	No	Yes	No[2]	Yes

[1] Vitamin D supplementation is indicated if there is insufficient exposure to sunlight.
[2] Fluoride supplementation is indicated with infant formulas only if water fluoride content is 0.3 ppm or less. (14)

TABLE 49-2. Recipe: Evaporated Whole Milk Infant Formula

Ingredients	Volume (ml)	Household Measure[1]
Evaporated whole milk	100	3.0 ounces
Water	130	4.5 ounces
Corn syrup	10	2.0 teaspoons

[1] Household measures approximately equal the volume in milliliters.

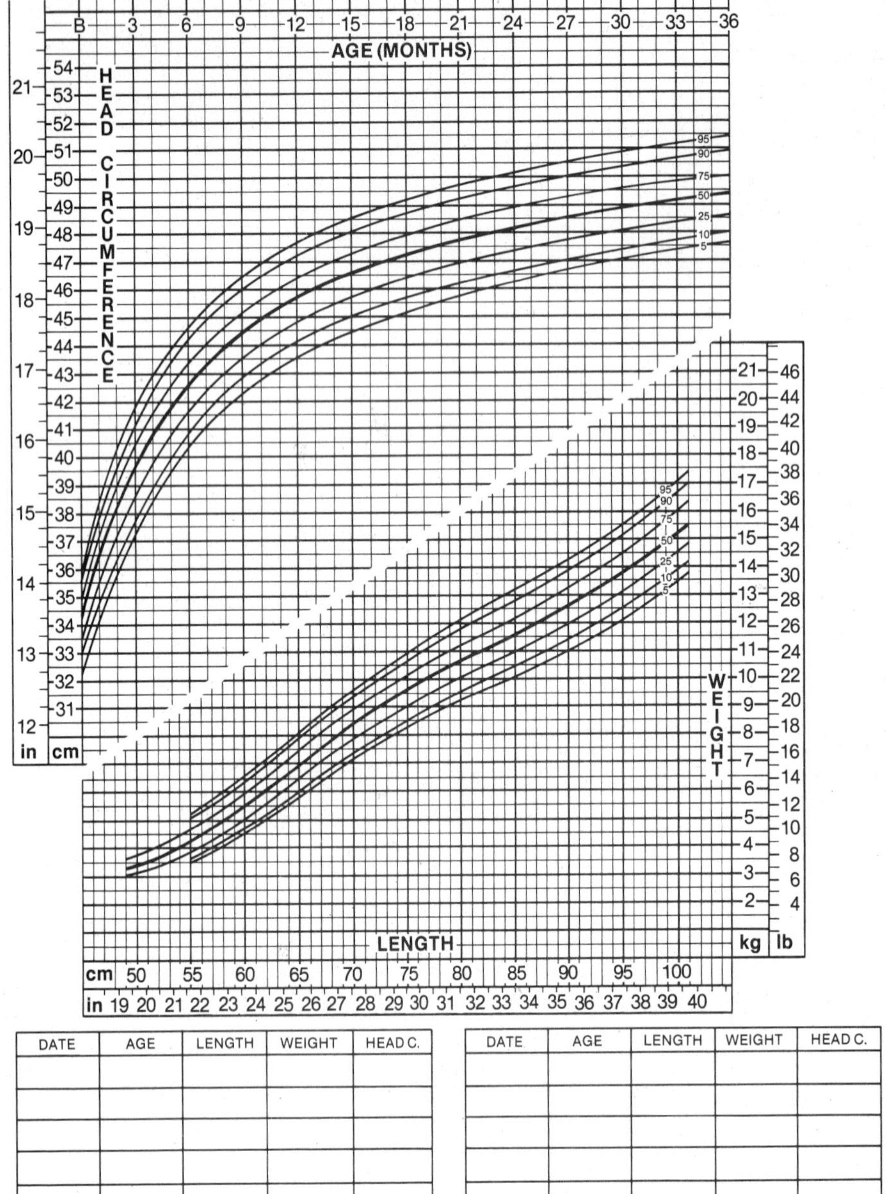

DATE	AGE	LENGTH	WEIGHT	HEAD C.

DATE	AGE	LENGTH	WEIGHT	HEAD C.

FIGURE 49-1 *Girls: Birth to 36 months, physical growth, NCHS percentiles; head circumference, length, and weight.* [Courtesy of Ross Laboratories, Columbus, Ohio.]

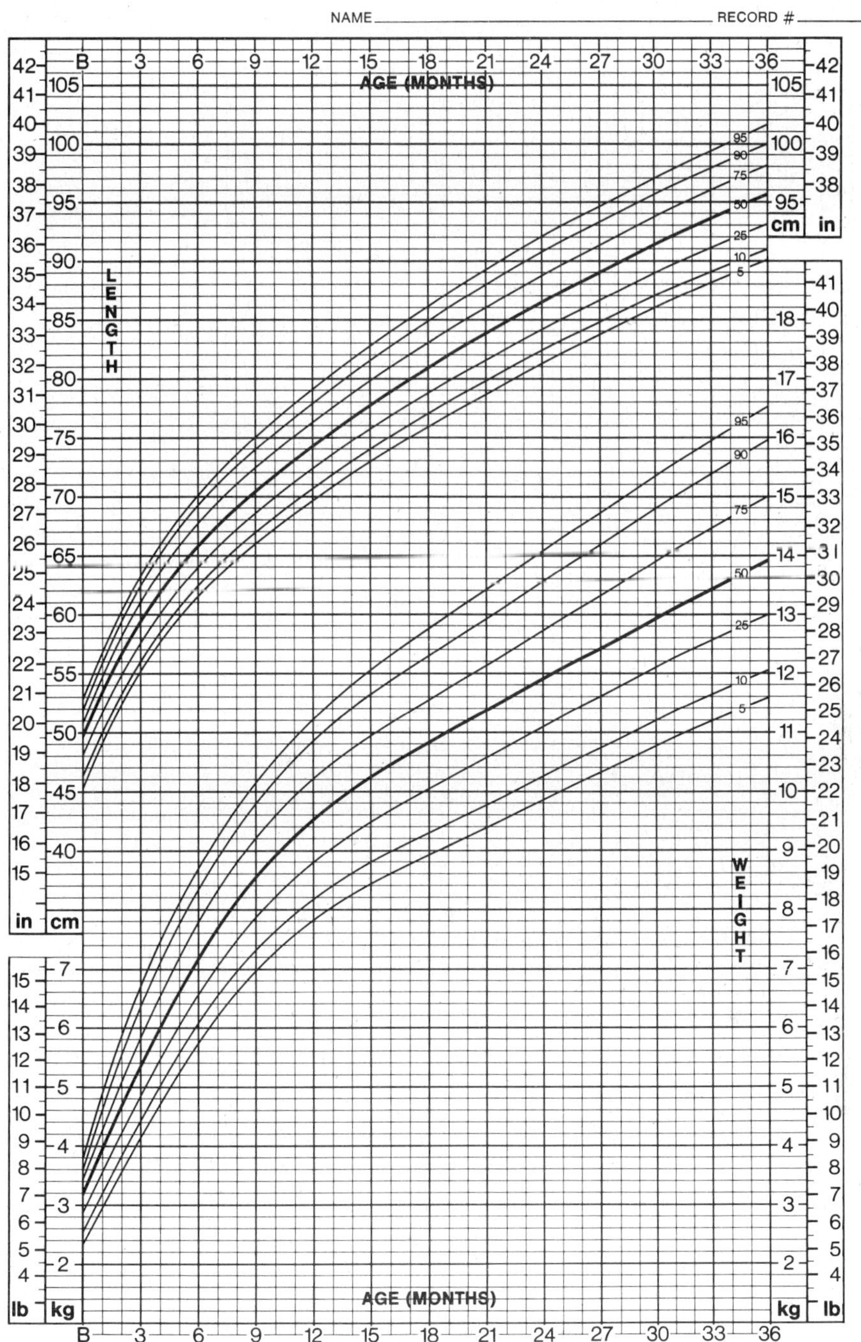

FIGURE 49-2 *Girls: Birth to 36 months, physical growth, NCHS percentiles; age, length, and weight.* [Courtesy of Ross Laboratories, Columbus, Ohio.]

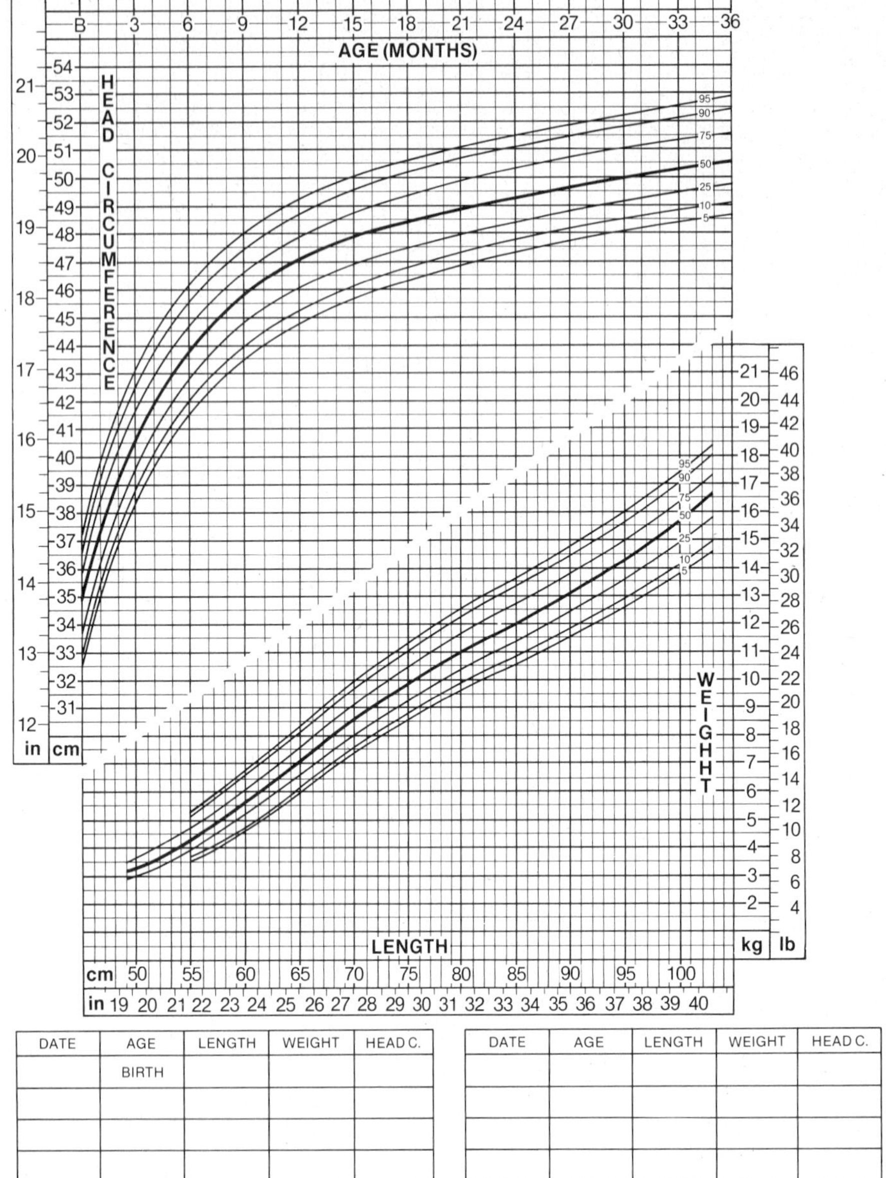

DATE	AGE	LENGTH	WEIGHT	HEAD C.
	BIRTH			

DATE	AGE	LENGTH	WEIGHT	HEAD C.

FIGURE 49-3 *Boys: Birth to 36 months, physical growth, NCHS percentiles; head circumference, length, and weight.* [Courtesy of Ross Laboratories, Columbus, Ohio.]

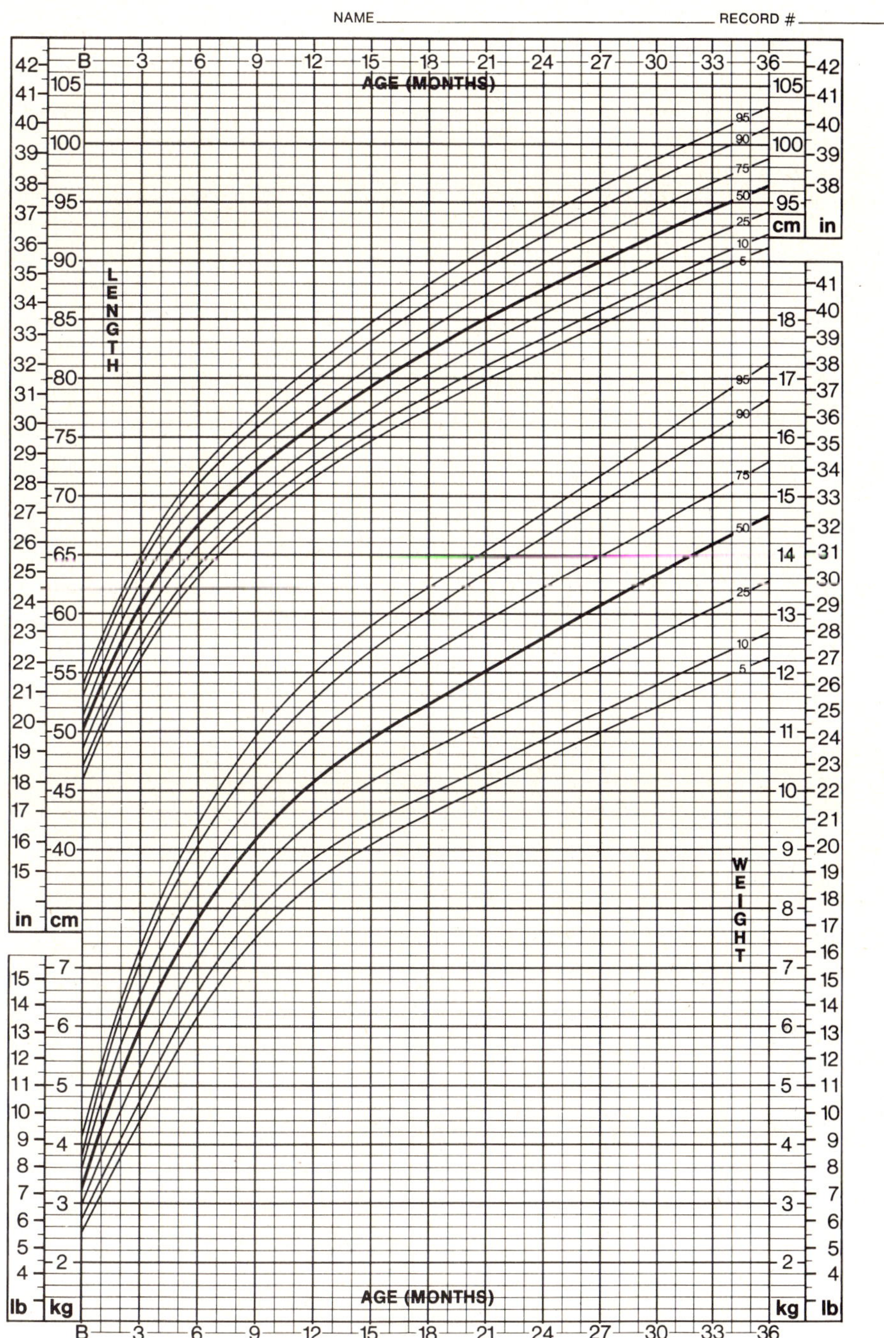

FIGURE 49-1 *Boys: Birth to 36 months, physical growth, NCHS percentiles; age, length, and weight.* [Courtesy of Ross Laboratories, Columbus, Ohio.]

REFERENCES CITED

1. Food and Nutrition Board. 1980. *Recommended dietary allowances.* 9th rev. ed. Washington, D.C.: National Academy of Sciences.
2. Wait, B.; Blair, R.; and Roberts, L. J. 1969. Energy intakes of well-nourished children and adolescents. *Am. J. Clin. Nutr.* 22:1383.
3. Committee on Nutrition, American Academy of Pediatrics; Nutrition Commission, Paediatric Society. 1979. Breast-feeding. *Pediatrics* 62:591.
4. Owen, A. L. 1979. *Feeding guide. A nutritional guide for the maturing infant.* Bloomfield, N.J.: Health Learning Systems.
5. Goldman, A. S., and Smith, C. W. 1973. Host resistance factors in human milk. *J. Pediatr.* 82:1082.
6. Gothefors, L., and Winberg, J. 1975. Host resistance factors. *Environ. Child Health* 21:260.
7. Breast feeding: The immunological argument. *Br. Med. J.* 1:1167.
8. Gothefors, L.; Carlsson, B.; Ahlstedt, S.; Hanson, L. A.; and Winberg, J. 1976. Influence of maternal gut flora and colostral and cord serum antibodies on presence of *Escherichia coli* in faeces of the newborn infant. *Acta Paediatr. Scand.* 65:225.
9. Mata, L. J., and Urrutia, J. J. 1971. Intestinal colonization of breast-fed children in a rural area of low socioeconomic level. *Ann. N.Y. Acad. Sci.* 176:93.
10. Cunningham, A. S. 1977. Morbidity in breast-fed and artificially fed infants. *J. Pediatr.* 90:726.
11. Cunningham, A. S. 1979. Mobidity in breast-fed and artificially fed infants. II. *J. Pediatr.* 95:685.
12. Anderson, T. A., and Fomon, S. J. 1974. Vitamins. In *Infant Nutrition,* ed., S. J. Fomon, p. 216. 2nd ed. Philadelphia: W. B. Saunders.
13. Lakdawala, D. R., and Widdowson, E. M. 1977. Vitamin D in human milk. *Lancet* 1:167.
14. Fomon, S. J.; Filer, L. J., Jr.; Anderson, T. A.; and Ziegler, E. E. 1979. Recommendations for feeding normal infants. *Pediatrics* 63:52.
15. McMillan, J. A.; Landaw, S. A.; and Oski, F. A. 1976. Iron sufficiency in breast-fed infants and the availability of iron from human milk. *Pediatrics* 58:686.
16. Bullen, J. J.; Rogers, H. J.; and Griffiths, E. 1972. Iron binding proteins and infection. *Br. J. Haematol.* 23:389.
17. Committee on Nutrition, American Academy of Pediatrics. 1978. Relationship between iron status and incidence of infection in infancy. *Pediatrics* 62:246.
18. Committee on Nutrition, American Academy of Pediatrics. 1979. Fluoride supplementation: Revised dosage schedule. *Pediatrics* 63:150.
19. Fomon, S. J.; Filer, L. J., Jr.; Ziegler, E. E.; Bergmann, K. E.; and Bergman, R. L. 1977. Skim milk in infant feeding. *Acta Paediatr. Scand.* 66:17.
20. Willis, N. H. 1971. *Basic infant nutrition,* pp. 53–57. Philadelphia: J. B. Lippincott.

OTHER REFERENCES

Jelliffe, D. B., and Jelliffe, E. F. P. 1977. "Breast is best": Modern meanings. *N. Eng. J. Med.* 297:912.

Children 6 to 24 Months

INDICATIONS FOR USE

This diet is indicated for children 6 to 24 months of age requiring no dietary modifications.

DESCRIPTION

Metabolic requirements in this age group reflect the decreased rate of growth after the first 6 months of life. Protein requirements remain at approximately 2 g per kilogram of body weight per day, but energy requirements decrease to 100 kcal per kilogram of body weight per day by the end of the first year. Most vitamin and mineral requirements increase for this age group (refer to Appendix 1).

Milk (breast, formula, or whole) remains the primary source of calories until approximately 18 months of age. Beikost (foods other than milk or formula) may be introduced at 4 to 6 months of age. (1)

GUIDELINES FOR NUTRITIONAL MANAGEMENT

Diets for this age group include foods from the basic four food groups. Foods should be pureed, minced, or soft, since children in this age group have not yet developed molars to thoroughly masticate their food. The food can be divided into three or more meals depending on the needs of the child.

Milk. Whole cow's milk may be substituted for breast milk or infant formula after 6 months of age when the child is consuming at least 200 g beikost (1.5 jars, 7 ounces, or $\frac{3}{4}$ to 1 cup strained food) daily. (1) Skim milk is not suitable for this age group as it supplies insufficient calories. (2) If fed *ad libitum,* 2% milk will probably provide sufficient calories. However, the large volume that the child will need to consume to achieve an adequate caloric intake may not be conducive to later nonweight-gaining eating habits. (1)

Goat's milk has been used for infant feeding. Infants receiving goat's milk as a major source of calories are likely to develop megaloblastic anemia as an expression of folate deficiency. If daily supplements of iron, vitamin C, vitamin D, and 50 μg folacin are provided, goat's milk is probably nutritionally adequate and may be more readily digested than cow's milk due to the nature of its fatty acid content. (3)

Breast-fed children receiving iron-fortified cereal will require only continued fluoride supplementation and, if there is inadequate exposure to sunlight, vitamin D supplementation. (1, 4) Children fed formula and solids require no supplementation. Children switched to whole cow's milk require no supplementation if they are receiving a dietary source of iron and vitamin C. (1)

The use of a bottle of milk, juice, or other sugar-containing beverage as a pacifier may contribute to development of "nursing bottle caries" and should be discouraged. (5)

Beikost. Beikost may be introduced at 4 to 6 months of age. (1) Children not receiving a supplemental source of iron should receive iron-fortified baby cereal as their first solid food. There is no prescribed order for introduction of fruits, vegetables, and meats. The consistency of beikost can gradually be advanced from strained foods at 6 months to table foods by 12 to 18 months of age. It is neither necessary nor advisable to add sugar or salt to the child's food. Honey should be avoided for the first year of life due to infants' sensitivity to botulism spores found in honey. (6) *Foods that may cause the child to choke, such as nuts, popcorn, and raw carrot, should be avoided.*

After introduction of solids, a maximum of 24 to 32 ounces per day of milk or formula is recommended. More than this may interfere with adequate solid food intake and cause iron deficiency anemia. (1)

Hospital diets. The appropriate diet for the hospitalized child will depend on the child's age, physical development, concurrent illness or dysfunction, and the types of food that were tolerated at home. The hospital diets for 6- to 24-month-old children are divided into three categories (Table 50-1):

1. *Baby soft diet 1.* This diet is designed for children approximately 4 to 6 months of age and includes strained foods appropriate for the child beginning to eat solid foods.
2. *Baby soft diet 2.* This diet is designed for children approximately 7 to 11 months of age and includes strained or ground foods and some finger foods such as toast, crackers, and bread appropriate for the child beginning to pick up and masticate foods. Finger foods that can easily be swallowed whole may choke the infant and need to be avoided.
3. *Finger food diet.* This diet is designed for children approximately 9 months of age and older and includes diced and soft whole foods appropriate for the child beginning to pick up and masticate semisoft chunks of food. Finger foods are important for development of "pincer grasp" and hand-to-mouth coordination.

Sample menu as served in hospital

Portion sizes are not identified because they vary considerably with age and from day to day. Formula and whole milk are provided for those children who are not breast fed. Salt is not placed on the trays.

Baby Soft Diet 1	Baby Soft Diet 2	Finger Food Diet
Breakfast	*Breakfast*	*Breakfast*
Infant rice cereal	Orange juice	Orange juice
Strained banana	Farina	Rice Krispies
Formula or whole milk	Scrambled egg	Hard-cooked egg
	Toast	Toast
	Formula or whole milk	Formula or whole milk
Lunch	*Lunch*	*Lunch*
Strained turkey	Junior or minced turkey	Hot dog on bun
Strained green beans	Whipped potato	Cooked carrot coins
Strained peaches	Asparagus puree	Vanilla pudding
Formula or whole milk	Custard	Formula or whole milk
	Formula or whole milk	Catsup

Dinner	*Dinner*	*Dinner*
Strained beef	Junior or minced beef	Diced roast beef
Whipped potato	Whipped potato	French-fried potatoes
Strained beets	Beet puree	Diced beets
Strained applesauce	Applesauce	Peeled apple
Formula or whole milk	Formula or whole milk	Formula or whole milk
		Margarine

NUTRIENT ADEQUACY

Actual nutrient intake depends upon the child's appetite, preferences, and ability to eat. Provided that the child consumes a wide variety of foods in adequate amounts, the diet will meet the recommended dietary allowances. Consistent plotting of the child's height and weight on a growth chart (Figures 49-1, 49-2, 49-3, and 49-4) provides the most reliable determination of adequate nutrient intake.

TABLES

TABLE 50-1. Hospital Diets for Children 6 to 24 Months

	Recommended Foods and Daily Intake		
Food Group	Baby Soft Diet 1 (4 to 8 months)	Baby Soft Diet 2 (7 to 11 months)	Finger Food Diet (9 to 24 months)
Milk and calcium equivalents	Breast milk or 24–32 ounces formula or whole cow's milk	Breast milk or 24–32 ounces formula or whole cow's milk, mild cheese	Breast milk or 24 ounces whole cow's milk, mild cheese, cottage cheese, ice cream
Meat and protein equivalents	2–4 tablespoons strained meat	2–8 tablespoons strained or ground meat, egg, fish (no bones), mild cheese, cottage cheese	4–8 tablespoons diced meat, egg, fish (no bones), mild cheese, cottage cheese, cooked dried beans, peas, or legumes, smooth peanut butter
Fruit and vegetable	2 or more tablespoons strained fruit, strained vegetables, whipped potatoes	4 or more tablespoons soft or strained fruit, fruit juice from a cup, diced or ground vegetables, whipped potatoes	4 ($\frac{1}{4}$–$\frac{1}{2}$ cup) servings fresh or canned fruit, fruit juices, cooked or raw vegetables
Grain	2 or more tablespoons infant cereals or finely milled, cooked cereals (Cream of Wheat, Cream of Rice)	4 or more tablespoons bread, crackers, cooked cereals, infant cereals, refined ready-to-eat cereals, zwieback	4 or more servings (1 serving = 1 slice bread; $\frac{1}{4}$–$\frac{1}{2}$ cup cereal, rice, or noodles; 1 ounce of crackers)

REFERENCES CITED

1. Fomon, S. J.; Filer, L. J., Jr.; Anderson, T. A.; and Ziegler, E. E. 1979. Recommendations for feeding normal infants. *Pediatrics* 63:52.
2. Fomon, S. J.; Filer, L. J., Jr.; Ziegler, E. E.; Bergmann, K. E.; and Bergmann, R. L. 1977. Skim milk in infant feeding. *Acta Paediatr. Scand.* 66:17.
3. Fomon, S. J. 1974. *Infant nutrition.* 2nd ed. Philadelphia: W. B. Saunders.
4. Committee on Nutrition, American Academy of Pediatrics. 1979. Fluoride supplementation: Revised dosage schedule. *Pediatrics* 63:150.
5. Wei, S. H. Y. 1974. Nutritional aspects of dental caries. In *Infant nutrition,* ed., S. J. Fomon, p. 345. 2nd ed. Philadelphia: W. B. Saunders.
6. Arnon, S. S.; Midura, T. F.; Damus, K.; Thompson, B.; Wood, R. M.; and Chin, J. 1979. Honey and other environmental risk factors for infant botulism. *J. Pediatr.* 94:331.

51 Children 2 to 11 Years

INDICATIONS FOR USE

This diet is indicated for children 2 to 11 years of age who require no dietary modifications.

DESCRIPTION

Growth during this age period has slowed dramatically from the first two years of life. Energy requirements reflect this with a decrease in caloric requirements per unit body weight. Total vitamin, mineral, and protein requirements increase. Refer to Appendix 1 for the recommended dietary allowances.

GUIDELINES FOR NUTRITIONAL MANAGEMENT

Food intake will vary considerably depending on age, growth, activity, and physical development. The diet should include a variety of foods from the four basic food groups in the minimum amounts listed in Table 51-1. These foods may be consumed in greater amounts or other foods added to supply sufficient calories to meet individual needs. By this age, use of skim or other low-fat milks in the diet is probably preferable to the use of whole milk. (1)

NUTRIENT ADEQUACY

Actual nutrient intake depends upon the child's appetite, preferences, and ability to eat. Provided that the child consumes a wide variety of foods in adequate amounts, the diet will meet the recommended dietary allowances. Consistent plotting of the child's height and weight on a growth chart (refer to Figures 51-1, 51-2, 51-3, and 51-4) provides the most reliable determination of adequate nutrient intake.

REFERENCE CITED

1. Fomon, S. J.; Ziegler, E. E.; and O'Donnell, A. M. 1974. Infant feeding in health and disease. In *Infant nutrition,* ed., S. J. Fomon, pp. 481–482. 2nd ed. Philadelphia: W. B. Saunders.

TABLES AND FIGURES

Table 51-1. Recommended Minimum Daily Intake from the Four Basic Food Groups for Children 2 to 11 Years

Food Group	Minimum Daily Amount
Milk and calcium equivalents	3 cups milk or equivalent[1]
Meat and protein equivalents	2 to 4 ounces meat or equivalent[1]
Fruit and vegetable	4 servings, including a dark green or dark yellow vegetable daily and a citrus fruit or juice daily
Grain	4 servings of whole grain or enriched breads and cereals

[1] Refer to Chapters 8 and 9 for listings of calcium and protein equivalents.

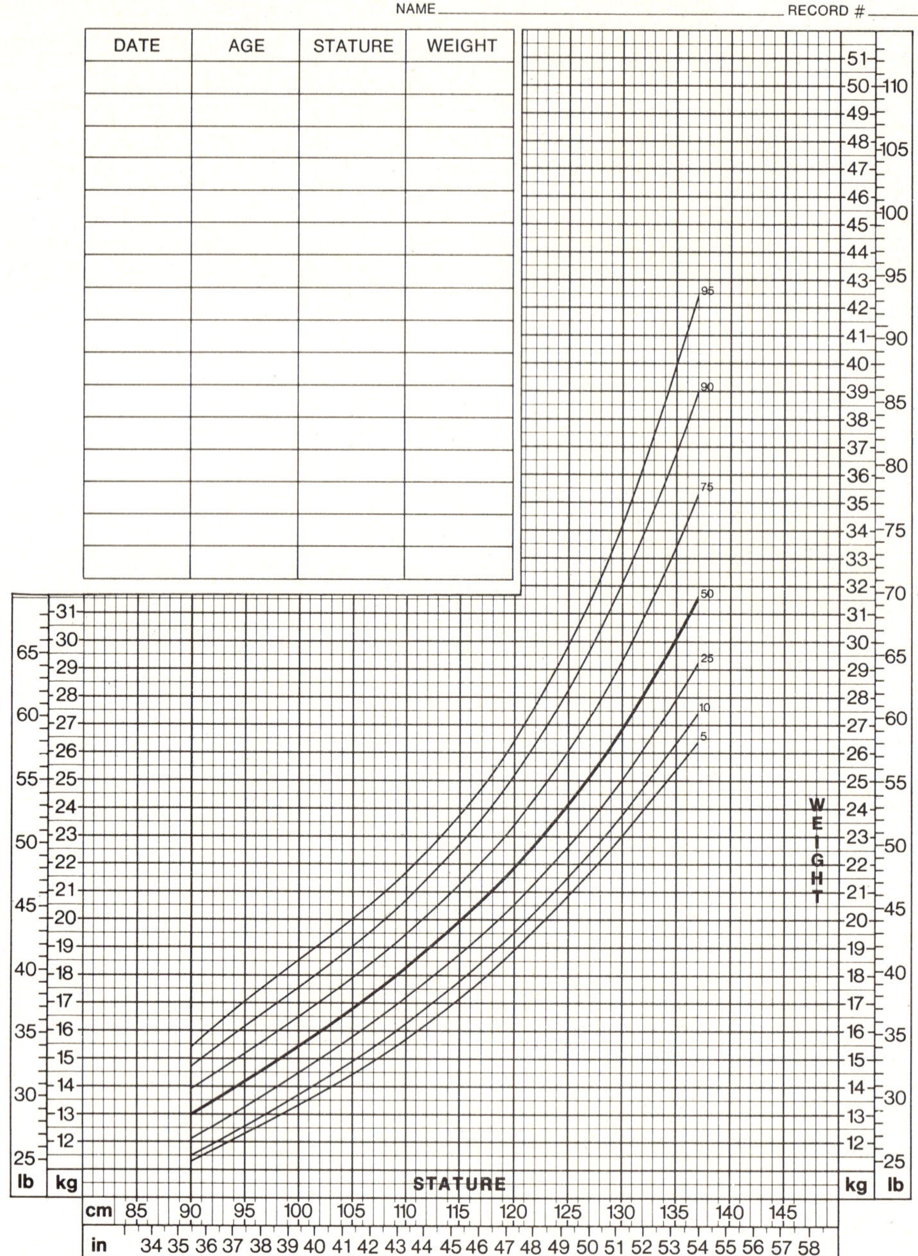

FIGURE 51-1 *Girls: Prepubescent, physical growth, NCHS percentiles.* [Courtesy of Ross Laboratories, Columbus, Ohio.]

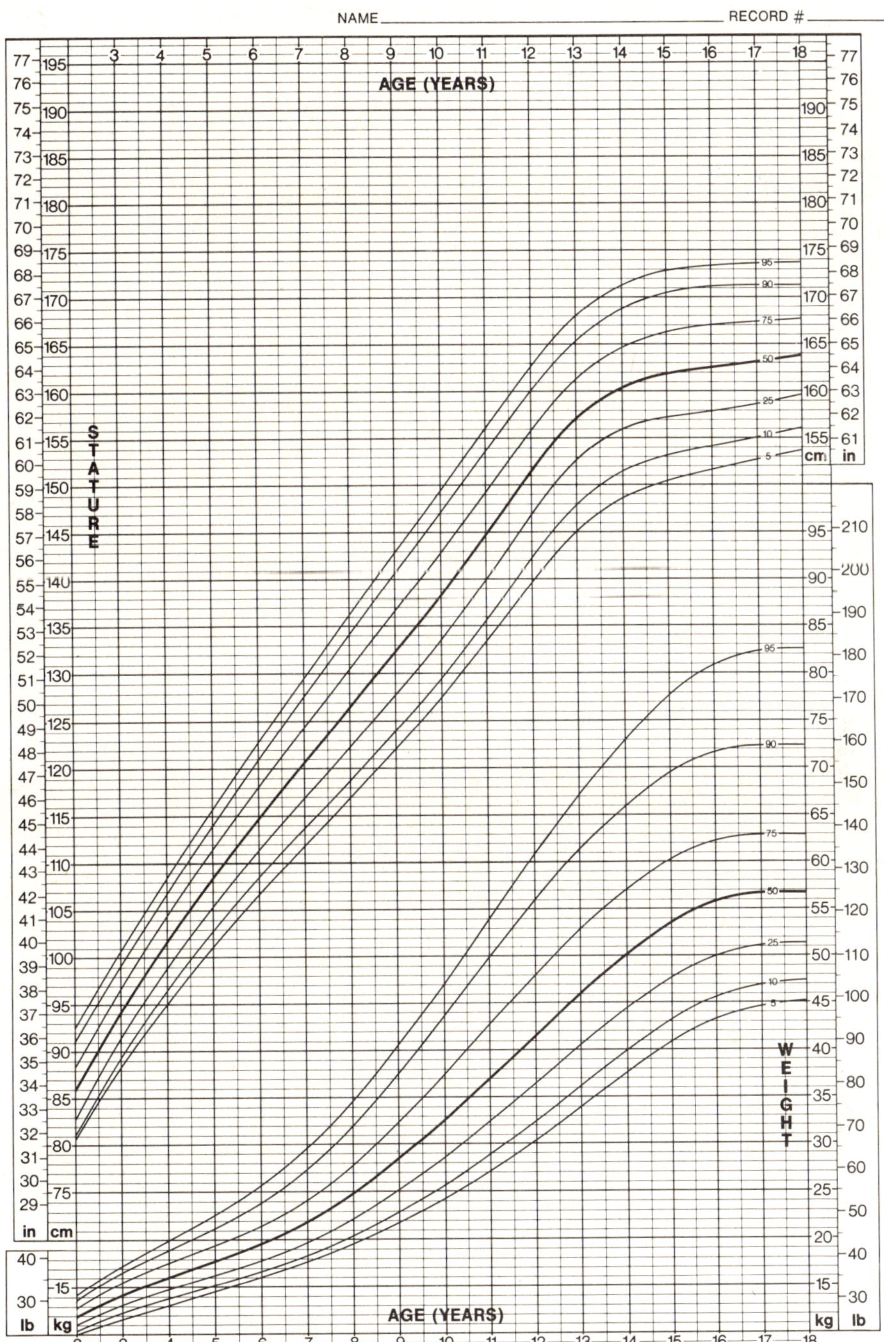

FIGURE 51-2 *Girls: 2 to 18 years, physical growth. NCHS percentiles.* [Courtesy of Ross Laboratories, Columbus, Ohio.]

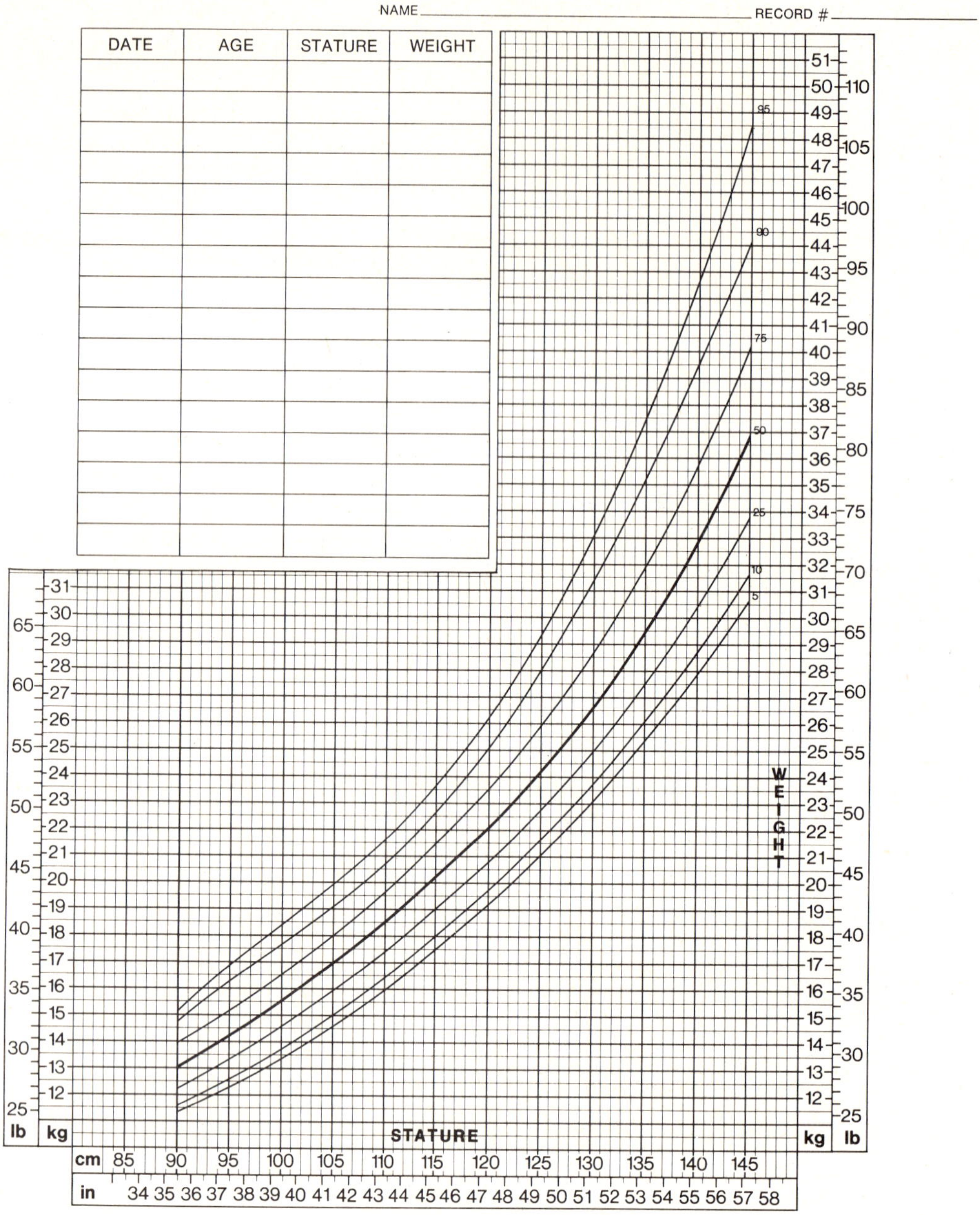

NAME ______________________ RECORD # ____________

DATE	AGE	STATURE	WEIGHT

STATURE

cm 85 90 95 100 105 110 115 120 125 130 135 140 145

in 34 35 36 37 38 39 40 41 42 43 44 45 46 47 48 49 50 51 52 53 54 55 56 57 58

WEIGHT

kg 12–51 lb 25–110

Percentiles: 95, 90, 75, 50, 25, 10, 5

FIGURE 51-3 *Boys: Prepubescent, physical growth. NCHS percentiles.* [Courtesy of Ross Laboratories, Columbus, Ohio.]

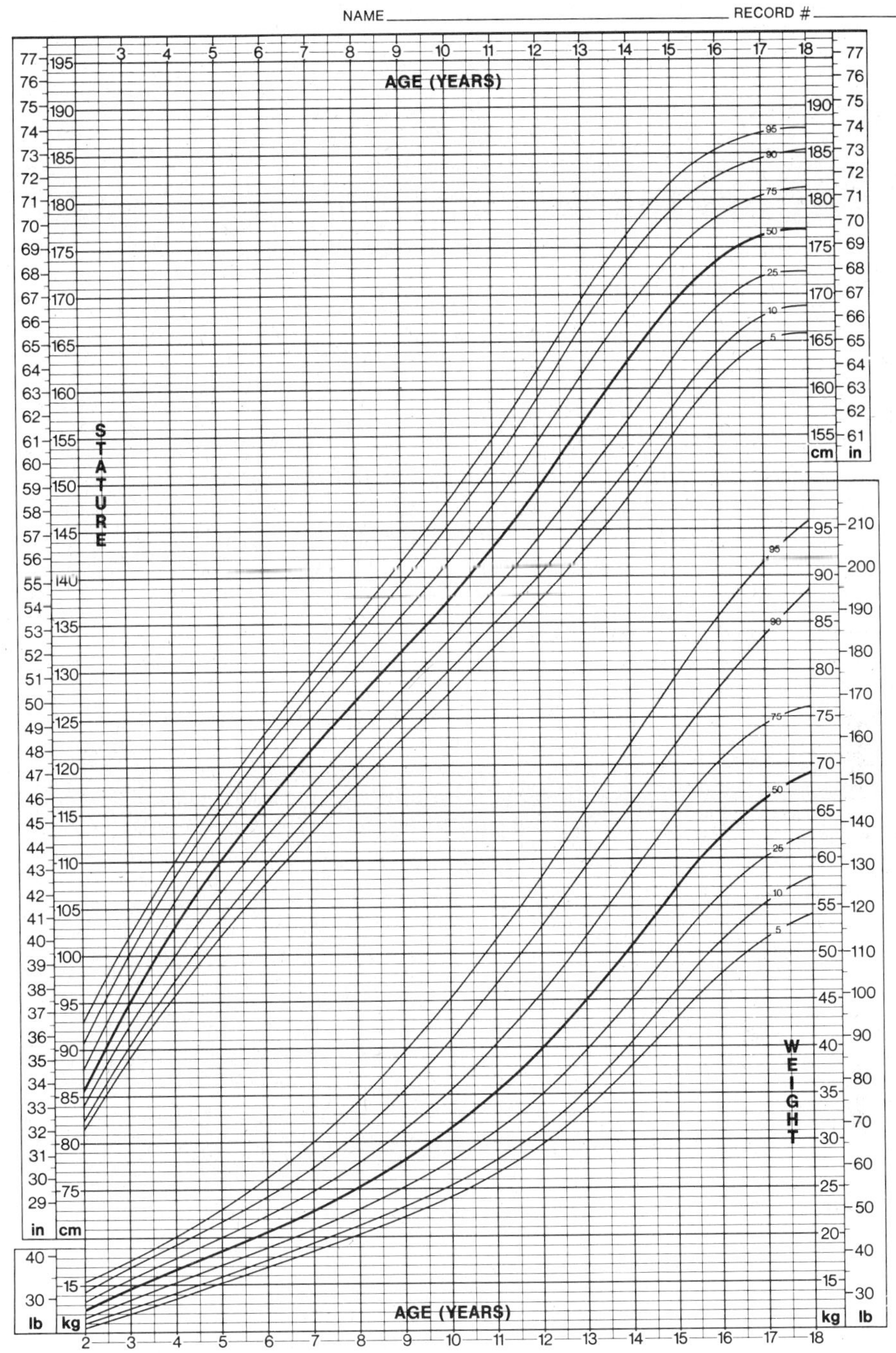

NAME ________________ RECORD # ________

AGE (YEARS)

STATURE

WEIGHT

AGE (YEARS)

FIGURE 51-4 *Boys; 2 to 18 years, physical growth, NCHS percentiles.* [Courtesy of Ross Laboratories, Columbus, Ohio.]

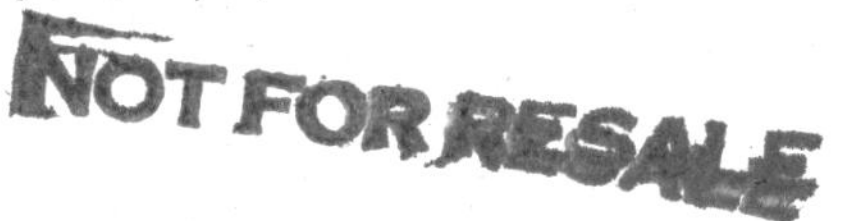

52 Adolescents 12 to 18 Years

INDICATIONS FOR USE

This diet is indicated for adolescents 12 to 18 years of age who require no dietary modifications.

DESCRIPTION

Adolescence is determined by physical growth and maturation rather than by chronological age. Adolescence generally occurs between the ages of 12 and 18 years. Nutritional needs for the adolescent are special due to the rapid physical growth that takes place during this period. This rapid growth results in an increased need for calories, protein, calcium, iron, and folate. The postmenarchial adolescent girl will also have increased requirements for iron due to menstrual blood loss. Refer to Appendix 1 for the recommended dietary allowances.

GUIDELINES FOR NUTRITIONAL MANAGEMENT

Food intake will vary considerably depending on age, growth, activity, and physical development. The diet should include a variety of foods from the basic four food groups in the minimum amounts listed in Table 52-1. These foods may be consumed in greater amounts or other foods added to supply sufficient calories to meet individual needs.

NUTRIENT ADEQUACY

Actual nutrient intake depends upon the individual's appetite, preferences, and ability to eat. Provided that the individual consumes a wide variety of foods in adequate amounts, the diet will meet the recommended dietary allowances with the possible exception of iron for the postmenarchial girl. Due to the documented poor food habits of teenagers, iron supplements for adolescent females may be necessary to meet nutrient needs. (1) Evaluation of height and weight (refer to Figures 51-1, 51-2, 51-3, and 51-4) are a good assessment of adequacy of calorie intake.

REFERENCE CITED

1. GAINES, E. G., and DANIEL, W. A., JR. 1974. Dietary iron intakes of adolescents. *J. Am. Dietet. A.* 65:275.

TABLES

TABLE 52-1. Recommended Minimum Daily Intake from the Four Basic Food Groups for Adolescents 11 to 18 Years

Food Group	Minimum Daily Amount
Milk and calcium equivalents	4 cups milk or equivalent[1]
Meat and protein equivalents	4 to 6 ounces meat or equivalent[1]
Fruit and vegetable	4 servings, including a dark green or dark yellow vegetable daily and a citrus fruit or juice daily
Grain	4 servings of whole grain or enriched breads and cereals

[1] Refer to Chapters 8 and 9 for listings of calcium and protein equivalents.

53 Weight Control for Infants, Children, and Adolescents

INDICATIONS FOR USE

Weight control is indicated for children who are obese. Although there is no precise definition of obesity for children, it has been suggested that values greater than +2 standard deviations for triceps and subscapular skinfold thickness can be considered evidence of obesity. (1) Growth charts (Figures 51-1, 51-2, 51-3, and 51-4) can be utilized as a guide for determining the degree of obesity.

DESCRIPTION

The primary goal of a weight control program for children is to establish appropriate eating habits early in life to prevent adult obesity and associated complications. Treatment and management of the obese child depends upon age and the degree of obesity:

Infants (at birth to 12 months). Treatment for the obese infant is not weight reduction but a slowing of the rate of weight gain to coincide with linear growth. (2) For normal growth and development, a daily intake of 115 kcal per kilogram of body weight is recommended for infants under 6 months and 105 kcal per kilogram of body weight for infants 6 to 12 months. (3)

Children (1 to 11 years). The emphasis for the obese child is to slow the rate of weight gain to coincide with linear growth. The markedly obese child will need special assistance and may require a patterned calorie-restricted diet. Energy and protein intake should be adequate for growth and development. (4)

Adolescents (12 to 18 years). Behavior modification techniques and moderate restriction of calories are recommended for the obese adolescent. (5, 6) The techniques and the degree of caloric restriction are based on individual needs.

Nutritional follow-up is a necessary part of all weight control programs.

GUIDELINES FOR NUTRITIONAL MANAGEMENT

Nutrient requirements are dependent upon the age, body size, activity, and nutritional status of the individual. The diet should include the amounts of food from each food group as listed in the section for each age group (Chapters 49–52). For an adolescent, an energy-controlled diet can be planned utilizing food exchange groups (Chapter 25).

Guidelines for nutritional management according to age group are as follows:

Infants (at birth to 12 months). The following feeding practices are potential means of slowing weight gain:

1. Breast feeding is advised compared with bottle feeding because the infant will normally stop sucking when satiated. (2, 7) With bottle feeding, there is often a tendency for the caretaker to encourage a satiated infant to finish a bottle.
2. When bottle feeding, the daily intake of formula should be limited to approximately 28–30 ounces per day. Water feedings can be added when necessary. (2) The use of skim or 2% milk is not advised during the first year of life.
3. Feeding each time the infant cries is discouraged. (2) The infant may be uncomfortable, tired, discovering his or her voice, or giving a signal of desire for physical contact.
4. Sweet desserts should be eliminated from the infant's diet.
5. Introduction of solid foods should be delayed until the infant is 5 to 6 months old.

Children (1 to 11 years). A general diet for age is recommended; emphasis is on the elimination of excess calories from fats and concentrated sweets. Any child old enough to understand the basic concepts being taught should be included in the counseling session. (4) The following recommendations may be advised:

1. Encourage daily exercise and active play. (8)
2. Substitute low-calorie snacks for high-calorie foods with little nutritive value.
3. Do not use food for bribery, punishment, or reward.
4. Encourage smaller portions and avoid second portions of high-calorie foods. Do not require the child to clean the plate at each meal.
5. Encourage the child to eat in one place and at specific times to control intake.
6. Slow the rate of eating by engaging in conversation with the child.
7. Encourage other members of the family to be supportive and alter their eating habits too.

Adolescents (12 to 18 years). Moderate restriction of calories is recommended. For some individuals, a more controlled diet of as few as 1400 kcal with a planned meal pattern may be necessary (Chapter 24). Behavior modification techniques are recommended:

1. Encourage regular exercise.
2. Substitute snacks of fresh fruits and vegetables for high-calorie snack foods and sweets.
3. Direct the adolescent's attention to some activity other than eating to deal with boredom, emotional stress, and fatigue.
4. Encourage the individual to eat more slowly, leave food on the plate,

cut food into smaller pieces, and use a smaller plate with smaller portions.

5. Control the eating pattern by eating only at specific times and in specific places. The type of food eaten should be planned in advance. Discourage skipping meals and eating heavily before bedtime.
6. A system of rewards (other than food) for weight loss may serve as reinforcement. (6)
7. Encourage family members to be supportive. Other overweight members of the family are advised to follow the recommended dietary regimen.

NUTRIENT ADEQUACY

A weight reduction diet can be planned to provide all nutrients needed for growth and development with the exception of iron for the postmenarchial girl. An iron supplement may be recommended.

REFERENCES CITED

1. Fomon, S. J. 1974. Normal growth, failure to thrive and obesity. In *Infant nutrition,* ed., S. J. Fomon, pp. 34–94. 2nd ed. Philadelphia: W. B. Saunders.
2. Taitz, L. S. 1977. Obesity in pediatric practice: Infantile obesity. *Pediatr. Clin. N. Am.* 24:107, 1977.
3. Food and Nutrition Board. 1980. *Recommended dietary allowances.* 9th rev. ed. Washington, D.C.: National Academy of Sciences.
4. Neumann, C. G. 1977. Obesity in pediatric practice: Obesity in the pre-school and school-age child. *Pediatr. Clin. N. Am.* 24:117.
5. Barnes, H. V., and Berger, R. 1975. An approach to the obese adolescent. *Med. Clin. N. Am.* 59:1507.
6. Gross, I.; Wheeler, M.; and Hess, K. 1976. The treatment of obesity in adolescents using behavioral self-control. *Clin. Pediatr.* 15:920.
7. Fomon, S. J. 1974. Voluntary food intake and its regulation. In *Infant nutrition,* ed., S. J. Fomon, pp. 20–33. 2nd ed. Philadelphia: W. B. Saunders.
8. Allen, D. W., and Quigley, B. M. 1977. The role of physical activity in the control of obesity. *Med. J. Aust.* 2:434.

ADDITIONAL REFERENCES

Bruch, H. 1976. The treatment of eating disorders. *Mayo Clin. Proc.* 51:266.

Fomon, S. J., and Ziegler, E. E. 1977. Skim milk in infant feeding. *Acta Paediatr. Scand.* 66:17.

Meyer, E. E., and Neumann, C. G. 1977. Management of the obese adolescent. *Pediatr. Clin. N. Am.* 24:123.

Weil, W. B., Jr. 1977. Current controversies in childhood obesity. *J. Pediatr.* 91:175.

REFERENCES FOR THE LAY PUBLIC

Refer to Chapter 24.

Children with Diabetes Mellitus

INDICATIONS FOR USE

This diet is indicated for the child with insulin-dependent diabetes mellitus. Clinical symptoms of the untreated disease include polyuria, polydipsia, polyphagia, weight loss, visual disturbances, fatigue, and muscle weakness. (1) Treatment involves the integration of insulin, diet, exercise, emotional support and guidance, and education. (1–4)

DESCRIPTION

The physiological rationale for dietary management and a complete description of dietary principles are included in Chapter 25.

Dietary management for children with diabetes is based on that for adults described in Chapter 25. The goals of diet therapy for children are to (1–6)

- Provide an appropriate level of energy intake that includes sufficient calories for normal growth and development.
- Prevent hyper- and hypoglycemia by maintaining blood glucose at as near the normal physiologic range as possible.
- Maintain or improve overall health by providing a nutritionally adequate diet.
- Prevent and/or delay the development and/or progression of complications of diabetes to the extent that they are related to metabolic control.
- Modify the diet as necessary for the treatment of existing hyperlipidemia, cardiovascular, renal, and other complications of diabetes and for the treatment of associated diseases.

As with adults, the translation of these goals into recommendations for dietary management requires flexibility and individualization. The physician, dietitian, child with diabetes, and family must work together to develop a realistic diet plan. Individual personality, life-style, physical condition, and diabetic state must be considered.

Appropriate caloric intake is of primary importance in providing for normal physical growth in children. Energy needs are determined by age, appetite, activity, and growth rate. A history of the child's previous intake is one of the best means of estimating caloric level. No attempt should be made to restrict total calories provided that weight is appropriate. (1–5) Weight and height status for age are evaluated on the basis of the National Center for Health Statistics Growth Charts (refer to Figures 49-1, 49-2, 49-3, and 49-4, and 51-1, 51-2, 51-3, and 51-4).

An estimate of the daily energy requirement for children under 12 years of age may be calculated on the basis of 1000 kcal plus 100 kcal for each year of age (e.g., 1500 kcal for a five-year-old child). (1, 2) An exception to the formula is the newly diagnosed diabetic who has lost a considerable amount of weight prior to diagnosis; such a child will generally have an increased appetite and increased energy requirement until weight has been regained and glucosuria controlled. The formula also does not give an accurate estimate of the energy needs of the adolescent.

Needs range widely among individuals within this age group, and boys require a greater intake than girls. A thorough diet history is valuable in helping to determine caloric requirement. As age and growth rate change, caloric intake should be reevaluated on each clinic visit to ensure appropriate growth. Hunger and appetite are good indicators of changing caloric needs. (5) The child and/or family should be educated to make appropriate dietary modifications on their own between clinic visits to ensure continued growth and development.

Daily activity in children is extremely variable. To maintain blood glucose levels within an acceptable range, the dietary program must be regarded as a baseline pattern that must be individually modified for variations in activity. (2, 3)

For dietary management during illness, refer to Chapter 25.

BASIC GUIDELINES FOR NUTRITIONAL MANAGEMENT

Based on diet history and the recommended dietary allowances, a diet pattern is calculated for each child. The pattern incorporates the dietary principles and the diabetic food exchange system described in Chapter 25.

Dietary emphasis is placed on consistent intake of carbohydrate, protein, and fat and on meal frequency. Three well-balanced meals plus snacks at midafternoon, bedtime, and often midmorning are encouraged to distribute food intake throughout the day. (1–5) Selection of a variety of foods should be encouraged.

NUTRIENT ADEQUACY

Provided that the child consumes a wide variety of foods from the diabetic food exchange system, the diet can be planned to meet the recommended dietary allowances for any age group. Evaluation of growth and development is important to assess the adequacy of caloric intake.

REFERENCES CITED

1. Drash, A. L. 1978. Managing the child with diabetes mellitus. *Postgrad. Med.* 63:85.
2. Bacon, G. E.; Spencer, M. L.; and Kelch, R. P. 1975. *A practical approach to pediatric endocrinology,* pp. 1–38. Chicago: Year Book Medical Publishers.
3. Lowrey, G. H. 1962. Management of the young diabetic patient. *J. Mich. State Med. Soc.* 61:1097.
4. Bloom, A. 1977. Some practical aspects of the management of diabetes. *Clin. Endocrinol. Metab.* 6:499.
5. Guthrie, R. A., and Jackson, R. L. 1975. Control of diabetes in children: Recent concepts concerning vascular complications and growth retardation. *Pediat. Ann.* 50:343.
6. American Diabetes Association. 1979. Principles of nutrition and dietary recommendations for individuals with diabetes mellitus: 1979. *Diabetes Care* 2:520.

ADDITIONAL REFERENCES

Birkbeck, J. A.; Truswell, A. S.; and Thomas, B. J. 1976. Current practice in dietary management of diabetic children. *Arch. Dis. Child.* 51:467.

Dorchy, H., and Loeb, H. 1977. Dietary management of diabetic children. *Arch. Dis. Child.* 52:252.

Koukal, S. M., and Parham, E. S. 1978. A family learning experience to serve the juvenile patient with diabetes. *J. Am. Dietet. A.* 72:411.

55 Galactosemia

INDICATIONS FOR USE

This diet is indicated from birth for the child with galactosemia. Although the incidence of galactosemia in the population is not known, it has been estimated to occur once in 10,000 to once in 187,000 births. (1)

Symptoms of untreated galactosemia include failure to thrive, liver disease, cataracts, and mental retardation. If the diet is instituted within the first weeks of life, all symptoms of the disease can usually be prevented. (2, 3) Although less rigid restriction of galactose in the diet for the older child and adult may be indicated, there is inadequate evidence at this time as to when the diet might be liberalized. (2, 4, 5)

DESCRIPTION

Galactosemia is a hereditary metabolic condition characterized by an inability to convert ingested galactose to glucose. Toxicity is associated with the accumulation of galactose and galactose metabolites in body tissues. Two types of galactosemia are now recognized, both of which involve an enzymatic defect in carbohydrate metabolism; these are transferase deficiency galactosemia and galactokinase deficiency galactosemia. (6)

Dietary management is based on elimination of galactose from the diet. Glucose can be converted to galactose by the body in sufficient quantities to fulfill the body's requirement for galactose. (1)

Galactose is a component of lactose; therefore, all milk products and products containing milk must be omitted. The diet consists of a milk substitute and all foods that do not contain physiologically available galactose. Soy-based formulas are often suggested for use as milk substitutes and have been used successfully in clinical management. (7, 8) Because soybeans contain appreciable amounts of two galactose-containing alpha-galactosides (stachyose and raffinose), some investigators advise against the use of these formulas. (9) However, research indicates that this galactose is probably physiologically unavailable and has no toxic effects. (7)

BASIC GUIDELINES FOR NUTRITIONAL MANAGEMENT

The child with galactosemia has the same nutritional needs for growth and development as do other children. The minimum amount of food to be consumed daily from each food group is the same as for the general diets for age (Chapters 49–52). A milk substitute should replace the recommended amount of milk-based foods. Nutramigen (Mead Johnson) contains minimal lactose and is used successfully as a milk substitute. (2) Soy-based formulas may also be prescribed with apparent safety. (2) Table 48-2 presents the nutrient composition of special infant formulas.

With the exception of milk products and foods containing them, the galactose-restricted diet allows most protein foods, fruits, vegetables, grain products, fats, and sugars. (10) Refer to Table 55-1 for foods to avoid. Because lactose is added during the processing of a wide variety of foods, labels of food products should be read carefully. Ingredients that indicate the presence of galactose include casein, curd, dry milk solids, butter, and whey. Food products that contain lactate, lactic acid, lactalbumin, and calcium compounds are acceptable. (11)

Organ meats such as liver, pancreas, and brain are galactose storing and should be avoided. Legumes, sugar beets, and lima beans are generally excluded because of their content of galactose-containing oligosaccharides; evidence to indicate whether or not this galactose is physiologically available is incomplete. (3, 11)

Medicines as well as foods must be monitored. Lactose and galactose are often used as ingredients in tablets and liquid medicine preparations.

NUTRIENT ADEQUACY

Provided that the child consumes a nutritionally complete milk substitute, the diet can be planned to meet the recommended dietary allowances for any age group. Children who do not drink recommended amounts of a milk substitute should receive calcium and vitamin D supplementation.

TABLES

TABLE 55-1. Foods to Avoid for a Galactose-Restricted Diet[1]

Food Group	Foods to Avoid
Milk and calcium equivalents	All milk and milk products
Meat and protein equivalents	Organ meats; legumes; all containing milk products
Fruit and vegetable	Green peas; sugar beets; lima beans
Grain	All containing milk products
Other	All containing milk products All products listing casein, curd, dry milk solids, butter, or whey on label

[1] Refer to Chapter 43 for a more complete listing of lactose-containing foods to avoid.

REFERENCES CITED

1. Ellis, G.; Wilcock, A. R.; and Goldberg, D. M. 1972. Experience of routine live-birth screening for galactosaemia in a British hospital, with emphasis on heterozygote detection. *Arch. Dis. Child.* 47:34.
2. Fomon, S. J., ed. 1974. *Infant nutrition,* pp. 200–202. 2nd ed. Philadelphia: W. B. Saunders.
3. Koch, R.; Donnell, G. N.; Wenz, E.; Fishler, K.; Graliker, B.; and Bergren, W. R. 1973. Galactosemia. In *Brennemann's practice of pediatrics.* New York: Harper & Row.
4. Clayton, B. 1975. Galactosaemia. *Practitioner.* 214:554.
5. Komrower, G. M., and Lee, D. H. 1970. Long-term follow-up of galactosaemia. *Arch. Dis. Child.* 45:367.
6. Cohn, R. M., and Segal, S. 1973. Galactose metabolism and its regulation. *Metabolism* 22:627.
7. Gitzelmann, R., and Auricchio, S. 1965. The handling of soya alpha-galactosides by a normal and a galactosemic child. *Pediatrics* 36:231.
8. Gitzelmann, R. 1966. The handling of soya alpha-galactosides by a normal and a galactosemic child. *Pediatrics* 37:531.
9. Schwartz, V. 1966. The handling of soya alpha-galactosides by a normal and a galactosemic child. *Pediatrics* 37:532.
10. Hardinge, M. G.; Swarner, J. B.; and Crooks, H. 1965. Carbohydrates in foods. *J. Am. Dietet. A.* 46:197.
11. Koch, R.; Acosta, P.; Donnell, G.; and Lieberman, E. 1965. Nutritional therapy of galactosemia. *Clin. Pediatr.* 4:571.

OTHER REFERENCES

Bureau of Public Health Nutrition. 1961. *Parents' guide for the galactose-free diet.* Berkeley.: California State Department of Public Health.

Cornblath, M., and Schwartz, R. 1976. *Disorders of carbohydrate metabolism in infancy,* pp. 294–321. 2nd ed. Philadelphia: W. B. Saunders.

Koch, R.; Acosta, P.; Ragsdale, N.; and Donnell, G. N. 1963. Nutrition in the treatment of galactosemia. *J. Am. Dietet. A.* 43:216.

Los Angeles Children's Hospital: Nutritional management of galactosemia. Evansville, Ind.: Mead Johnson Laboratories.

56

Glycogen Storage Diseases

INTRODUCTION

Glycogen is the principal storage form of carbohydrate in humans. (1) Disorders of glycogen metabolism result from genetic deficiencies of a variety of enzymes involved in glycogen synthesis and degradation. (1) Classified by their enzymatic abnormality, eight types of glycogen storage disease have been identified. Types I, III, and V, briefly described in Table 56-1, may be amenable to diet therapy. (1–4)

Type I (Von Gierke's disease)

INDICATIONS FOR USE

This diet is indicated for individuals with Type I glycogen storage disease.

DESCRIPTION

Due to either a deficiency or a decreased activity of glucose-6-phosphatase, glucose formation from glycogen or gluconeogenesis is obstructed, making glycogen stores in the liver and renal convoluted tubules metabolically unavailable. (2, 6) Severe hypoglycemia may be present. Clinically detected hypoglycemia is generally infrequent, although plasma glucose levels may be very low. (2, 4) As the child grows older, the plasma glucose levels rise toward normal. (2) Increased plasma lactate levels, ketosis, hyperlipidemia, growth retardation, and hepatic enlargement are often present. (1, 2, 6)

The diet is individualized to prevent hypoglycemic reactions. Children with severe hypoglycemia may require feedings every three to four hours. (3, 4) Some children may benefit from continuous intragastric feeding (7) or from continual intragastric feeding at night combined with frequent feeding during the day. (8)

Appropriate caloric intake is provided to avoid any excessive fat or glycogen accumulation that would result in hepatic enlargement. (4) Fifty to seventy percent of the total calories should come from carbohydrate with a minimum of 15% from protein. (2) Fat intake, particularly saturated fat, should be reduced to prevent hyperlipidemia. (2) The carbohydrate source should be from glucose or its polymers: dextromaltose, starch, or glycogen. (4) Galactose, fructose, lactose, and sucrose are avoided as the liver is unable to convert these to glucose. (2, 9)

GUIDELINES FOR NUTRITIONAL MANAGEMENT

The following criteria are used when planning a diet to control Type I:

- Provide a diet appropriate for age (Chapters 49–52).
- Avoid galactose, fructose, lactose, sucrose, and excess saturated fat. Table 56-2 lists foods to use and foods to avoid to achieve a galactose-, fructose-, lactose-, sucrose-, and saturated fat-restricted diet.
- Read labels carefully to ensure that galactose, fructose, lactose, or sucrose have not been added to the product.

NUTRIENT ADEQUACY

Provided that a fortified milk substitute is consumed in sufficient amounts, the diet can be planned to meet the recommended dietary allowances for all age groups, for all nutrients except vitamin C. Vitamin C supplementation is necessary. If a fortified milk substitute is not used, calcium and vitamin D must also be supplemented.

Type III (Cori–Forbes's disease)

INDICATIONS FOR USE

This diet is indicated for individuals with Type III glycogen storage disease.

DESCRIPTION

In Type III glycogen storage disease the debranching enzyme amylo-1,6-glucosidase is inactive. (1) The glycogen molecule is not degraded beyond the branching points, resulting in polysaccharide accumulation in the liver and muscle. (2, 10) During long periods of fasting, plasma glucose levels are decreased. (4)

The goal of the diet is to prevent hypoglycemia and progressive hepatic enlargement. (10)

GUIDELINES FOR NUTRITIONAL MANAGEMENT

The following are criteria used when planning a diet to control Type III:

- Provide a diet appropriate for age (Chapters 49–52).
- Prevent hypoglycemia by avoiding long periods of fasting.
- Provide a night feeding including protein to help maintain plasma glucose levels.
- Prevent hepatic enlargement by avoiding excessive calories from any source. Starch should provide the majority of the carbohydrate. (3, 4)

NUTRIENT ADEQUACY

This diet can be planned to meet the recommended dietary allowances for all age groups provided that a variety of foods from the basic four food groups is consumed.

Type V (McArdle's disease)

INDICATIONS FOR USE

This diet is indicated for individuals with Type V glycogen storage disease.

DESCRIPTION

Type V glycogen storage disease is a rare disease in which a deficiency of the enzyme myophosphorylase impairs breakdown of muscle glycogen. (10) The child is generally symptom free until the teenage years, at which time muscle fatigue and cramping may be noted. (4) The ingestion of glucose or fructose during exercise may help to prevent symptoms. (2)

GUIDELINES FOR NUTRITIONAL MANAGEMENT

The following are criteria used when planning a diet to decrease symptoms of Type V:

- Plan a diet appropriate for age (Chapters 49–52).
- If successful in preventing symptoms, provide glucose or fructose for ingestion during exercise.

NUTRIENT ADEQUACY

This diet can be planned to meet the recommended dietary allowances for all age groups provided that a variety of foods from the basic four food groups is consumed.

TABLES

TABLE 56-1. Description of the Three Types of Glycogen Storage Disease Amenable to Diet Therapy (2, 4, 5)

	Type I (Von Gierke)	Type III (Cori–Forbes)	Type V (McArdle)
Enzymatic defect	Glycose-6-phosphatase	Amylo-1,6-glucosidase	Myophosphorylase
Glycogen structure	Normal	Abnormal	Normal
Plasma glucose	Very low	Low	Normal
Plasma lactate	High	Normal to high	Low
Organs involved	Intestines; kidney; liver	Kidney; liver; red blood cells; white blood cells	Liver; muscle; red blood cells; white blood cells
Other abnormalities	Hepatomegaly; growth retardation; increased pyruvate; increased urate; increased free fatty acids; increased lipids	Hepatomegaly; fasting hypoglycemia; weakness; increased lipids	Myopathy; muscle weakness and cramping after exertion

TABLE 56-2. Foods Allowed and Foods to Avoid to Achieve a Galactose, Fructose, Lactose, Sucrose, and Saturated Fat Restricted Diet (4)[1]

Food Group	Foods Allowed	Foods to Avoid
Milk and calcium equivalents	Pregestimil (Mead Johnson) refer to Table 48-2 for nutrient composition	All milk including lactose-hydrolyzed milk; cheese spreads; ice cream; yogurt; custard; natural cheeses such as cheddar, brick, Parmesan; Swiss may be used in limited amounts
Meat and protein equivalents	Eggs, beef, lamb, pork, veal, chicken, turkey, fish	Meats such as luncheon meats in which sugar, milk, or milk products are used in processing; liver, brains, sugar-cured bacon, peanuts, peanut butter, legumes
Fruit and vegetable	Asparagus, cauliflower, wax beans, green beans, celery, lettuce, spinach, white potatoes	All fruits, all fruit juices, other vegetables including any vegetables in which sugar, lactose, milk, or milk products have been added in processing
Grain	Bread made without milk or sugar, saltine crackers, unsweetened cooked cereals other than instant, puffed rice, puffed wheat, shredded wheat, macaroni, noodles, spaghetti, rice	Prepared mixes, breads, cereals, rolls and other baked products made with milk or sugar
Other		
Beverage	Diet carbonated beverages, coffee, tea, broth, unsweetened Kool-Aid	Regular carbonated beverages; regular fruit flavored drinks; milk beverages
Fat	Oil, margarine containing no milk solids, vinegar-oil salad dressing without sugar	Margarine containing milk solids; butter; cream; cream cheese; shortening; salad dressings made with milk or sugar
Sweet	Non-nutritive artificial sweeteners, dextrose, artificially sweetened gelatin	Candy, jam, jelly, honey, brown or white sugar, fructose, sucrose, lactose, all desserts prepared with these sweeteners or with fruit or fruit juices
Miscellaneous	Soups made with allowed ingredients	Catsup, chili sause and other sauces containing sugar

[1] This food list is not comprehensive. Product labels must be read to determine whether individual products are acceptable.

REFERENCES CITED

1. Howell, R. R. 1978. The glycogen storage diseases. In *The metabolic basis of inherited disease,* eds., J. B. Stanbury, J. B. Wyngaarden, and D. S. Fredrickson, pp. 137–159. 4th ed. New York: McGraw-Hill.
2. Drash, A. L., and Field, J. B. 1971. The glycogen storage diseases. *Disease-a-Month,* October 3, 1971.
3. Holtzman, N. A.; Batshaw, M. L.; and Valle, D. L. 1980. Genetic aspects of human nutrition. In *Modern nutrition in health and disease,* eds., R. S. Goodhart and M. E. Shils, pp. 1217–1218. 6th ed. Philadelphia: Lea & Febiger.
4. Cornblath, M., and Schwartz, R. 1976. *Disorders of carbohydrate metabolism in infancy,* pp. 231–293. 2nd ed. Philadelphia: W. B. Saunders.
5. DiMauro, S., and Eastwood, A. B. 1977. Disorders of glycogen and lipid metabolism. *Adv. Neurol.* 17:123.
6. Harper, H. A.; Rodwell, V. W.; and Mayes, P. A. 1977. *Review of physiological chemistry,* p. 265. 16th ed. Los Altos, Calif.: Lange Medical Publishers.
7. Burr, I. M.; O'Neill, J. A.; Karzon, D. T.; Howard, L. J.; and Greene, H. L. 1974. Comparison of the effects of total parenteral nutrition, continuous intragastric feeding, and portacaval shunt on a patient with Type I glycogen storage disease. *J. Pediatr.* 85:792.
8. Greene, H. L.; Slonim, A. E.; O'Neill, J. A., Jr.; and Burr, I. M. 1976. Continuous nocturnal intragastric feeding for management of Type I glycogen storage disease. *N. Eng. J. Med.* 294:423.
9. Fernandes, J. 1974. The effect of disaccharides on the hyperlactacidaemia of glucose-6-phosphatase-deficient children. *Acta Paediatr. Scand.* 63:695.
10. Senior, B., and Sadeghi-Nejad, A. 1976. The glycogenoses and other inherited disorders of carbohydrate metabolism. *Clin. Perinatol.* 3:79.

OTHER REFERENCES

Hardinge, M. G.; Swarner, J. B.; and Crooks, H. 1965. Carbohydrate in foods. *J. Am. Dietet. A.* 46:197.

Phenylketonuria

INDICATIONS FOR USE

A diet low in phenylalanine is indicated for infants and children with phenylketonuria (PKU).

PKU can be identified by screening newborn infants using the Guthrie bacterial inhibition assay test. Compulsory PKU screening programs for infants exist in more than 40 states. For example, in Michigan, mandatory screening for PKU became effective on August 1, 1965. States without mandatory testing often have voluntary detection programs.

A preliminary diagnosis of PKU can be made within the first 12 to 24 hours of life with a blood specimen even from an unfed infant. Diagnosis of classical PKU is usually confirmed during the first 14 days of life by blood phenylalanine levels greater than 20 mg/100 ml. Normal blood phenylalanine levels are 1–3 mg/100 ml.

At University Hospital, a diet low in phenylalanine is prescribed immediately after laboratory diagnosis and is maintained for at least the first three years of life. Symptoms of untreated disease include seizures and delayed development associated with microcephaly. A musty odor may be noted in the untreated infant or adult. PKU untreated by six months of age will generally be associated with mental retardation.

Almost one half of positive newborn tests reveal variants with hyperphenylalaninemia (levels of less than 10 mg/100 ml) who do not require dietary treatment. Variants of the disease may exhibit some of the same clinical characteristics as classical phenylketonurics but respond poorly to reduced dietary phenylalanine intake. (1) Some variants are without apparent mental disability or other clinical problems and may not require treatment. (2)

An individual with PKU will always possess the inborn error of metabolism. After diet termination, the blood phenylalanine will rise above normal. Since this is an inherited disorder, men and women with PKU who have reached the age of reproduction need genetic counseling. In addition to potentially inheriting the defect, the fetus of the woman with PKU will be exposed to her elevated levels of phenylalanine, which cross the placental barrier and cause *in utero* brain damage. (3) A carefully controlled low phenylalanine diet for the entire nine months of pregnancy and prior to conception may decrease the risk of brain damage. (3–5)

DESCRIPTION

Classical PKU is an autosomal recessive defect affecting the metabolism of the essential amino acid, phenylalanine. A deficiency of the hepatic enzyme, phenylalanine hydroxylase, and possibly a deficiency of a related co-factor or coenzyme results in the accumulation of phenylalanine and metabolites in the blood and urine. Classical PKU is treated primarily with dietary restriction of phenylalanine. (6, 7) The etiology and treatment of the symptoms in atypical PKU is less well defined. (8) Atypical PKU may result from brain hydroxylase dysfunction due to a deficiency of cofactors or co-enzymes such as dihydropteridine reductase or biopterin involved in phenylalanine, tyrosine, dopamine, and tryptophan metabolism. (9–12) The role of tyrosine and/or biopterin supplementation is under investigation. (8)

The goals of nutritional management are to:

- Provide a diet in which phenylalanine is limited to the amount necessary for normal physical growth and brain development.
- Maintain a blood phenylalanine level 5–10 mg/100 ml and prevent urinary excretion of phenylketones. Maintenance of blood phenylalanine levels below 4 mg/100 ml may be inadequate to support growth and development. (13)
- Supply adequate energy, protein, and all other nutrients to meet nutritional needs and to allow for normal growth and development.
- Educate the family on the management of PKU utilizing a health care team, which includes physician, dietitian, psychologist, and nurse clinician.

To meet these goals, dietary management is individualized for each infant and child. The diet is prescribed in terms of total milligrams of phenylalanine per 24 hours. Classical or severe PKU frequently requires the limitation of phenylalanine to approximately 250–350 mg/24 hr. Patients with less severe enzyme deficiency can ingest upwards of 350 mg/24 hr. Mildly affected individuals with PKU can tolerate more phenylalanine with increasing age. A diet allowing phenylalanine of less than 200 mg/24 hr should be avoided, as it may endanger normal growth and lead to symptoms of hypophenylalanemia and negative nitrogen balance. (8)

Blood phenylalanine levels tend to increase during acute febrile or infectious conditions. Protein is catabolized during the infectious process so that amino acids may be supplied for use in other metabolic pathways. (14) Phenylalanine levels are elevated due to the protein breakdown. Careful dietary attention must be given to provide an adequate phenylalanine intake.

GUIDELINES FOR NUTRITIONAL MANAGEMENT

Phenylalanine occurs in proteins of both animal and plant origin, although the proportion of phenylalanine in vegetable and fruit protein is less than in seed, meat, milk, and egg protein. (7) The diet for PKU is planned using a variety of phenylalanine-containing foods, a variety of free foods with negligible phenylalanine, and formulas with modified phenylalanine content.

Dietary management is facilitated by use of the two formulas Lofenalac and Phenyl-Free (formerly Product 3229) (refer to Tables 57-1 and 48-2 for nutrient composition). The protein in Lofenalac is an enzymatic hydrolysate of casein and selected amino acids, processed to remove 95% of the phenylalanine. At standard dilution, Lofenalac contains 4 mg phenylalanine per ounce. Phenyl-Free is phenylalanine free.

Procedures to follow when planning a low phenylalanine diet are as follows:

1. After diagnosis, Lofenalac is used alone without added natural protein until blood phenylalanine levels fall within an acceptable therapeutic range. This period generally does not exceed five to seven days.

2. When blood phenylalanine levels are stable, regular infant formula or diluted evaporated milk (refer to Table 57-1 for nutrient compo-

sition) is added to the diet. It is essential to include a source of natural protein in the infant's diet to ensure the consumption of dietary factors that may not be present in the synthesized amino acid mixtures.

The amount of Lofenalac and regular infant formula in the diet is determined by the total volume of formula the infant is consuming per day, the kilocalorie requirement for age, and the dietary phenylalanine prescription. The diet is adjusted (generally on a biweekly basis) based on weight gain of the infant and quantitative blood phenylalanine determinations. Changes in the dietary phenylalanine prescription are made in increments of 25–50 mg/24 hr. Infants with milk PKU and a high milligram allowance of phenylalanine daily often require a large intake of regular infant formula.

Phenylalanine intake should be within plus or minus 10 mg of the dietary phenylalanine prescription. Families are instructed to measure accurately and to keep accurate diaries of food intake. The Lofenalac and regular infant formula are given separately, not mixed together, so that phenylalanine intake can be monitored accurately. To allow for maximum protein utilization, the regular infant formula is usually given in two feedings, spaced 12 hours apart.

3. Solid foods may be introduced early. Rice cereal is usually the first solid to be introduced due to its low phenylalanine content and because rice is less allergenic than other grains. Strained fruits, strained meat and vegetable dinners, and strained vegetables are gradually added (refer to Tables 57-2, 57-3, and 57-4 for nutrient composition of infant, toddler and junior foods). At University Hospital, Gerber infant foods are used as they have been analyzed specifically for phenylalanine content. Early introduction of meat–vegetable dinners may simplify meal planning for infants with mild PKU who have a high phenylalanine allowance by permitting them to be maintained on a single formula (Lofenalac) and solids.

4. At approximately four to five months of age, as more solids have been incorporated into the diet, the infant is weaned completely off the regular infant formula feedings. This prevents the infant from acquiring a preference for the regular formula over the Lofenalac.

5. At approximately one year of age, for infants on diets highly restricted in phenylalanine, Lofenalac may be replaced by Phenyl-Free. The use of Phenyl-Free allows a greater variety and quantity of regular foods to be used while keeping within the dietary phenylalanine prescription. Phenyl-Free should not be used for routine diets of PKU infants below 6–12 months of age.

   Added kilocalories are supplied by free foods listed in Table 57-5. Parents are cautioned not to overfeed the child with free foods. Overfeeding with free foods could result in decreased appetite, inadequate consumption of phenylalanine-containing foods, and failure to meet the daily dietary phenylalanine prescription with decreased growth and development.

   Due to the high carbohydrate content of the low-phenylalanine diet, a dental hygiene program is encouraged early in the child's life to prevent excessive formation of dental caries.

   During most illnesses, it is important to maintain the total prescribed amount of dietary phenylalanine per 24 hours. If solids are not consumed during periods of acute illness, limited quantities of milk or diluted skim milk are suggested. Clear liquids, jello, and carbonated beverages are recommended to provide fluid for hydration without adding significant phenylalanine. When diarrhea and dehydration are of clinical concern during illness, routine management as employed with any infant may be necessary.

Four case examples with dietary calculations follow:

Example 1

Fourteen-day-old male newly diagnosed with classical PKU.
WEIGHT: 3.4 kg
DIETARY PRESCRIPTION: Lofenalac only, as much as desired

Food Item	Serving Size: Weight (g)	Serving Size: Household Measure	kcal	Protein (g)	Phenylalanine (mg)
Lofenalac	As desired				
Total					

Example 2

Twenty-one-day-old infant with classical PKU consuming 24 ounces formula per day.
WEIGHT: 3.8 kg
DIETARY PRESCRIPTION: 310 mg phenylalanine per 24 hours

Food Item	Serving Size: Weight (g)	Serving Size: Household Measure	kcal	Protein (g)	Phenylalanine (mg)
Lofenalac	360	12 ounces	240	8.4	48
Enfamil	360	12 ounces	240	6.0	264
Total			480	14.4	312

Example 3

Twenty-one-day-old infant with classical PKU consuming 24 ounces formula per day and rice cereal.
WEIGHT: 3.8 kg
DIETARY PRESCRIPTION: 310 mg phenylalanine per 24 hours

Food Item	Serving Size: Weight (g)	Serving Size: Household Measure	kcal	Protein (g)	Phenylalanine (mg)
Lofenalac	390	13 ounces	260	9.1	52
Enfamil	330	11 ounces	220	5.5	242
Rice cereal, dry[1]	4	2 tablespoons	18	0.4	18
Total			498	15.0	312

[1] Data for Gerber products used.

Example 4

Six-month-old infant with classical PKU consuming 30 ounces Lofenalac per day and baby foods.
WEIGHT: 7.0 kg
DIETARY PRESCRIPTION: 320 mg phenylalanine per 24 hours

Food Item	Serving Size		kcal	Pro-tein (g)	Phenyl-alanine (mg)
	Weight (g)	Household Measure			
Lofenalac	900	30 ounces	600	21.0	120
Rice cereal, dry[1]	6	3 tablespoons	27	0.6	27
Strained baby dinner, beef with vegetables[1]	42	3 tablespoons	33	2.4	115
Strained green beans[1]	28	2 tablespoons	8	0.4	17
Strained sweet potatoes[1]	42	3 tablespoons	24	0.6	34
Strained applesauce[1]	42	3 tablespoons	18	0.1	4
Strained Dutch apple dessert[1]	42	3 tablespoons	30	0.0	3
Total			740	25.1	320

[1] Data for Gerber products used.

NUTRIENT ADEQUACY

Lofenalac alone will meet the recommended dietary allowances for infants from birth to six months except for phenylalanine and iron. If the water supply is not fluoridated, fluoride should be added to both Lofenalac and Phenyl-Free. With the addition of infant formula and iron-fortified infant cereal to the diet, the requirements for phenylalanine and iron are met. Lofenalac and regular infant formula will meet the recommended dietary allowances for infants from birth to six months except for iron. Iron-fortified formula or cereal included in the diet will meet the requirement for iron.

Upon discontinuation of regular infant formula, a diet of Lofenalac and infant foods will meet the recommended dietary allowances, provided that sufficient variety and quantity of infant foods are consumed.

A diet of Phenyl-Free and solid foods will meet the recommended dietary allowances provided that sufficient variety and quantity of foods are consumed.

TABLES

TABLE 57-1. Protein, Phenylalanine, and Leucine Content of Infant Formulas and Milk

Food Item	Serving Size		kcal	Protein (g)	Phenylalanine (mg)	Leucine (mg)
	Weight (g)	Household Measure				
Enfamil	946	1 quart	640	14.4	698	1421
	30	1 ounce	20	0.5	22	44
Lofenalac	946	1 quart	640	20.8	110	1939
	30	1 ounce	20	0.7	4	61
Phenyl-Free	946	1 quart	800	40.0	0	3400
(Product 3229)	30	1 ounce	25	1.3	0	106
MSUD Diet	946	1 quart	640	11.0	740	0
(powder diluted to 20 kcal per ounce)	30	1 ounce	20	0.3	23	0
Milk						
Chocolate	30	1 ounce	26	1.0	48	97
Evaporated, diluted 1:1 with water	30	1 ounce	21	1.0	52	105
Skim	30	1 ounce	11	1.0	50	102
Whole, 3.5% fat	30	1 ounce	19	1.0	49	98

TABLE 57-2. Phenylalanine and Leucine Content of Some Strained Baby Foods

Food Item	Serving Size				Phenylalanine		Leucine	
	Weight (g)	Household Measure	kcal	Protein (g)	Avg. (mg)	Gerber (mg)	Avg. (mg)	Gerber (mg)
Meat or protein equivalents								
Plain meat								
Beef	14	1 tablespoon	15	1.9	75	75	156	142
Beef with beef heart	14	1 tablespoon	13	1.8	75	75	144	143
Chicken	14	1 tablespoon	19	2.0	80	86	151	145
Egg yolks	14	1 tablespoon	29	1.4	59	58	121	118
Ham	14	1 tablespoon	16	2.0	76	85	159	154
Lamb	14	1 tablespoon	15	2.0	79	91	159	163
Liver (beef)	14	1 tablespoon	14	2.0	98	116	189	176
Pork	14	1 tablespoon	18	2.0	81	85	161	158
Turkey	14	1 tablespoon	16	2.0	84	85	163	156
Veal	14	1 tablespoon	14	1.9	75	78	149	148
Dinners								
Beef and egg noodles	14	1 tablespoon	8	0.3	15	17	27	30
Beef with vegetables	14	1 tablespoon	11	0.8	31	38	61	66
Chicken with noodles	14	1 tablespoon	7	0.3	14	15	26	28
Chicken soup, cream of	14	1 tablespoon	8	0.4	15	15	24	28
Chicken with vegetables	14	1 tablespoon	11	0.9	34	39	70	70
Cottage cheese with pineapple	14	1 tablespoon	17	0.9	42	45	80	85
Ham with vegetables	14	1 tablespoon	11	0.9	32	37	67	71
Macaroni and cheese	14	1 tablespoon	8	0.4	19	19	33	33
Macaroni, tomato, and beef	14	1 tablespoon	8	0.3	14	14	26	25
Turkey and rice	14	1 tablespoon	7	0.3	11	12	22	22
Turkey with vegetables	14	1 tablespoon	12	0.8	33	42	63	67
Veal with vegetables	14	1 tablespoon	10	0.8	33	39	67	65
Vegetables and bacon	14	1 tablespoon	10	0.2	9	9	15	15
Vegetables and beef	14	1 tablespoon	8	0.3	10	8	19	16
Vegetables and chicken	14	1 tablespoon	6	0.3	11	13	19	22
Vegetables and ham	14	1 tablespoon	7	0.3	9	9	18	17
Vegetables and lamb	14	1 tablespoon	7	0.3	11	11	21	20
Vegetables and liver	14	1 tablespoon	6	0.3	15	15	27	27
Vegetables and turkey	14	1 tablespoon	6	0.2	9	9	18	18
Fruit								
Applesauce	14	1 tablespoon	6	0.03	NA	1	NA	NA
Applesauce and apricots	14	1 tablespoon	6	0.03	NA	2	NA	NA
Applesauce and pineapple	14	1 tablespoon	5	0.01	NA	2	NA	NA
Apricots with tapioca	14	1 tablespoon	9	0.04	NA	1	NA	NA
Banana and pineapple with tapioca	14	1 tablespoon	10	0.03	NA	1	NA	NA
Banana with tapioca	14	1 tablespoon	8	0.06	NA	2	NA	NA
Peaches	14	1 tablespoon	10	0.07	NA	3	NA	NA
Pears	14	1 tablespoon	6	0.04	NA	2	NA	NA
Pears and pineapple	14	1 tablespoon	6	0.04	NA	1	NA	NA
Plums with tapioca	14	1 tablespoon	10	0.01	NA	1	NA	NA
Prunes with tapioca	14	1 tablespoon	10	0.09	NA	2	NA	NA

[Continued]

TABLE 57-2. Phenylalanine and Leucine Content of Some Strained Baby Foods [*Concluded*]

	Serving Size				Phenylalanine		Leucine	
Food Item	Weight (g)	Household Measure	kcal	Protein (g)	Avg. (mg)	Gerber (mg)	Avg. (mg)	Gerber (mg)
Vegetable								
Beans, green	14	1 tablespoon	4	0.2	8	9	12	12
Beets	14	1 tablespoon	5	0.2	3	3	7	6
Carrots	14	1 tablespoon	4	0.1	3	3	5	4
Corn, creamed	14	1 tablespoon	8	0.2	7	10	20	20
Garden vegetables	14	1 tablespoon	5	0.3	13	17	20	23
Peas	14	1 tablespoon	6	0.5	20	22	34	32
Spinach, creamed	14	1 tablespoon	5	0.4	14	20	32	33
Squash	14	1 tablespoon	3	0.1	4	5	7	7
Sweet potatoes	14	1 tablespoon	8	0.2	9	11	11	12
Grain								
Cereal and egg yolks	14	1 tablespoon	7	0.3	13	13	25	25
Grits and egg yolks	14	1 tablespoon	11	0.3	14	14	26	26
Mixed cereal with applesauce and bananas	14	1 tablespoon	12	0.2	9	9	13	12
Oatmeal with applesauce and bananas	14	1 tablespoon	10	0.2	9	11	14	15
Rice with applesauce and bananas	14	1 tablespoon	11	0.2	8	3	17	6
Dessert								
Cherry vanilla pudding	14	1 tablespoon	10	0	NA	1	NA	NA
Chocolate custard pudding	14	1 tablespoon	12	0.3	12	17	26	NA
Cottage cheese with pineapple	14	1 tablespoon	10	0.4	15	19	26	NA
Dutch apple	14	1 tablespoon	10	0	NA	1	NA	NA
Orange pudding	14	1 tablespoon	11	0.2	6	8	16	NA
Peach cobbler	14	1 tablespoon	9	0	NA	2	NA	NA
Vanilla custard pudding	14	1 tablespoon	12	0.2	10	14	8	NA

NA = not available

TABLE 57-3. Phenylalanine and Leucine Content of Some Junior Foods

Food Item	Serving Size				Phenylalanine		Leucine	
	Weight (g)	Household Measure	kcal	Protein (g)	Avg. (mg)	Gerber (mg)	Avg. (mg)	Gerber (mg)
Meat or protein equivalents								
Plain								
Beef	14	1 tablespoon	15	2.1	80	79	166	152
Chicken	14	1 tablespoon	21	2.1	86	NA	162	NA
Chicken sticks	10	1 stick	19	1.5	67	66	114	112
Ham	14	1 tablespoon	18	2.2	82	90	173	163
Lamb	14	1 tablespoon	16	2.2	85	95	171	173
Meat sticks	10	1 stick	18	1.3	61	58	104	104
Turkey	14	1 tablespoon	18	2.2	91	95	175	175
Turkey sticks	10	1 stick	18	1.4	61	62	107	109
Veal	14	1 tablespoon	16	2.2	84	89	169	169
Dinners								
Beef and egg noodles	14	1 tablespoon	8	0.4	17	18	30	31
Beef with vegetables	14	1 tablespoon	12	0.9	34	40	67	70
Chicken and noodles	14	1 tablespoon	7	0.3	13	13	24	23
Chicken and vegetables	14	1 tablespoon	13	1.0	39	46	79	87
Ham with vegetables	14	1 tablespoon	11	0.9	32	38	68	72
Macaroni and cheese	14	1 tablespoon	9	0.4	19	19	33	33
Macaroni, tomato, and beef	14	1 tablespoon	8	0.4	16	14	28	25
Split pea and ham	14	1 tablespoon	10	0.5	22	21	35	33
Turkey and rice	14	1 tablespoon	7	0.3	11	12	21	23
Turkey with vegetables	14	1 tablespoon	13	0.8	35	38	67	69
Veal with vegetables	14	1 tablespoon	10	0.9	34	42	68	69
Vegetables with bacon	14	1 tablespoon	10	0.3	11	12	18	21
Vegetables and beef	14	1 tablespoon	8	0.3	12	12	23	23
Vegetables and chicken	14	1 tablespoon	7	0.3	11	11	19	20
Vegetables and ham	14	1 tablespoon	7	0.3	13	14	26	27
Vegetables and lamb	14	1 tablespoon	7	0.3	12	10	22	18
Vegetables and liver	14	1 tablespoon	6	0.3	12	13	23	25
Vegetables and turkey	14	1 tablespoon	7	0.3	9	10	19	19
Fruit								
Applesauce	14	1 tablespoon	5	0	NA	1	NA	NA
Applesauce and apricot	14	1 tablespoon	7	0	NA	2	NA	NA
Applesauce and pineapple	14	1 tablespoon	6	0	NA	2	NA	NA
Apricots with tapioca	14	1 tablespoon	9	0	NA	1	NA	NA
Banana and pineapple with tapioca	14	1 tablespoon	9	0	NA	1	NA	NA
Banana with tapioca	14	1 tablespoon	10	0.1	NA	2	NA	NA
Peaches	14	1 tablespoon	10	0.1	NA	3	NA	NA
Pears	14	1 tablespoon	6	0	NA	2	NA	NA
Pears and pineapple	14	1 tablespoon	6	0	NA	1	NA	NA
Plums with tapioca	14	1 tablespoon	11	0	NA	1	NA	NA
Prunes with tapioca	14	1 tablespoon	10	0.1	NA	2	NA	NA
Fruit juice								
Apple	16	1 tablespoon	8	0	NA	1	NA	NA
Apple/cherry	16	1 tablespoon	6	0	NA	1	NA	NA

[*Continued*]

TABLE 57-3. Phenylalanine and Leucine Content of Some Junior Foods [*Concluded*]

Food Item	Serving Size				Phenylalanine		Leucine	
	Weight (g)	Household Measure	kcal	Protein (g)	Avg. (mg)	Gerber (mg)	Avg. (mg)	Gerber (mg)
Apple/grape	16	1 tablespoon	7	0	NA	1	NA	NA
Mixed fruit	16	1 tablespoon	7	0	NA	1	NA	NA
Orange	16	1 tablespoon	7	0.1	NA	1	NA	NA
Orange/apple	16	1 tablespoon	7	0.1	NA	1	NA	NA
Orange/apple/banana	16	1 tablespoon	7	0.1	NA	1	NA	NA
Orange/apricot	16	1 tablespoon	7	0.1	NA	1	NA	NA
Orange/pineapple	16	1 tablespoon	7	0.1	NA	1	NA	NA
Prune/orange	16	1 tablespoon	11	0.1	NA	1	NA	NA
Vegetable								
Beans, green	14	1 tablespoon	4	0.2	7	NA	11	NA
Beans, green, creamed	14	1 tablespoon	5	0.1	6	9	11	15
Carrots	14	1 tablespoon	5	0.1	4	3	5	4
Corn, creamed	14	1 tablespoon	9	0.2	7	10	20	20
Mixed vegetables	14	1 tablespoon	6	0.2	8	10	13	12
Spinach, creamed	14	1 tablespoon	6	0.4	17	21	38	35
Squash	14	1 tablespoon	3	0.1	4	5	7	7
Sweet potatoes	14	1 tablespoon	9	0.2	9	11	11	12
Cereal, dry								
Barley, dry	2	1 tablespoon	9	0.3	16	15	19	20
Cereal and egg yolks	14	1 tablespoon	7	0.3	13	13	25	25
High protein, dry	2	1 tablespoon	9	0.9	45	44	71	68
High protein with apples and oranges, dry	2	1 tablespoon	9	0.6	NA	32	NA	50
Mixed cereal, dry	2	1 tablespoon	9	0.3	16	15	25	24
Mixed cereal with applesauce and bananas	14	1 tablespoon	12	0.2	9	10	12	13
Mixed cereal with bananas, dry	2	1 tablespoon	9	0.3	13	12	23	23
Oatmeal, dry	2	1 tablespoon	10	0.3	13	19	26	27
Oatmeal with applesauce and bananas	14	1 tablespoon	11	0.2	10	11	14	16
Oatmeal with bananas, dry	2	1 tablespoon	9	0.3	15	15	23	23
Rice, dry	2	1 tablespoon	9	0.2	9	9	13	14
Rice with bananas, dry	2	1 tablespoon	10	0.2	10	10	20	20
Rice mixed with fruit	14	1 tablespoon	12	0.1	8	9	14	15
Teething biscuit	11	1 biscuit	43	1.2	57	NA	161	NA
Dessert								
Cherry vanilla pudding	14	1 tablespoon	10	0	NA	1	NA	NA
Chocolate custard pudding	14	1 tablespoon	13	0.3	12	17	27	NA
Cottage cheese with pineapple	14	1 tablespoon	11	0.4	15	19	26	NA
Dutch apple	14	1 tablespoon	10	0	NA	1	NA	NA
Peach cobbler	14	1 tablespoon	10	0	NA	2	NA	NA
Vanilla custard pudding	14	1 tablespoon	13	0.2	11	14	8	NA

NA = not available

TABLE 57-4. Phenylalanine and Leucine Content of Some Toddler Foods

Food Item	Serving Size: Weight (g)	Serving Size: Household Measure	kcal	Protein (g)	Phenylalanine: Avg. (mg)	Phenylalanine: Gerber (mg)	Leucine: Avg. (mg)	Leucine: Gerber (mg)
Meat or protein equivalents, dinners								
Beef and rice	14	1 tablespoon	12	0.7	28	NA	56	NA
Beef lasagna	14	1 tablespoon	11	0.6	26	25	46	49
Beef stew	14	1 tablespoon	7	0.7	29	29	55	55
Chicken stew	14	1 tablespoon	11	0.7	30	32	58	60
Spaghetti, tomato, and meat	14	1 tablespoon	11	0.8	34	NA	59	NA
Vegetables and ham	14	1 tablespoon	10	0.6	26	NA	46	NA
Vegetable and turkey	14	1 tablespoon	11	0.7	29	NA	56	NA

NA = not available

TABLE 57-5. Free Foods with Negligible Phenylalanine Content

Beverages
- Carbonated drinks
- Fruit-flavored drinks, powdered or canned
- Lemonade
- Limeade

Fats
- Butter, margarine, diet margarine
- Rich's Whipped Topping
- Shortening

Sweets
- Candies: cream mints, fondant, gum drops, hard candies, jelly beans, lollipops
- Jam, jelly
- Jello Quick
- Popsicles
- Sugars
- Syrups

Miscellaneous
- Cornstarch, tapioca
- Hunt's lemon pudding (canned)
- Seasonings: herbs, pepper, salt, spices
- Vinegar

REFERENCES CITED

1. Kaufman, S.; Holtzman, N. A.; Milstien, S.; Butler, I. J.; and Krumholz, A. 1975. Phenylketonuria due to a deficiency of dihydropteridine reductase. *N. Eng. J. Med.* 293:785.
2. Tourian, A. Y., and Sidbury, J. B. 1978. Phenylketonuria. In *The metabolic basis of inherited disease.* eds., J. B. Stanbury, J. B. Wyngaarden, and D. S. Fredrickson, pp. 240–255. 4th ed. New York: McGraw-Hill.
3. Komrower, G. M.; Sardharwalla, I. B.; Coutts, J. M. J.; and Ingham, D. 1979. Management of maternal phenylketonuria: An emerging clinical problem. *Br. Med. J.* 1:1383.
4. Nielsen, K. B.; Wamberg, E.; and Weber, J. 1979. Successful outcome of pregnancy in a phenylketonuric woman after low-phenylalanine diet introduced before conception. *Lancet* 1:1245.
5. Zaleski, L. A.; Casey, R. E.; and Zaleski, W. 1979. Maternal phenylketonuria: Dietary treatment during pregnancy. *Can. Med. Assoc. J.* 121:1591.
6. Koch, R.; Blaskovics, M.; Wenz, E.; Fishler, K.; and Schaeffler, G. 1974. Phenylalaninemia and phenylketonuria. In *Heritable disorders of amino acid metabolism: Patterns of clinical expression and genetic variation,* ed., W. L. Nyhan, pp. 109–140. New York: John Wiley.
7. Management of newborn infants with PKU. DHEW Publication No. (HSA) 78-5211, 1978.
8. Personal communication with R. J. Allen, M.D., Professor of Pediatric Neurology, University of Michigan Medical School, Ann Arbor, Mich., February 1980.
9. Firgaira, F. A.; Cotton, R. G. H.; and Danks, D. M. 1979. Dihydropteridine reductase deficiency diagnosis by assays on peripheral blood cells. *Lancet* 2:1260.
10. Danks, D. M.; Bartholome, K.; Clayton, B. E.; Curtius, H.; Gröbe, H.; Kaufman, S.; Leeming, R.; Pfleiderer, W.; Rembold, H.; and Rey, F. 1978. Malignant hyperphenylalaninaemia–Current status (June 1977). *J. Inher. Metab. Dis.* 1:49.
11. Kaufman, S.; Berlow, S.; Summer, G. K.; Milstien, S.; Schulman, J. D.; Orloff, S.; Spielberg, S.; and Pueschel, S. 1978. Hyperphenylalaninemia due to a deficiency of biopterin: A variant form of phenylketonuria. *N. Eng. J. Med.* 299:673.
12. Niederwieser, A.; Curtius, H.-Ch.; Bettoni, O.; Bieri, J.; Schircks, B.; Viscontini, M.; and Schaub, J. 1979. Atypical phenylketonuria caused by 7,8-dihydrobiopterin synthetase deficiency. *Lancet* 1:131.
13. Hsia, D. Y.-Y. 1965. Forum: Nutrition in prevention and treatment of specific disease: Hereditary metabolic diseases. *Proceedings Western Hemisphere Nutrition Congress,* Council on Foods and Nutrition. American Medical Association, Chicago: November 8–11, 1965.
14. Wannemacher, R. W., Jr. 1974. Amino acid losses and plasma changes during infection. In *Proceedings of collaborative study of children treated for phenylketonuria,* ed., P. B. Acosta. Sixth Nutritionists' Conference, March 1974.

OTHER REFERENCES

Allen, R. J., and Schwartz, E. 1976. Clinical study of diet discontinuation in PKU—A ten-year review. In *Summary of proceedings of collaborative study of children treated for phenylketonuria.* Twelfth General Medical Conference, 1976.

REFERENCES FOR THE LAY PUBLIC

Acosta, P. B., and Wenz, E. 1977. *Management of PKU for infants and pre-school children.* DHEW Publication No. (HSA) 77-5209.

1978. *Living with PKU.* Denver: University of Colorado Medical Center.

Schuett, V. E. 1977. *Low-protein cookery for phenylketonuria.* Madison: University of Wisconsin Press.

58

Maple Syrup Urine Disease

INDICATIONS FOR USE

The diet is indicated for infants and children with classical maple syrup urine disease (MSUD). Diagnosis is confirmed by plasma levels of leucine, isoleucine, and valine each greater than 10 mg/100 ml. Normal values are leucine 1.5–3.0 mg/100 ml, isoleucine 0.8–1.5 mg/100 ml, and valine 2.0–3.0 mg/100 ml. The infant appears normal at birth, but, after ingestion of milk or other protein-containing foods, the inborn error of metabolism becomes apparent. Symptoms of untreated disease include poor sucking ability, vomiting, lethargy, convulsions, muscle hypertonicity, and the presence of keto acids in the urine, giving the characteristic maple syrup odor. The diet must be continued for life, although it may be possible to allow less stringent control with increasing age. (1) Prompt medical and dietary intervention is crucial to prevent irreversible neurological damage to the infant.

Several variant forms of MSUD have been identified that are generally less severe than classical MSUD and that occasionally are episodic. (2) In one form, the infant responds to a limited protein intake and supplemental thiamin. (3) Thiamin pyrophosphate is a co-enzyme involved in the oxidative decarboxylation of the branched-chain amino acids. In episodic forms, abnormalities are often present during stress, such as infections.

DESCRIPTION

MSUD is a rare, autosomal recessive disease, also known as branched-chain ketoaciduria. An enzymatic defect is present in the second step of the metabolism of leucine, isoleucine, and valine, the essential branched-chain amino acids. The transamination process is intact, but the oxidative decarboxylation step is impaired. (1) Excessive levels of the branched-chain amino acids and metabolites accumulate in body fluids.

The treatment for MSUD is restriction of the three essential branched-chain amino acids in the diet. Because it is generally representative of the levels of all three essential branched-chain amino acids, the leucine level in the blood and in foodstuffs is used for monitoring the individual with MSUD. However, blood levels of the three branched-chain amino acids may vary. Individualization of the diet and supplementation or restriction of individual branched-chain amino acids may be necessary.

Plasma leucine levels above 10 mg/100 ml are frequently accompanied by neurologic symptoms. The effect of each individual amino acid may be different and unrelated to these numerical blood levels. (4) Since secondary metabolic pathways can be affected, the central nervous system effects are not directly proportional to the amino acid blood levels. (4)

The goals of nutritional management are to

- Provide a diet in which the essential branched-chain amino acids are limited to the amounts required to maintain normal growth and development of central nervous system. (5, 6)
- Maintain a blood leucine level of 5–10 mg/100 ml. (7)
- Supply adequate energy, protein, and all other nutrients to meet nutritional needs and to allow for normal growth and development.
- Educate the family on the management of MSUD using a health care

team approach, including physician, dietitian, psychologist, and nurse clinician.

Dietary management is individualized depending on age and blood levels of leucine, isoleucine, and valine. The diet is prescribed in milligrams of leucine per 24 hours and generally allows 300–800 mg per 24 hours. (8) Frequent home-administered tests for the presence of leucine ketoacids in urine and blood samples are utilized to monitor control. Dietary modifications are made based on blood and urine values, height and weight, and the presence of neurological symptoms.

During illness or febrile conditions, efforts must be made to supply adequate amino acids and fluids to prevent tissue catabolism. Careful adherence to the dietary prescription is absolutely necessary.

GUIDELINES FOR NUTRITIONAL MANAGEMENT

The amount of branched-chain amino acids in the diet is controlled by calculating the leucine content of the diet. The leucine content is representative of the total amount of essential branched-chain amino acids present in foods. Because branched-chain amino acids are widely distributed in foods, the MSUD diet places extreme limitations on food intake. The diet is largely synthetic, low in protein, high in carbohydrates, especially sugars, and high in fat. (8)

Synthetic formulas used for the MSUD diet are MSUD Amino Acids added to Product 80056 and MSUD Diet Powder (refer to Tables 48-2 and 57-1). MSUD Amino Acids[1] is a purified amino acid mixture void of leucine, isoleucine, and valine. Product 80056 is a carbohydrate, fat, vitamin, and mineral preparation. MSUD Diet Powder is an amino acid, carbohydrate, fat, vitamin, and mineral preparation free of leucine, isoleucine, and valine. These formulas must be supplemented with natural whole protein to supply a source of the essential branched-chain amino acids.

Since the incidence of MSUD is low, experience with nutritional treatment is not yet standardized and requires a high degree of individualization and continual monitoring. The following procedure is provided as a general guideline. Blood leucine levels, urinary ketoacid levels, the presence of neurological symptoms, and growth and development must be monitored to make appropriate dietary adjustments. Procedures to follow when planning a low-leucine diet are as follows:

1. After diagnosis, the MSUD Amino Acids–Product 80056 formula or MSUD Diet Powder is used without an added source of whole protein until blood levels of the three branched-chain amino acids are within a normal range. During acute, catastrophic bouts of illness, dialysis may be necessary to reduce blood levels. (9)

   Method 1. MSUD Amino Acids–Product 80056 formula. The amount of Product 80056 provided is based on appetite and calorie requirements for growth. Product 80056 is mixed with water to provide a formula of 20 kcal per ounce. MSUD Amino Acids, supplied in an amount guided by the recommended dietary allowances for protein, are added to the Product 80056 formula.

[1] MSUD Amino Acids is available from Grand Island Biochemical Company, 3175 Staley Road, Grand Island, New York 14072, Med. No. 69243.

Method 2. MSUD Diet Powder. The amount of MSUD Diet Powder provided is based on the recommended dietary allowances for protein. One hundred grams of the powder provides 8.2 g protein void of leucine, isoleucine, and valine. The powder is diluted with water to provide a formula of 20 kcal per ounce. The dilution may be modified for variations of individual intake.

2. When the blood levels of the branched-chain amino acids are within normal range, a source of natural protein, such as infant formula or diluted evaporated milk, is added to the diet to provide a source of branched-chain amino acids. The amount added is based on the dietary leucine prescription. The milk may be mixed with the MSUD Amino Acids–Product 80056 formula or the MSUD Diet Powder formula. The amount of leucine per ounce of the mixture is calculated so that leucine intake can be monitored.

   Families are instructed to measure and weigh formulas and foods carefully and to keep accurate diet diaries, recording leucine and protein intake.

3. Solid foods are added early. Rice cereal is usually added first as it is less allergenic than other cereal grains. When the infant has refused a portion of the formula containing whole protein, an appropriate amount of rice cereal is given to reach the prescribed leucine level.

4. Other foods are added in the sequence of fruits, meat–vegetable combinations, and vegetable items. Fruits contain negligible quantities of the branched-chain amino acids and are considered free foods in the diet. Other foods with negligible leucine content—free foods—are included to supply adequate calories (Table 58-1). The leucine content of some foods is listed in Tables 57-2, 57-3, and 57-4. When the exact value for leucine content is not available, leucine content is estimated by utilizing the ratio of milligrams leucine per gram protein of various food proteins (refer to Table 58-2). (8) To estimate the leucine content of a food item, the number of grams of protein in the serving is multiplied by the number of milligrams of leucine per gram of protein contained in that food item. One ounce of beef containing 8 g of protein would contain

   $$8 \text{ g protein} \times 82 \text{ mg leucine/g protein} = 656 \text{ mg leucine}$$

   Due to the highly refined carbohydrate content of the MSUD diet, a dental hygiene program is encouraged early in the child's life to prevent excessive formation of dental caries.

Three case examples with dietary calculations follow demonstrating both methods 1 and 2 for each case:

Example 1

Twenty-one-day-old infant newly diagnosed with classical MSUD.
WEIGHT: 3.8 kg
DIETARY PRESCRIPTION: 0 leucine until blood levels return to normal

METHOD 1: MSUD Amino Acids–Product 80056 formula.
Amounts provided will vary depending on the infant's intake. Adjustments will have to be made to be certain that the infant is obtaining adequate amino acids in the amount of formula being consumed.

Method 2: MSUD Diet Powder formula.
MSUD Diet Powder is diluted to 20 kcal per ounce and provided as desired.

Example 2

Four-week-old infant with classical MSUD consuming 28 ounces formula and rice cereal.
Weight: 4.6 kg
Dietary prescription: 425 mg leucine

Method 1: MSUD Amino Acid-Product 80056 formula.

Food Item	Serving Size		kcal	Protein (g)	Leucine (mg)
	Weight (g)	Household Measure			
MSUD Amino Acids (11.5 g) and Product 80056 (90 g) diluted to 20 kcal/ounce	735	24.5 ounces	490	11.5	0
Evaporated whole milk diluted 1:1 with water	105	3.5 ounces	74	3.5	368
Rice cereal, dry[1]	8	4 tablespoons	36	0.8	56
Total			600	15.8	424

[1] Data for Gerber products used.

Method 2: MSUD Diet Powder formula.

Food Item	Serving Size		kcal	Protein (g)	Leucine (mg)
	Weight (g)	Household Measure			
MSUD Diet Powder diluted to 20 kcal/ounce	735	24.5 ounces	490	7.4	0
Evaporated whole milk diluted 1:1 with water	105	3.5 ounces	74	3.5	368
Rice cereal, dry[1]	8	4 tablespoons	36	0.8	56
Total			600	11.7	424

[1] Data for Gerber products used.

Example 3

Six-month-old infant with classical MSUD consuming 28 ounces formula and baby foods.
Weight: 7.0 kg

Method 1: MSUD Amino Acids–Product 80056 formula.

Food Item	Serving Size: Weight (g)	Serving Size: Household Measure	kcal	Protein (g)	Leucine (mg)
MSUD Amino Acids (17 g) and Product 80056 (100 g) diluted to 28 ounces	840	28 ounces	490	17.0	0
Rice cereal, dry[1]	12	6 tablespoons	54	1.2	84
Strained baby dinner, chicken with vegetables[1]	56	4 tablespoons	44	3.6	280
Strained green beans[1]	28	2 tablespoons	8	0.4	24
Strained creamed corn[1]	28	2 tablespoons	16	0.4	40
Strained apple-sauce[1]	42	3 tablespoons	18	0.1	—
Sugar	8	2 teaspoons	30	—	—
Margarine	10	2 pats	72	—	—
Total			732	22.7	428

[1] Data from Gerber products used.

Method 2: MSUD Diet Powder formula.

Food Item	Serving Size: Weight (g)	Serving Size: Household Measure	kcal	Protein (g)	Leucine (mg)
MSUD Diet Powder diluted to 20 kcal/ ounce	840	28 ounces	560	8.4	0
Rice cereal, dry[1]	12	6 tablespoons	54	1.2	84
Strained baby dinner, chicken with vegetables[1]	56	4 tablespoons	44	3.6	280
Strained green beans[1]	28	2 tablespoons	8	0.4	24
Strained creamed corn[1]	28	2 tablespoons	16	0.4	40
Strained apple-sauce[1]	42	3 tablespoons	18	0.1	—
Sugar	8	2 teaspoons	30	—	—
Total			730	14.1	428

[1] Data from Gerber products used.

NUTRIENT ADEQUACY

One hundred grams of Product 80056 will meet the recommended dietary allowances for the infant from birth to 6 months of age except for protein. (10) The protein requirement is met by MSUD amino acids and the sources of natural whole protein added to the diet. Adequate sodium will need to be supplied in the preparation of the feedings. (10) Vitamin–mineral supplementation is necessary for the older child. (8)

One quart of MSUD Diet Powder formula will meet the recommended dietary allowances for the infant except for protein. (10) Adequate protein is supplied by the addition of small amounts of natural whole protein to the diet. To reach the RDA, vitamin–mineral supplementation is necessary for the infant consuming less than one quart of formula and for the older child. (8)

TABLES

TABLE 58-1. Free Foods with Negligible Leucine Content

Beverage
Carbonated drinks
Fruit juices
Fruit-flavored drinks, powdered or canned
Lemonade
Limeade
Fat
Butter, margarine
Mayonnaise[1]
Rich's Whipped Topping
Salad dressing (except those containing cheese)
Sweet
Candies: cream mints, fondant, gum drops, hard candies, jelly beans, lollipops
Fruit float
Fruit butters (e.g., apple, cherry)
Honey
Hunt's lemon pudding (canned)
Jam, jelly
Marshmallows
Popsicles
Rennet Danish dessert
Sugars
Syrups
Miscellaneous
Cornstarch
Fruit
Low-protein bread
Low-protein pasta
Seasonings: herbs, pepper, salt, spices
Vinegar

[1] Limit amounts used during a day due to the egg.

TABLE 58-2. Protein–Leucine Ratios (Milligrams Leucine Per Gram Protein) of Various Types of Protein Foods (8)[1]

Food	Leucine (mg/g protein)
Beef	82
Chicken	72
Eggs (chicken)	88
Gelatin	34
Halibut	76
Lamb	77
Liver (beef or chicken)	92
Milk, cow's	98
Peanuts	70
Pork	74
Salmon	76
Shrimp	76
Turkey	77
Veal	73
Corn	130
Oats	75
Potatoes	50
Rice	86
Wheat flour	
White	77
Whole grain	67

REFERENCES CITED

1. Snyderman, S. E. 1978. The treatment of branched-chain ketoacidemia. In *Diet therapy for MSUD and organic acidurias.* Amino Acid Subcommittee, Nutriture Committee, American Academy of Pediatrics.
2. Zipf, W. B.; Hieber, V. C.; and Allen, R. J. 1979. Valine-toxic intermittent maple syrup urine disease: A previously unrecognized variant. *Pediatrics* 63:286.
3. Scriver, C. R.; Clow, C. L.; Mackenzie, S.; and Delvin, E. 1971. Thiamine-responsive maple-syrup-urine disease. *Lancet* 1:310.
4. Communication with R. J. Allen, M.D., Professor of Pediatric Neurology, University of Michigan Medical School, Ann Arbor, Mich. April 1980.
5. Westall, R. G. 1963. Dietary treatment of a child with maple syrup urine disease (branched-chain ketoaciduria). *Arch. Dis. Child.* 38:485.
6. Bell, L.; Chao, E.; and Milne, J. 1979. Dietary management of maple-sirup-urine disease: Extension of equivalency systems. *J. Am. Dietet. A.* 74:357.
7. Allen, R. J.; Frey, H. J.; Fleming, L. M.; and Owings, C. L. 1972. Semi-quantitation of leucine, isoleucine, and valine by thin-layer chromatography in management of maple-syrup urine disease. *Clin. Chem.* 18:413.
8. Noel, M. B.; Stanley, P. B.; Girz, J. C.; and Allen, R. J. 1976. Dietary treatment of maple sirup urine disease (branched-chain ketoaciduria). *J. Am. Dietet. A.* 69:62.
9. Allen, R. J.; Bauer, R. C.; Fleming, L. M.; and Frey, H. J. 1971. Peritoneal dialysis in the modification of neurologic and metabolic abnormalities of branched-chain ketoaciduria (MSUD). Read by title, Society for Pediatric Research, April 1971.
10. Mead Johnson. 1979. *Products for dietary management of inborn errors of metabolism and other special feeding problems.* Evansville, Ind.: Mead Johnson.

OTHER REFERENCES

Dancis, J., and Levitz, M. 1978. Abnormalities of branched-chain amino acid metabolism. In *The metabolic basis of inherited disease,* eds., J. B. Stanbury, J. B. Wyngaarden, and D. S. Fredrickson, pp. 397–410. 4th ed. New York: McGraw-Hill.

Menkes, J. H.; Hurst, P. L.; and Craig, J. M. 1954. A new syndrome: Progressive familial infantile cerebral dysfunction associated with an unusual urinary substance. *Pediatrics* 14:462.

Ketogenic

INDICATIONS FOR USE

The ketogenic diet, either the traditional or the medium-chain triglyceride form, may be indicated as an adjunct to drug therapy for children with seizure disorders for whom medications alone have failed to control seizure activity. (1, 2) The diet is usually more effective in children under age ten. (3) Disadvantages of the traditional ketogenic diet are elevated lipids, possible renal calculi, loss of appetite, and poor acceptance by the child and family. (4, 5) The use of medium-chain triglycerides in the diet prevents lipid elevation and increases acceptability but may cause diarrhea, nausea, abdominal cramps, or mild hypoglycemia. (5) The anticonvulsant effect of the ketogenic diet may diminish over time. (6)

DESCRIPTION

In 1924 it was reported that fasting and the resulting ketosis decreased the frequency of seizures in epileptic children. (7) The ketogenic diet was developed to promote ketosis without starvation. (8) The anticonvulsant effect appears to be associated with elevation of ketone bodies in plasma, particularly beta-hydroxybutyrate and acetoacetate. (1) Ketonemia may have a direct anticonvulsant effect or may act by inducing secondary changes in cerebral metabolism. (1, 3)

The original ketogenic diet restricted protein to 1 g per kilogram body weight and allowed only 10–15 g carbohydrate per day. (8) The discovery that medium-chain triglycerides were more ketogenic than dietary fats has allowed the diet to be liberalized with increased amounts of carbohydrate and protein when MCT oil is used. (5)

The goals of the ketogenic diet are to

- Provide a diet with sufficient fat and sufficient restriction of carbohydrate and protein so that fat is incompletely oxidized and that the ketone bodies, acetone, acetoacetate, and beta-hydroxybutyrate, are formed.
- Provide sufficient calories, protein, and other nutrients required for normal growth and development.

GUIDELINES FOR NUTRITIONAL MANAGEMENT

Fasting prior to starting the traditional or MCT ketogenic diet is sometimes recognized. (1, 3) At University Hospital children are not fasted prior to initiation of the diet. A strongly positive urine reaction should be obtained with ketotest tablets during treatment.

Regardless of which diet is used, care must be taken to eliminate sources of sugar that are not calculated as part of the diet. This includes sugars in medications, syrups, sugar-coated pills, and toothpastes. At least 32 ounces of fluid should be provided each day to help maintain adequate hydration.

Traditional Ketogenic Diet (9)

The traditional ketogenic diet supplies approximately 90% of dietary calories from fat. Protein is provided in the amount of 1 g per kilogram body weight per day. A 4:1 ketogenic-to-antiketogenic ratio is used in planning the diet to achieve the ketogenic effect. Fat is ketogenic; protein and carbohydrate are antiketogenic. Calculation of the diet is made by using the dietary unit. One unit of the 4:1 ratio diet contains 4 g of fat and 1 g of carbohydrate and protein combined. One unit provides 40 kcal: 36 kcal from fat and 4 kcal from carbohydrate and protein.

The diet is planned using ketogenic food exchange groups listed in Tables 59-1 and 59-2. (Food composition tables could also be used.) A milk group is not included because of milk's high carbohydrate and protein content; whipping cream is used as a substitute. The carbohydrate food group is divided into three sections; the allowed number of exchanges from the carbohydrate group should be divided equally among these three. Lipomul, a fat emulsion, is used to meet the dietary fat prescription when adequate fat from other food sources is not consumed; 1 tablespoon (15 ml) provides 10 g of fat (refer to Chapter 3 for more complete nutrient content of Lipomul).

The procedure for calculating a traditional ketogenic diet is as follows:

Steps	*Example*
1. Establish calorie requirement using recommended dietary allowances.	Two-year-old child WEIGHT: 13 kg CALORIE REQUIREMENT: 1300 kcal
2. Determine total number of dietary units allowed. $\frac{\text{kcal requirement}}{\text{40 kcal/unit}} = \text{Total units}$	$\frac{\text{1300 kcal}}{\text{40 kcal/unit}} = \text{32.5 units}$
3. Determine the amount of fat to be provided daily. Total units × 4 g fat/unit = Daily g fat	32.5 × 4 g fat/unit = 130 g fat daily
4. Determine the amount of protein allowed in the diet. 1 g protein per kg body weight × kg body weight = Daily g protein	1 g protein/kg body weight × 13 kg = 13 g protein daily
5. Determine the amount of carbohydrate allowed in the diet. Total units − g protein = Daily g carbohydrate	32.5 − 13 g protein = 19.5 g carbohydrate daily
6. Using the calculated prescription for daily fat, protein, and carbohydrate, plan the diet using the nutrient values of the food groups listed in Table 59-1.	Daily dietary prescription: Carbohydrate: 19.5 g Protein: 13 g Fat: 130 g

Food Group	Amount Per Day	Carbohydrate (g)	Protein (g)	Fat (g)
Fat	11 exchanges	—	—	55
Meat	1½ exchanges	—	11	7.5
Carbohydrate	1½ exchanges	15	—	—
Whipping cream	½ cup	4	2	45
Lipomul	2 tablespoons + 2 teaspoons	—	—	27
Total		19	13	134.5

7. Divide the diet into three meals with the food groups evenly distributed among meals. Lipomul is provided between meals as it may influence the flavor of other foods and may decrease appetite.

Sample Pattern	Sample Menu
Breakfast	*Breakfast*
½ carbohydrate exchange	Puffed Wheat, 6 tablespoons
½ protein exchange	Hard-cooked egg, ½
3 fat exchanges	Margarine, 3 teaspoons
¼ cup whipping cream	Whipping cream, ¼ cup
	Artificially sweetened lemonade, ½ cup
Midmorning	*Midmorning*
2 teaspoons Lipomul	Lipomul, 2 teaspoons in artificially sweetened beverage
Lunch	*Lunch*
½ carbohydrate exchange	Pear half, 1 tablespoon
½ protein exchange	Tuna fish, 2 tablespoons
4 fat exchanges	Mayonnaise, 4 teaspoons
2 tablespoons whipping cream	Whipping cream, 2 tablespoons
	Artificially sweetened gelatin, ½ cup
Midafternoon	*Midafternoon*
1 tablespoon Lipomul	Lipomul, 1 tablespoon in artificially sweetened beverage
Dinner	*Dinner*
½ carbohydrate exchange	Carrots, cooked, ½ cup
½ protein exchange	Cheese, ½ ounce
4 fat exchanges	Margarine, 2 teaspoons
2 tablespoons whipping cream	Mayonnaise, 2 teaspoons
	Whipping cream, 2 tablespoons
	Celery, raw
Evening	*Evening*
1 tablespoon Lipomul	Lipomul, 1 tablespoon in artificially sweetened beverage

Medium-Chain Triglyceride Ketogenic Diet (5, 6)

The MCT ketogenic diet provides 50–70% of calories from MCT oil (refer to Chapter 3 for nutrient content). Protein is provided to meet the recommended dietary allowances for age. Total carbohydrate and protein in the diet supplies no more than 29% of total calories. Remaining calories are provided in the form of dietary fat. The ketogenic or the diabetic food exchange groups can be used for planning the diet.

MCT oil contains 8.3 kcal/g and weighs 14 g per tablespoon (15 ml). MCT oil is initially provided at an amount equal to 60% of calories. Urine testing for ketones is utilized to determine if an increased or decreased amount of MCT oil is appropriate. The oil is usually blended with skim milk and flavorings or juices or is used in cooking. The MCT oil should be taken with other foods and consumed slowly throughout the meal to prevent abdominal cramps and nausea.

The diet is planned with at least three well-balanced meals per day. Equal amounts of carbohydrate, protein, and fat at each meal are not necessary. The MCT oil is divided evenly among meals.

The procedure for calculating an MCT ketogenic diet is as follows:

Steps	***Example***
1. Establish calorie requirement.	Two-year-old child WEIGHT: 13 kg CALORIE REQUIREMENT: 1300 kcal
2. Determine the amount of MCT oil to be included in the diet.	
60% of total kcal = Kilocalories from MCT oil	$.60 \times 1300 \text{ kcal} = 780 \text{ kcal}$
$\frac{\text{Kilocalories from MCT oil}}{8.3 \text{ kcal/g MCT oil}}$ = Grams MCT oil	$\frac{780 \text{ kcal}}{8.3 \text{ kcal/g MCT oil}} = 94 \text{ g MCT oil}$
$\frac{\text{Grams MCT oil}}{14 \text{ g/tablespoon MCT oil}}$ = Tablespoon MCT oil	$\frac{94 \text{ g MCT oil}}{14 \text{ g/tablespoons MCT oil}} = 6.7 \text{ tablespoons MCT oil}$ = 6 tablespoons + 2 teaspoons MCT oil
3. Determine the number of calories to come from other foods.	
Total kilocalories − kilocalories from MCT oil = Kilocalories from other foods	1300 kcal − 780 kcal = 520 kcal from other foods
4. Determine the number of calories allowed from carbohydrate and protein.	
29% of total kilocalories	$.29 \times 1300$ kcal = 377 kcal from carbohydrate and protein
5. Determine the amount of protein to be included in the diet. Use RDA for age.	23 g protein (RDA for two-year-old child)
Calculate the number of calories to come from protein.	
Grams protein × 4 kcal/g = Kilocalories from protein	$23 \text{ g} \times 4 \text{ kcal/g} = 92$ kcal from protein

6. Determine the maximum amount of carbohydrate allowed in the diet.

(Kilocalories from carbohydrate + protein) − kilocalories from protein = Kilocalories from carbohydrate

377 kcal − 92 kcal = 283 kcal

$$\frac{\text{Kilocalories from carbohydrate}}{4 \text{ kcal/g carbohydrate}} = \text{Grams carbohydrate}$$

$$\frac{285 \text{ kcal}}{4 \text{ kcal/g}} = 71 \text{ g carbohydrate}$$

7. Determine the minimum amount of dietary fat to be provided in the diet.

Kilocalories from other foods − (kilocalories from protein + kilocalories from carbohydrate) = Kilocalories from fat

520 kcal − (92 kcal + 285 kcal) = 143 kcal

$$\frac{\text{Kilocalories from fat}}{9 \text{ kcal/g fat}} = \text{Grams fat}$$

$$\frac{143 \text{ kcal}}{9 \text{ kcal/g}} = 16 \text{ g fat}$$

8. Using food exchange groups, plan the diet according to the calculated prescription.

Daily dietary prescription:
MCT oil: 95 g; 6.7 tablespoons (6 tablespoons + 2 teaspoons)
Carbohydrate: ≤71 g
Protein: 23 g
Fat: ≥16 g

Food Group[1]	Amount Per Day	Carbohydrate (g)	Protein (g)	Fat (g)	MCT (g)
Milk, skim	1½	18	12	—	—
Vegetable	1	5	2	—	—
Fruit	1½	15	—	—	—
Bread	2	30	4	—	—
Meat	1	—	7	5	—
Fat	3	—	—	15	—
MCT oil	6 tablespoons + 2 teaspoons				94
Total		68	25	20	94

[1] Diabetic food exchange groups used; refer to Chapter 25.

9. Divide food into at least three meals per day.

Sample Pattern	Sample Menu
Breakfast	*Breakfast*
½ Skim milk exchange	Skim milk, ½ cup
1 Fruit exchange	Banana, ½
½ Bread exchange	Puffed Wheat, ½ cup
2 tablespoons MCT oil	MCT oil, 2 tablespoons mixed into the skim milk
	Artificially sweetened lemonade, ½ cup
Lunch	*Lunch*
½ Skim milk exchange	Skim milk, ½ cup
½ Fruit exchange	Pear, ½ small
½ Bread exchange	Bread, ½ slice
½ Meat exchange	Tunafish, 2 tablespoons
1 Fat exchange	Salad dressing, 2 teaspoons
2 tablespoons + 1 teaspoon MCT oil	MCT oil, 2 tablespoons + 1 teaspoon mixed into tuna or skim milk
	Artificially sweetened beverage, ½ cup
Dinner	*Dinner*
½ Skim milk exchange	Skim milk, ½ cup
1 Vegetable exchange	Carrots, cooked, ½ cup
½ Bread exchange	Potatoes, mashed, ¼ cup
½ Meat exchange	Beef, cooked, ½ ounce
1 Fat exchange	Margarine, 1 teaspoon
2 tablespoons + 1 teaspoon MCT oil	MCT oil, 2 tablespoons + 1 teaspoon mixed into potatoes or skim milk
	Artificially sweetened lemonade, ½ cup
Evening	*Evening*
½ Bread exchange	Graham crackers, 1 square
1 Fat exchange	Margarine, 1 teaspoon
	Artificially sweetened beverage, 1 cup

NUTRIENT ADEQUACY

The ketogenic diet is deficient in vitamin D, vitamin E, B vitamins, iron, and calcium and may be deficient in others. (1, 6) Protein may be deficient in the traditional ketogenic diet. Nonsugar-containing vitamin–mineral and calcium supplements are recommended. (1) The iodine requirement can be met by adding ⅛ teaspoon of iodized salt to the diet per day. (6)

TABLES

TABLE 59-1. Nutrient Content of One Exchange, Traditional Ketogenic Diet

Food Exchange Group	Amount	Carbohydrate (g)	Protein (g)	Fat (g)	kcal
Fat	1 exchange	—	—	5	45
Meat	1 exchange	—	7	5	73
Carbohydrate	1 exchange	10	—	—	40
I Bread/cereal					
II Fruit					
III Vegetable					
Whipping cream, unwhipped	1 cup (8 fluid ounces)	8	5	90	862
Lipomul	1 tablespoon (15 ml)	—	—	10	90

Table 59-2. Traditional Ketogenic Diet Food Exchange System

Group	Food Item	One Exchange (serving size)
Fat	Avocado	1/8
	Avocado, mashed	2 tablespoons
	Butter, lard, margarine	1 teaspoon
	Cream cheese	1 tablespoon
	Fried bacon rinds	8 pieces or 1/2 cup
	Lipomul	1/2 tablespoon
	Oil, vegetable	1 teaspoon
	Olives	3 large or 5 small
	Salad dressings	
	Mayonnaise	1 teaspoon
	Mayonnaise types (Thousand Island, Russian)	2 teaspoons
	Vinegar/oil types	2 teaspoons
	Shortening or hydrogenated fats	1 teaspoon
	Sour cream	2 tablespoons
Meat	Bacon, crisp	3 slices
	Cheese, unprocessed	1 ounce
	Clams, oysters, shrimp, lobster, crab	5 small or 1 ounce
	Egg	1
	Frankfurters, all meat	1
	Lunchmeat, all meat	1 ounce
	Meat, cooked (beef, fish, lamb, pork, poultry, veal, wild game)	1 ounce or 1/4 cup
	Sardines	3
	Sausage, ground	2 links
	Sausage, Vienna, all meat	3
Carbohydrate I		
Bread and cereal	Bread, thin or diet	1 slice
	Biscuit, roll, muffin, 2 in. diameter	1
	Bun, hamburger or weiner	1/2 bun
	Corn bread, 1 1/2 in. cube	1
	English muffin, small	1
	Melba toast	3 slices
	Pancake, 4 in. diameter	1
	Tortilla, 6 in. diameter	1
	Waffle, 3 in. square	1
	Cereal, cooked	1/3 cup
	Cereal, flakes	1/2 cup
	Cereal, puffed	3/4 cup
	Crackers, 2 in. square	3
	Grits, cooked	1/3 cup
	Macaroni, noodles, rice, spaghetti, cooked	1/4 cup
	Popcorn, popped	1 cup
	Cornstarch	1 1/2 tablespoons
	Flour	1 1/2 tablespoons
	Tapioca	1 1/2 tablespoons

[*Continued*]

TABLE 59-2. Traditional Ketogenic Diet Food Exchange System [*Continued*]

Group	Food Item	One Exchange (serving size)
Carbohydrate II		
Fruit	Apple	½ large or 1 small 2 in.
	Apple juice, cider	⅓ cup (3 ounces)
	Applesauce	½ cup
	Apricots, fresh	2 medium
	Apricots, dried or canned	4 halves
	Banana	3 inch long (½ small)
	Berries	
	Blackberries	½ cup
	Blueberries	½ cup
	Raspberries	½ cup
	Strawberries	¾ cup
	Cantaloupe, 6 in. diameter	¼
	Cherries	10 large or 15 small
	Dates	2 small
	Figs, fresh or dried	1
	Fruit cocktail	½ cup
	Grapefruit	½
	Grapefruit juice	½ cup (4 ounces)
	Grapefruit sections	½ cup
	Grapes	12
	Grape juice	¼ cup (2 ounces)
	Guava	½ medium
	Honeydew melon, 6 in. diameter	⅛
	Lemon	1 large
	Lime	1 medium
	Mango	½ small
	Nectarine	1 small
	Orange	1 small
	Orange juice	½ cup (4 ounces)
	Orange sections	½ cup
	Papaya	¾ cup
	Peach	1 medium
	Peach halves	2
	Peach slices	½ cup
	Pear	½ large or 1 small
	Pear halves	2 small
	Persimmon	1 medium
	Pineapple	½ cup or 1½ rings
	Pineapple juice	⅓ cup (3 ounces)
	Plums	2 medium
	Prunes, dried	2 medium
	Prune juice	¼ cup (2 ounces)
	Raisins	½ ounce or 2 tablespoons

Table 59-2. Traditional Ketogenic Diet Food Exchange System [*Continued*]

Group	Food Item		One Exchange (serving size)
	Rhubarb		1 cup
	Tangerine		1 medium
	Tomato juice		1 cup (8 ounces)
	Watermelon, 3 in. × $\frac{1}{2}$ in. slice		1
	Watermelon diced		1 cup
Carbohydrate III Vegetable			
	Alfalfa sprouts	Kohlrabi	$\frac{2}{3}$ cup cooked or raw
	Artichoke	Mushrooms	
	Asparagus	Okra	
	Bamboo shoots	Onions	
	Bean sprouts	Pea pods	
	Beans, string or green	Pepper, green and pimiento	
	Beans, wax	Pickles, unsweetened	
	Beets	Rutabaga	
	Broccoli	Sauerkraut	
	Brussels sprouts	Squash, summer	
	Cabbage	Tomatoes	
	Carrots	Tomato juice	
	Cauliflower	Tomato sauce, unsweetened	
	Celery	Turnips	
	Chard	Vegetable juice	
	Cucumber	Zucchini	
	Eggplant		
	Greens: beet, collard, dandelion, kale, mustard, spinach, turnip		
	Mixed vegetables		$\frac{1}{2}$ cup
	Water chestnuts		5
	Corn		$\frac{1}{4}$ cup
	Beans and peas, dried, cooked		$\frac{1}{3}$ cup
	Parsnips		$\frac{1}{2}$ cup
	Peas, green		$\frac{1}{3}$ cup
	Potatoes, sweet or yam		$\frac{1}{4}$ cup
	Potatoes, white		$\frac{1}{3}$ cup or $\frac{1}{2}$
	Pumpkin		$\frac{1}{2}$ cup
	Squash, winter		$\frac{1}{3}$ cup
Free foods	Artificial sweeteners (check for "no calories")		As desired
	Clear bouillon		
	Clear broth		
	Cocoa (unsweetened plain)		
	Coffee		
	Dietetic carbonated beverages (1 kcal per 6 ounces)		

TABLE 59-2. Traditional Ketogenic Diet Food Exchange System [*Concluded*]

Group	Food Item	One Exchange (serving size)
	D'zerta gelatin	
	Extracts	
	Mustard	
	Pepper	
	Pickles, sour and dill	
	Salt	
	Spices	
	Tea	
	Unflavored gelatin	
	Unsweetened Kool-Aid	
	Unsweetened lemonade	
	Vegetables	
	Chicory	
	Chinese cabbage	
	Chives	
	Endive	
	Escarole	
	Lettuce	
	Parsley	
	Radishes	
	Romaine	
	Watercress	
	Vinegar	
	Water	

REFERENCES CITED

1. Dodson, W. E.; Prensky, A. L.; DeVivo, D. C.; Goldring, S.; and Dodge, P. R. 1976. Management of seizure disorders: Selected aspects. Part II. *J. Pediatr.* 89:695.
2. Communication with R. J. Allen, M.D., Professor Pediatric Neurology, University of Michigan Medical School, Ann Arbor, Mich., February 1980.
3. Huttenlocher, P. R. 1976. Ketonemia and seizures: Metabolic and anticonvulsant effects of two ketogenic diets in childhood epilepsy. *Pediatr. Res.* 10:536.
4. Dekaban, A. S. 1966. Plasma lipids in epileptic children treated with the high fat diet. *Arch. Neurol.* 15:177.
5. Huttenlocher, P. R.; Wilbourn, A. J.; and Signore, J. M. 1971. Medium-chain triglycerides as a therapy for intractable childhood epilepsy. *Neurology* 21:1097.
6. Signore, J. M. 1973. Ketogenic diet containing medium-chain triglycerides. *J. Am. Dietet. A.* 62:285.
7. Hoeffel, G., and Moriarty, M. 1924. The effect of fasting on the metabolism of epileptic children. *Am. J. Dis. Child.* 28:16.
8. Peterman, M. G. 1924. The ketogenic diet in the treatment of epilepsy. *Am. J. Dis. Child.* 28.28.
9. Mike, E. M. 1965. Practical guide and dietary management of children with seizures using the ketogenic diet. *Am. J. Clin. Nutr.* 17:399.

OTHER REFERENCES

Appleton, D. B., and DeVivo, D. C. 1974. An animal model for the ketogenic diet. *Epilepsia* 15:211.

PART XIII
Test

Allergy Elimination

INDICATIONS FOR USE

Elimination diets are indicated when an individual is suspected of having a food allergy. (1, 2)

PURPOSE OF TEST

Elimination diets are used along with the individual's history to identify food allergy. (2, 3) Diagnosis of food allergy with the use of elimination diets must be made with caution as adverse reactions to foods may result from various other causes including intestinal enzyme deficiency, chemical or parasitic food contaminants, or psychological factors. (4) Adverse reactions from these causes may also respond to elimination diets and show increased severity when the offending food is reintroduced.

DESCRIPTION

Allergy elimination diets are designed to eliminate foods suspected of causing food allergy and then to systematically challenge the individual with the suspected foods. If the addition of a new food to the baseline diet is correlated with exacerbation of symptoms and symptoms subside when the food is removed from the diet, a food allergy may be present. Retesting is done to confirm the reaction.

GUIDELINES FOR NUTRITIONAL MANAGEMENT

The individual is maintained on a baseline diet, allergy I or allergy II, for 5 to 14 days.

- *Allergy I* (Table 60-1) eliminates the most common food allergens from the diet. It should not be used when a cereal sensitivity is suspected as it includes rice.
- *Allergy II* (Table 60-2) is devoid of all cereals as well as milk, eggs, and certain other items; it allows a more liberal selection of meat and vegetables than does the allergy I diet.

Foods are reintroduced into the diet one at a time, generally one new food every other day. Common food allergens such as milk, eggs, and wheat are generally the first foods added. A new food is added in large servings with meals and between meals. The individual is instructed to keep a food diary (Table 60-3) when new foods are being added to the diet.

If the new food does not induce allergic symptoms, it is considered a part of the diagnostic elimination diet, and the addition of another food is ordered by the physician. If a food produces an allergic reaction, it is eliminated from the diet. After the reaction subsides, other foods are added. Unless the initial reaction was violent, the suspected food is added once or twice more, at perhaps weekly intervals, to substantiate the apparent hypersensitivity.

The following are initial sample menus for allergy I and II diets.

Sample Menus

Allergy I

Breakfast

Unsweetened apricots
Unsweetened cranberry juice
Puffed Rice
Rice wafers
Water

Lunch

Roast lamb
Rice
Sliced beets
Carrot sticks
Unsweetened peaches
Rice wafers
Unsweetened pear nectar
Water

Supper

Roast lamb
Baked sweet potato
Shredded lettuce
  with corn oil and vinegar
Rice wafers
Fresh pear
Unsweetened apricot nectar
Water

Allergy II

Breakfast

Unsweetened apple juice
Unsweetened pineapple
Hash brown potatoes
Bacon
Water

Lunch

Hamburger patty
French fries
Asparagus cuts with milk-free
  margarine
Carrot sticks
Unsweetened apricots
Unsweetened pear nectar

Supper

Roast turkey
Baked potato with free margarine
Sliced beets
Shredded lettuce
  with corn oil and vinegar
Unsweetened baked apple
Unsweetened cranberry juice

TABLES

TABLE 60-1. Allergy I Diet: Foods Allowed and Foods to Avoid

Food Group	Foods Allowed	Foods to Avoid
Milk and calcium equivalents	None	All
Meat and protein equivalents	Lamb	All other
Fruit and vegetable	Unsweetened or artificially sweetened fruits and their juices: apricots, cranberries, peaches, pears	All other
	Beets; carrots; Swiss chard; lettuce; oyster plant (salsify); sweet potato	
Grain	Rice; rice wafers; Puffed Rice and other rice cereals that do not contain any food listed in foods to avoid	
Other		
Fat	Olive oil; vegetable oil; shortening	All other
Sweet	Sugar	All other
Miscellaneous	Salt; tapioca; vanilla extract (synthetic); water; white vinegar	All other including coffee, tea, carbonated beverages, chewing gum, and all medications except those ordered by the physician

Table 60-2. Allergy II Diet: Foods Allowed and Foods to Avoid

Food Group	Foods Allowed	Foods to Avoid
Milk and calcium equivalents	None	All
Meat and protein equivalents	Bacon; beef; chicken; ham; lamb; turkey; pork	All other
Fruit and vegetable	Unsweetened fruits and their juices: apples, apricots, cranberries, peaches, pears, pineapple, plums, prunes	All other
	Artichokes; asparagus; beets; carrots; Swiss chard; lettuce; lima beans; peas; spinach; squash; string beans; sweet potatoes; white potatoes	
Grain	None	All
Other		
Beverage	Water; ginger ale not artificially sweetened; coffee, tea	All other including coffee, tea, and carbonated beverages
Fat	Margarine with no milk products added; olive oil; vegetable oil; shortening	All other
Sweet	Maple syrup, sugar	All other
Miscellaneous	Jello (not red); salt; tapioca; vanilla extract; white vinegar	All other

TABLE 60-3. Food Diary Form for Use with Allergy Elimination Diets

Date	Location	Service

Reg. No.

Name

Address

Food Diary Sheet

INSTRUCTIONS: Avoid duplication in recording foods. Indicate by circle, days on which symptoms occur. On back of sheet record in detail the menu immediately preceding onset of allergic symptoms, giving date, time of day or any special circumstances which you can associate. BRING THIS RECORD ON EACH RETURN VISIT.

Month Day																														
List Each Food One Time Only	S	M	T	W	T	F	S	S	M	T	W	T	F	S	S	M	T	W	T	F	S	S	M	T	W	T	F	S	S	
Symptom Record																														
At the end of each day record degree of symptoms as follows: 1. No symptoms 2. Mild symptoms 3. Average symptoms 4. Increased symptoms 5. Much worse																														

205341 University of Michigan—University Hospital

REFERENCES CITED

1. Communication with K. Matthews, M.D., Professor of Internal Medicine, Head of Division of Allergy, University Hospital, University of Michigan, Ann Arbor, Mich., January 1980.
2. SHELDON, J. M.; LOVELL, R.; and MATTHEWS, K. 1967. *A manual of clinical allergy,* pp. 196–225. Philadelphia: W. B. Saunders.
3. MAY, C. D. 1975. Food allergy: A commentary. *Pediatr. Clin. N. Am.* 22:217.
4. MAY, C. D. 1974. Food allergy. In *Infant nutrition,* ed., S. J. Fomon, pp. 435–458. 2nd ed. Philadelphia: W. B. Saunders.

Low Calcium (140 mg), Low Phosphorus (500–700 mg)

INDICATIONS FOR USE

A low-calcium, low-phosphorus test diet is indicated during the evaluation of calcium balance and diagnosis of hypercalciurias. (1–3)

The individual is served this diet for three days prior to and during the 24 hour urine collection. (4, 5) This diet is nutritionally inadequate and should not be used as a therapeutic calcium-restricted diet.

PURPOSE OF TEST

The 24 hour urine analysis for calcium in combination with a low-calcium test diet is used to diagnose absorptive, resorptive, and renal hypercalciurias and to determine calcium balance. (1–3) Individuals with normal calcium excretion will have a 24 hour urinary excretion of under 150 mg of calcium. (1, 3, 6) Urinary calcium may be elevated in the presence of the following (2, 3, 7, 8):

Absorptive hypercalciuria:	An enhanced intestinal absorption of calcium
Resorptive hypercalciuria:	An excessive skeletal mobilization of calcium
Renal hypercalciuria:	An impairment in the renal tubular reabsorption of calcium

DESCRIPTION

Calcium intake is limited to 140 mg per day and should remain as constant as possible during the test period. Phosphorus intake is also limited, as phosphorus appears to combine with calcium in the gastrointestinal tract and influences calcium excretion. (5, 6, 9)

GUIDELINES FOR NUTRITIONAL MANAGEMENT

A 140 mg calcium, 500–700 mg phosphorus diet is planned using the calcium-restricted food exchange system (Tables 35-1 and 35-2) and the phosphorus-restricted food exchange system (Tables 39-2 and 39-3). The calculation of a sample menu is demonstrated in Table 61-1.

Because the diet is limited, fats and sugar are used generously to maintain adequate calorie intake.

Product labels must be read carefully to avoid foods that have been fortified with calcium or calcium-containing ingredients.

Depending on the calcium content of the water supply, the use of distilled water for drinking and cooking may be necessary. Information regarding the calcium content of the water supply can be obtained from the local public health or water department. For example, Ann Arbor city water contains approximately 28 mg of calcium per liter. (10)

TABLES

TABLE 61-1. Sample Menu for a Low-Calcium, Low-Phosphorus Diet

Food Item	Serving Size: Weight (g)	Serving Size: Household Measure	Calcium (mg)	Phosphorus (mg)
Breakfast				
Orange juice	120	½ cup	13	22
Farina	123	1 cup	5	15
Bread, milk free	23	1 slice	4	18
Butter	10	2 teaspoons	2	2
Jelly	20	1 tablespoon	4	2
Coffee or tea	240	1 cup	5	10
Sugar, white	24	2 tablespoons	0	0
Lunch				
Baked pork chop	56	2 ounces	8	108
Lettuce	55	1 cup	11	14
French dressing	14	1 tablespoon	2	2
Pineapple, canned	100	1 large slice	11	7
Bread, milk free	46	2 slices	8	36
Butter	10	2 teaspoons	2	2
Jelly	20	1 tablespoon	4	2
Coffee or tea	240	1 cup	5	10
Sugar, white	24	2 tablespoons	0	0
Supper				
Roast beef	84	3 ounces	12	174
Baked potato	100	1 medium	9	65
Sliced beets	83	½ cup	16	19
Baked peeled apple	150	1 medium	9	15
Bread, milk free	23	1 slice	4	18
Butter	10	2 teaspoons	2	2
Jelly	20	1 tablespoon	4	2
Coffee or tea	240	1 cup	5	10
Sugar, white	24	2 tablespoons	0	0
Total			145	555
Diet Prescription			140	500-700

REFERENCES CITED

1. Fuss, M.; Verbeelen, D.; Geurts, J.; Simon, J.; Bergans, A.; DeBacker, M.; Six, R.; and Corvilain, J. 1978. The use of a test for the differential diagnosis of hypercalciuria. *Eur. Urol.* 4:324.
2. Pak, C. Y. C.; Kaplan, R.; Bone, H.; Townsend, J.; and Waters, O. 1975. A simple test for the diagnosis of absorptive, resorptive and renal hypercalciurias. *N. Eng. J. Med.* 292:497.
3. Pak, C. Y. C.; Ohata, M.; Lawrence, E. C.; and Snyder, W. 1974. The hypercalciurias. Causes, parathyroid functions, and diagnostic criteria. *J. Clin. Invest.* 54:387.
4. *Diagnostic procedures manual.* 1978, rev. Ann Arbor: University Hospital, University of Michigan.
5. Communication with A. B. French, M.D., Professor of Internal Medicine, University Hospital, University of Michigan, Ann Arbor, Mich., August 1979.
6. Communication with J. Konnak, M.D., Department of Urology, University Hospital, University of Michigan, Ann Arbor, Mich., August 1979.
7. Peacock, M.; Hodgkinson, A.; and Nordin, B. E. C. 1967. Importance of dietary calcium in the definition of hypercalciuria. *Br. Med. J.* 3:469.
8. Parfitt, A. M.; Higgins, B. A.; Nassim, J. R.; Collins, J. A.; and Hilb, A. 1964. Metabolic studies in patients with hypercalciuria. *Clin. Sci.* 27:463.
9. Communication with S. S. Fajans, M.D., Professor of Internal Medicine, Head, Division of Endocrinology and Metabolism and Director, Metabolism Research Unit, University Hospital, University of Michigan, Ann Arbor, Mich., October 1979.
10. Communication with Ann Arbor Water Department, July 1979.

Colon Examination

INDICATIONS FOR USE

The preparatory diet for a colon examination is indicated at least 24 hours prior to the barium enema or sigmoidoscopy examination. (1)

PURPOSE OF TEST

The purpose of the barium enema examination is to detect mucosal abnormalities, structural defects, and masses or obstructions in the colon. X rays of the colon are taken after barium has been introduced by means of an enema. The sigmoidoscopy provides direct examination of the sigmoid, rectum, and anus by introduction of a lighted scope. (1)

DESCRIPTION

Elimination of all fecal material from the colon is the goal of preparation for the barium enema and the sigmoidoscopy examinations. Standard preparation consists of a clear liquid diet the entire day prior to the examination. This residue-free diet regimen is accompanied by an enema and/or laxative as directed by the physician. (1) Further instructions on the preparation of the patient can be found in the *Diagnostic Procedures Manual.* (1)

GUIDELINES FOR NUTRITIONAL MANAGEMENT

A clear liquid diet is used at least 24 hours prior to the examination (Chapter 11). Individuals with insulin-dependent diabetes mellitus should be provided with a clear liquid diet following the guidelines in Chapter 25.

REFERENCES CITED

1. *Diagnostic procedures manual.* 1978, rev. Ann Arbor: University Hospital, University of Michigan.

Fat Load (100 g Fat)

INDICATIONS FOR USE

The 100 g fat-load diet is indicated for use in diagnosing fat malabsorption. The diet is used for a period of five days including the two days prior to stool collection and during the three days of stool collection. (1)

PURPOSE OF TEST

The purpose of the 100 g fat-load test is to diagnose fat malabsorption. Stools are collected for three days for fecal fat analysis. Greater than 5 g of fat excreted in the stools per day while following this test diet indicates fat malabsorption.

DESCRIPTION

For each of the five days on the diet, the individual is provided with a diet containing approximately 100 g of fat. Due to variation in food composition and variation in measurement of the portion sizes, the actual fat content of the diet may vary by 75–125 g. Accurate test results are still obtained with this degree of variation.

GUIDELINES FOR NUTRITIONAL MANAGEMENT

Using the diabetic food exchange system (Tables 25-4 and 25-5), a diet containing approximately 100 g of fat is planned. The types of fat used should be as close to the individual's normal eating pattern as possible with a mixture of saturated and unsaturated fats. (1, 2) Medium-chain triglyceride oil should not be used as part of the 100 g of fat provided.

After each meal the fat intake of the individual is estimated, and replacements are provided for fat not eaten. For example, at University Hospital, the estimated fat consumed per meal is recorded on a nutrient intake form posted at the bedside, and the estimated fat consumed per day is recorded in the individual's chart at the end of the five-day period.

REFERENCES CITED

1. Communication with A. B. French, M.D., Professor of Internal Medicine, University Hospital, University of Michigan, Ann Arbor, Mich., January 1980.
2. WEIJERS, H. A., and VAN DE KAMER, J. H. 1953. Coeliac disease. III. Excretion of unsaturated and saturated fatty acids by patients with coeliac disease. *Acta Paediatr.* 42:97.

5-Hydroxyindoleacetic Acid (5-HIAA)

INDICATIONS FOR USE

The preparatory diet is indicated 72 hours prior to and during the 24 hour urine collection for 5-hydroxyindoleacetic acid (5-HIAA) analysis. (1) False positive or false negative results can occur from the ingestion of serotonin-containing foods, use of certain drugs, or presence of untreated celiac disease, tropical sprue, or Whipple's disease. (2)

PURPOSE OF TEST

Quantitative urine analysis for 5-HIAA is used as an aid in the diagnosis of carcinoid tumors. (1) The carcinoid tumors arising from the argentaffin cells of the gastrointestinal mucosa produce excessive amounts of serotonin. Since the bulk of urinary 5-HIAA is derived from serotonin, the amount of 5-HIAA excreted reflects the degree of serotonin secretion. (1) The normal range of urinary 5-HIAA is 3–10 mg per 24 hours; in carcinoid syndrome the levels can reach 25–1000 mg per 24 hours. (2–4)

DESCRIPTION

The consumption of foods that contain serotonin can cause an elevation in urinary 5-HIAA. (2, 4) Foods known to contain serotonin should be avoided prior to and during testing for urinary 5-HIAA to prevent false positive results.

GUIDELINES FOR NUTRITIONAL MANAGEMENT

The following foods are known to contain serotonin and should be avoided for 72 hours prior to testing and during the 24 hour urine collection (1, 5–14):

avocado	pineapple	pawpa (cariaca papaya)
banana	plantain	tomato
eggplant	plum, red	
passion fruit	plum, blue-red	

REFERENCES CITED

1. *Diagnostic procedures manual.* 1978, rev. Ann Arbor: University Hospital, University of Michigan.
2. KOWLESSAR, O. D. 1978. The carcinoid syndrome. In *Gastrointestinal disease: Pathophysiology, diagnosis, management,* eds., M. H. Sleisinger and J. S. Fordtrap, pp. 1190–1201. Vol. II. 2nd ed. Philadelphia: W. B. Saunders.
3. BATSAKIS, J. G. 1979. *Laboratories handbook, 1979–80.* Stow, Ohio: Lexi-Comp.
4. SPIRO, H. M. 1977. *Clinical gastroenterology,* pp. 580–585. 2nd ed. New York: Macmillan.
5. UDENFRIEND, S.; LOVENBERG, W.; and SJOERDSMA, A. 1959. Physiologically active amines in common fruits and vegetables. *Arch. Biochem. Biophys.* 85:487.
6. FOY, J. M., and PARRATT, J. R. 1960. A note on the presence of noradrenaline and 5-hydroxytryptamine in plantain (*Musa sapientum,* var. *paradisiaca*). *J. Pharm. Pharmacol.* 12:360.
7. WEST, G. B. 1958. Tryptamines in edible fruits. *J. Pharm. Pharmacol.* 10:589.
8. MARSHALL, P. B. 1959. Catechols and tryptamines in the "matoke" banana *(Musa paradisiaca). J. Pharm. Pharmacol.* 11:639.
9. WAALKES, T. P.; SJOERDSMA, A.; CREVELING, C. R.; WEISSBACH, H.; and UDENFRIEND, S. 1958. Serotonin, norepinephrine, and related compounds in bananas. *Science* 127:648.
10. BRUCE, D. W. 1961. Carcinoid tumours and pineapples. *J. Pharm. Pharmacol.* 13:256.
11. BRUCE, D. W. 1960. Serotonin in pineapple. *Nature* 188:147.
12. FOY, J. M., and PARRATT, J. R. 1961. 5-Hydroxytryptamine in pineapples. *J. Pharm. Pharmacol.* 13:382.
13. WEST, G. B. 1959. Tryptamines in tomatoes. *J. Pharm. Pharmacol.* 11:319.
14. WEST, G. B. 1959. Indole derivatives in tomatoes. *J. Pharm. Pharmacol.* 11:275T.

Glucose Tolerance Test

INDICATIONS FOR USE

Dietary preparation is indicated for at least three days prior to the oral glucose tolerance test (OGTT) for individuals whose carbohydrate intake has been determined to be inadequate.

PURPOSE OF TEST

The purpose of the OGTT is to determine the response of an individual to a known glucose load, and is used in the diagnosis of diabetes mellitus with or without associated reactive hypoglycemia and to confirm diagnoses of reactive functional hypoglycemia and alimentary hyperinsulinism with hypoglycemia. (1)

Diagnosis of diabetes can often be made without use of the OGTT; for example, when obvious symptoms of diabetes are present in conjunction with elevated plasma glucose levels. However, in the absence of such signs and symptoms, the standardized OGTT may be utilized to make a clinical diagnosis. (2) A variety of metabolic disturbances and conditions such as illness, trauma, intake of certain drugs, physical inactivity, and low carbohydrate intake can impair glucose tolerance. Therefore, it is imperative that elevated OGTT values be demonstrated on more than one occasion before a clinical diagnosis of diabetes is made. (2)

DESCRIPTION

The OGTT is performed in the morning after at least three days of unrestricted diet and activity. After an overnight fast, a fasting blood glucose sample is obtained and a standardized glucose load of 75 g (for children 1.75 g per kg ideal body weight, up to a maximum of 75 g) is administered. Blood samples for plasma glucose determinations are obtained at specified intervals thereafter.

For detailed information regarding test procedure and interpretation of results refer to reference number 2.

GUIDELINES FOR NUTRITIONAL MANAGEMENT

For a minimum of three days prior to the OGTT, the individual should consume an unrestricted diet containing at least 150 g carbohydrate per day. (2) A well balanced diet with representation from all food groups is recommended. At University Hospital, a diet containing at least 250 g carbohydrate is provided. Ambulatory care patients are provided with a list of the carbohydrate content of common foods and/or a sample menu to follow. For inpatients a record is kept of all carbohydrate consumed, making sure the daily total is at or above 250 g. This information is recorded in the patient's medical record.

The individual fasts for at least 10 hours yet no more than 16 hours prior to the test; water is allowed during this period. (2) After administration of the glucose load, the individual continues to fast until the completion of the test.

REFERENCES CITED

1. *Diagnostic procedures manual,* 1978, rev. Ann Arbor: University Hospital, University of Michigan.
2. National Diabetes Data Group: Classification and diagnosis of diabetes mellitus and other categories of glucose intolerance. 1979. *Diabetes* 28:1039.

Intraesophageal pH Reflux

INDICATIONS FOR USE

A pH-controlled diet is indicated during 24 hour pH monitoring of the distal esophagus. (1–3)

PURPOSE OF TEST

The purpose of the intraesophageal pH reflux test is to identify abnormal esophageal reflux or motor function. (1–4)

DESCRIPTION

An intraesophageal pH electrode is positioned 5 cm above the lower esophageal sphincter. (2, 4, 5) Normally, intraesophageal pH should be greater than 4.0; a pH of less than 4.0 indicates gastric acid regurgitation. (2–4)

GUIDELINES FOR NUTRITIONAL MANAGEMENT

A diet is served excluding foods and beverages having a pH value of less than 5.0. (2, 4) Smoking and foods and beverages that stimulate gastroesophageal reflux are also excluded. (2, 5–7) Table 66-1 lists foods allowed and foods to avoid. A pH meter may be used to test desired foods that are not listed. Mechanical soft or liquid foods may be more acceptable for individuals bothered by the presence of the intraesophageal tube.

The following is a sample menu.

SAMPLE MENU

Breakfast	*Lunch*	*Supper*
Puffed Wheat	Chicken consomme	Roast beef
Scrambled egg	Sliced turkey	Whipped potato
Toast	Bread	Asparagus
Margarine	Margarine	Dinner roll
Milk	Peas	Margarine
Cereal grain beverage	Vanilla pudding	Vanilla ice cream
Nondairy creamer	Milk	Milk
Sugar	Cereal grain beverage	Cereal grain beverage
Salt	Sugar	Sugar
	Salt	Salt

TABLES

TABLE 66-1. Foods Allowed and Foods to Avoid for pH Control During pH Monitoring of the Distal Esophagus (8–12)

Food Group	Foods Allowed	Foods to Avoid
Milk and calcium equivalents	Fresh, evaporated, or dried milk; cream; ice cream	Acidophilus milk; buttermilk; sour cream; yogurt
Meat and protein equivalents	Meat; poultry; fish; eggs; frankfurters	Cheese
Fruit and vegetable	Asparagus; cauliflower; corn; cucumbers; peas; potatoes; spinach; squash; sweet potatoes; turnips	All fruits and their juices; beets; red cabbage; carrots; olives; onions; pickles; pimiento; rhubarb; sauerkraut; tomatoes; all tomato products
Grain	All except those prepared with foods to avoid	None except those prepared with foods to avoid
Other		
Beverage	Water; cereal grain beverage	Beer; carbonated beverages; coffee; decaffeinated coffee; fruit-flavored beverages; fruit punch and juices; tea; wine
Fat	Butter; margarine; oil; shortening	Mayonnaise; salad dressing
Sweet	Sugar; desserts made with allowed ingredients	All desserts made with fruits; chocolate; jam, jelly
Miscellaneous	Salt	Catsup; mustard; peppermint; vinegar

REFERENCES CITED

1. Orringer, M. B. 1976. Esophageal function tests in the modern age of esophageal surgery. Editorial. *Ann. Thorac. Surg.* 22:204.
2. Johnson, L. F., and DeMeester, T. R. 1974. Twenty-four hr pH monitoring of the distal esophagus. *Am. J. Gastroenterol.* 63:325.
3. Hill, J. L.; Pelligrini, C. A.; Burrington, J. D.; Reyes, H. M.; and Demeester, T. R. 1977. Technique and experience with 24-hour esophageal pH monitoring in children. *J. Pediatr. Surg.* 12:877.
4. Communication with M. B. Orringer, M.D., Associate Professor of Surgery, Director, Thoracic Surgery Esophageal Clinic, University Hospital, University of Michigan, Ann Arbor, Mich., July 1979.
5. Price, S. F.; Smithson, K. W.; and Castell, D. O. 1978. Food sensitivity in reflux esophagitis. *Gastroenterology* 75:240.
6. Cohen, S., and Booth, G. H. 1975. Gastric acid secretion and lower-esophageal-sphincter pressure in response to coffee and caffeine. *N. Eng. J. Med.* 293:897.
7. Stanciu, C., and Bennett, J. R. 1972. The effect of smoking on gastroesophageal reflux. *Gut* 13:318.
8. *Handbook of food preparation,* 1971. p. 21. 6th ed. Washington, D.C.: American Home Economics Association.
9. Pierpaoli, P. G. 1972. Drug therapy and diet. *Drug Intelligence and Clinical Pharmacy* 6:89.
10. Lopez, A. 1975. *Complete course in canning,* p. 106. 10th ed. Cleveland: Publication of the Canning Trade.
11. Weast, R. L., ed. 1979. *CRC handbook of chemistry and physics,* p. D-149. 60th ed. Cleveland: Chemical Rubber Publishing Company.
12. The use of pH meter with the assistance of R. Schneider, Perfusionist, University Hospital, University of Michigan, Ann Arbor, Mich., August 1979.

Oral Cholecystogram

INDICATIONS FOR USE

Contrary to previous practice, which indicated the use of a light, fat-free meal the evening prior to the oral cholecystogram (1), present findings conclude that dietary restrictions prior to ingestion of the contrast medium are not necessary. (2, 3) Some radiologists believe that, if a fat-free preparation diet is used, the gallbladder is not stimulated to contract, bile accumulates, and the gallbladder is not prepared to receive the dye. (3, 4)

PURPOSE OF TEST

The purpose of the oral cholecystogram is to radiographically visualize the size, shape, and position of the gallbladder, the presence of calculi, and the gallbladder's ability to concentrate the dye.

DESCRIPTION

The contrast medium is administered orally, absorbed from the intestine, transported through the portal venous system, and concentrated in the gallbladder. (4)

GUIDELINES FOR NUTRITIONAL MANAGEMENT

No restriction on size or content of the supper meal is necessary the evening prior to the oral cholecystogram. Nothing by mouth except moderate amounts of water is allowed following the supper meal prior to the examination.

REFERENCES CITED

1. Saxton, H. M., and Strickland, B. 1972. *Practical procedures in diagnostic radiology,* p. 92. 2nd ed. New York: Grune and Stratton.
2. Parkin, G. J. S. 1974. Dietary preparation for oral cholecystography—A critical reappraisal. *Br. J. Radiol.* 47:452.
3. Communication with M. Childress, M.D., Department of Diagnostic Radiology, University Hospital, University of Michigan, Ann Arbor, Mich., June 1979.
4. Watson, J. C. 1974. *Patient care and special procedures in radiologic technology,* p. 100. 4th ed. Saint Louis, Mo.: C. V. Mosby.

68

10 mEq (230 mg) Sodium

INDICATIONS FOR USE

The 10 mEq (230 mg) sodium test diet is indicated when plasma renin activity needs to be measured. (1–5) The diet is monitored during the three-day test.

PURPOSE OF TEST

The purpose of this test is to diagnose low renin hypertension (1), hyporeninemic hypertension (1, 5), and primary aldosteronism. (2, 3, 4, 7) The diagnosis of primary aldosteronism consists of two phases: a 10 mEq (230 mg) sodium intake for three days designed to stimulate renin secretion and a 120–150 mEq (3000–3500 mg) sodium intake for the second three days to suppress aldosterone secretion. (3, 6, 7) The high sodium intake is achieved by supplementation of known sodium intake level diet with sodium chloride capsules. (7)

Individuals receive approximately 10 mEq (230 mg) of sodium for three days. On the fourth day, plasma renin activity is measured after two hours of upright posture. Normal supine renin is 1.0–10.0 mg/ml per hour, and upright normal values are 2.5–30.0 mg/ml per hour. (1, 2, 4–6)

GUIDELINES FOR NUTRITIONAL MANAGEMENT

This diet is highly restricted in sodium content, with severe limitation upon types and amounts of food. Food should be measured. The sodium-restricted exchange system (Tables 41-1 and 41-2) serves as a guideline for meal planning. If a more exact control of sodium intake is required for a research purpose, a clinical research center should be utilized where foods are especially prepared, served, and analyzed.

Sodium contained in drinking water varies, and its sodium content needs to be counted as part of the 10 mEq of sodium allowed. For example, tap water at University Hospital contains approximately 1 mEq sodium (20 mg) per quart. (8) Medications containing sodium such as antacids may interfere with test results.

REFERENCES CITED

1. McDonald, W. J.; Cohen, E. L.; and Conn, J. W. 1977. Renin reactivity, renin activity and renin concentration in patients with normal and low renin essential hypertension. *J. Clin. Endocrinol. Metab.* 45:685.
2. Hollenberg, N. K.; Chenitz, W. R.; Adams, D. F.; and Williams, G. H. 1974. Reciprocal influence of salt intake on adrenal glomerulosa and renal vascular responses to angiotensin II in normal man. *J. Clin. Invest.* 54:34.
3. Conn, J. W., and Hinerman, D. L. 1977. Spironolactone-induced inhibition of aldosterone biosynthesis in primary aldosteronism: Morphological and functional studies. *Metabolism* 26:1293.
4. Mendelsohn, F. A. O.; Johnston, C. I.; Doyle, A. E.; Scoggins, B. A.; Denton, D. A.; and Coghlan, J. P. 1972. Renin, angiotensin II, and adrenal corticosteroid relationships during sodium deprivation infusion in normotensive and hypertensive man. *Circ. Res.* 31:728.
5. Crane, M. G.; Harris, J. J.; and Johns, V. J., Jr. 1972. Hyporeninemic hypertension. *Am. J. Med.* 52:457.
6. Communication with R. Grekin, M.D., University Hospital, University of Michigan, Ann Arbor, Mich., July 1979.
7. *Diagnostic procedure manual.* 1978, rev. Ann Arbor: University Hospital, University of Michigan.
8. Communication with Ann Arbor Water Department, July 1979.

Upper Gastrointestinal Examination (UGI)

INDICATIONS FOR USE

The dietary preparation indicated for the upper gastrointestinal examination (UGI) consists only of taking nothing by mouth after 10 P.M. the evening prior to the examination.

PURPOSE OF TEST

The purpose of the UGI examination is to detect mucosal abnormalities, structural defects, and masses or obstructions in the upper gastrointestinal tract. The barium swallow and small bowel examination are included in the UGI. (1)

DESCRIPTION

The upper gastrointestinal tract must be empty to accommodate the barium meal, provide accurate radiographic representation of the structure being examined, and avoid complications if the patient is nauseated. (2, 3)

GUIDELINES FOR NUTRITIONAL MANAGEMENT

Nothing is taken by mouth after 10 P.M. the evening prior to the examination.

REFERENCES CITED

1. *Diagnostic procedures manual.* 1978, rev. Ann Arbor: University Hospital, University of Michigan.
2. French, R. M. 1975. *Guide to diagnostic procedures.* 4th ed. New York: McGraw-Hill.
3. Watson, J. C. 1974. *Patient care and special procedures in radiologic technology,* pp. 98–99. 4th ed. Saint Louis, Mo.: C. V. Mosby.

PART XIV
Other

70

Research

INDICATIONS FOR USE

Research diets are indicated for individuals on approved research protocols designed to study the metabolism of one or more nutrients or when it is desirable to control the variable of dietary intake. Diets are planned and implemented in a clinical research center. They may be for one meal or any other length of time.

DESCRIPTION

Because a high degree of accuracy and control is required, a specialized dietary service and a trained research staff are necessary. The Clinical Research Center at University Hospital is such a setting. Research dietitians, laboratory personnel, nurses, and kitchen personnel trained in research techniques contribute to an environment in which research diets can be developed and served and adherence closely monitored.

Diets are developed by research dietitians in response to the dietary requirements of approved research protocols. A computer nutrient data base is used to calculate the nutrient content of the diets. The data are updated by analysis of foods in the research laboratory, food company information, and various food composition tables. Foods and beverages are weighed to the nearest gram on Mettler balances. Individuals on very restrictive constant and metabolic diets may be required to rinse their dishes with distilled water and to consume the rinse. Food consumption is monitored and recorded after each meal. Absolute patient compliance is important to the success of the research protocol. Dietitians are notified when individuals do not comply, and appropriate food replacements or adjustment are made within 24 hours.

Research diets are divided into three types. Table 70-1 compares the three. The three types are as follows:

A nutrient-controlled diet is the least precisely calculated research diet. It is used when a high degree of accuracy and consistency are not necessary. Nutrient-controlled diets are calculated using food exchange lists or standard food composition tables. The majority of food used is obtained from the hospital's central food production area. Food and fluids are weighed or measured to meet the specific requirements. The menus change from day to day. Actual level of daily nutrient intake will vary. Tap water is used for drinking. Feces and urine are not analyzed in relation to the nutrient intake. Examples of nutrient-controlled diets routinely served are

diabetic
hyperlipoproteinemia
controlled calories, fat, carbohydrate, protein
purine free
pH > 5
low calcium, low oxalate

A constant diet is a more precisely calculated and consistent research diet. Although the constant diet is not a true metabolic balance diet, it offers a high degree of consistency. It is usually repeated daily for the duration of a study. If the study is of long duration, the diet becomes very monotonous. When mineral determination is important, distilled or deionized water is used. Feces and urine are often analyzed. Food aliquots may be analyzed for certain nutrients. The constant diet can be served as solid foods, oral formulas, or tube feedings.

Solid food constant diet. The majority of food items are prepared in the hospital's central food production area. Only foods that give consistent data on nutrient analysis are used. It is often necessary to use special food items not prepared in the hospital's central production area. These foods are prepared in the Clinical Research Center. Although the constant diet is usually repeated daily for the duration of the study, a two- to three-day rotation can be devised. The constant diet is developed to be compatible with the patient's personal food preferences and eating patterns, but it is nevertheless very monotonous. It is most successful for short periods and with complete cooperation from the individual. Examples of constant diets routinely served are

isocaloric 20 mEq sodium, 1000 mg calcium, 1000 mg phosphorus, and 60 mEq potassium
3500 kcal, 2% protein
10 mEq sodium, 100 mEq potassium
copper controlled

Formula constant diet. A formula diet is used when a diet is required that can be easily reproduced with little variability in nutrient content or when the nutrients required are impossible to meet with standard solid food items. Pharmaceutical nutritional products are often used in combination with analyzed food items. At University Hospital, formulas are designed to be used enterally. Examples of formula diets served are

isocaloric 75% carbohydrate, 25% protein, 0% fat or
isocaloric 50% carbohydrate, 2% protein, 48% fat

A metabolic balance diet offers the strictest control of any type of solid food diet. This type of diet is not available at University Hospital. A balance study technique is necessary based on having a precisely measured dietary intake (food and fluids) and output (urine and feces). With an extremely consistent intake, any changes in balance may be attributed to the disease, procedure, or medication under study. The foods used are purchased in large quantities from a reliable source that guarantees the food to be of the same lot number. This reduces variations in nutrient composition that might occur due to soil, climate, geographic location, variety, method of preservation, or storage. All foods must be prepared according to standard metabolic research methods. At spaced intervals during the study, one or more food aliquots are prepared by the metabolic kitchen staff and are sent to the laboratory for nutrient analysis to assure constancy.

NUTRIENT ADEQUACY

The purpose and duration of the study determines the nutrient content of the diet. Deficits of one or more nutrients may be important for the results of the study. All protocols are approved through a committee, and any known nutrient deficit is identified.

TABLES

TABLE 70-1. Description of Three Types of Research Diets

Variables	Nutrient Controlled	Constant: Solid Food	Constant: Formula	Metabolic
Source of nutrient calculations	Food exchange groups Standard tables Laboratory analysis	Laboratory analyzed nutrient data Manufacturer's data *USDA Handbook #8*	Laboratory analyzed nutrient data Manufacturer's data *USDA Handbook #8*	Laboratory analyzed nutrient data Manufacturer's data *USDA Handbook #8*
Measurements of foods and beverages	Household measures Mettler balance (g)	Mettler balance (g)	Mettler balance (g)	Mettler balance (g)
Food sources	Varied	Varied	Constant	Constant
Menu variations	Varies daily	Constant	Constant	Constant
Water source	Tap water	Distilled or deionized water	Distilled or deionized water	Distilled or deionized water
Food refusals	Estimated, sometimes replaced	Unacceptable Weighed, calculated, and possibly analyzed, replaced	Unacceptable Weighed, calculated, and possibly analyzed, replaced	Unacceptable Weighed, calculated, analyzed
Laboratory analysis of diet	No	Sometimes	Sometimes	Always
Advantages	Flexible; high food variety	Calculated nutrient intake is accurate and consistent Calculations are done one time	Calculated nutrient intake is very accurate and consistent Calculations are done one time Easy to replicate Manufacturer's analysis of pharmaceutical products reliable	Most reliable and consistent data
Disadvantages and limitations	Degree of inconsistency and variation in nutrient intake Requires daily calculation	Lack of food variety Requires constant monitoring to ensure complete intake Requires research dietary facilities	Lack of variety Requires constant monitoring to ensure complete intake Requires a research kitchen or formula room Not similar in consistency to normal dietary intake; therefore, may not be appropriate to the objectives and future application of some protocols	Lack of variety and flexibility Requires constant monitoring of dietary intake Requires a metabolic research kitchen and specially trained personnel Requires analysis of all intake and excreta

REFERENCES

HJORTLAND, M. C.; DUDDLESON, W. A.; PORTER, C.; and FRENCH, A. B. 1966. Using the computer to calculate nutrients in metabolic diets. *J. Am. Dietet. A.* 49:316.

MANALO, R., and JONES, J. E. 1966. The content of constant diets. A comparison between analyzed and calculated values. *Am. J. Clin. Nutr.* 18:339.

SAMPSON, A. G.; SPRAGUE, R. G.; and WOLLAEGER, E. E. 1952. Dietary techniques for metabolic balance. *J. Am. Dietet. A.* 28:912.

U.S. Department of Health, Education, and Welfare, Public Health Service, National Institutes of Health. 1974. *Clinical center diet manual.* DHEW Publication No. (NIH) 74-229, Reprinted January 1974.

U.S. Department of Health, Education, and Welfare, Public Health Service, National Institutes of Health. 1969. *A dietetic manual for metabolic kitchen units.* March 1969.

71 Historical

ACID ASH DIET

The acid ash diet was used for treatment of urinary magnesium ammonium phosphate stones. These stones precipitate in an alkaline solution. The principle of the diet was to produce an acidic urine by consuming only those foods that produce an acidic residue after digestion. Table 71-1 lists foods that produce an acid ash residue due to their chlorine, sulfur, and phosphorus content. The pH of a food before digestion does not correlate well with the pH residue after digestion. Today, drug therapy is the preferred treatment.

ALKALINE ASH DIET

The alkaline ash diet was used for treatment of urinary uric acid or cystine stones. These stones precipitate in acidic solutions. The principle of the diet was to produce an alkaline urine using those foods, such as milk and most fruits and vegetables, that produce an alkaline residue after digestion. Table 71-2 lists foods that produce an alkaline ash residue due to their sodium, potassium, calcium, and magnesium content. The diet has been replaced by drug therapy that is used to alkalinize the urine and/or decrease the stone-forming substrate.

GIOVANNETTI–MAGGIORE RENAL DIET

The Giovannetti–Maggiore renal diet was one of the original diets proposed for the treatment of renal disease. The diet was restricted to 1.0–1.5 g nitrogen, 25–40 mEq sodium, and 35–50 mEq potassium per day. This diet is severely inadequate in nutrients. It has been replaced by dialysis, kidney transplant, and, when appropriate, diets with moderate protein, sodium, potassium, and fluid restrictions. (Refer to Chapters 26 and 27.)

KEMPNER (rice–fruit) SEMISTARVATION DIET

The Kempner diet was introduced in 1944 for the treatment of hypertension. The basic diet consisted of rice, sugar, fruit, fruit juices, vitamins, and iron. It contained approximately 15–25 g protein, 4–6 g fat, and 11–18 mEq sodium. Currently, drug therapy, moderate sodium restriction, and calorie restriction when appropriate are used in the treatment of hypertension. (Refer to Chapters 24 and 41.)

PURINE-RESTRICTED DIET

A restricted purine diet was used in the treatment of gout and may now be used only as an adjunct to drug therapy. Table 71-3 lists foods high in purine. Drug therapy with allopurinol or uricosuric drugs, probenecid and sulfinpyrazone, is the treatment of choice. Allopurinol inhibits the action of xanthine oxidase, an enzyme in the hypoxanthine to uric acid pathway. Uricosuric drugs increase the renal clearance of uric acid by inhibiting the renal tubular reabsorption of uric acid. (1–4)

A diet restricted in purines may be of significance in the treatment of hyperuricosuria in patients with calcium oxalate nephrolithiasis (5) and of therapeutic benefit to some individuals with Lesch–Nyhan syndrome (6, 7) or with complete adenine phosphoribosyltransferase deficiency. (8) Further investigations need to be completed to confirm these.

SIPPY DIET

The Sippy diet was based on the hypothesis that the presence of food in the stomach dilutes and neutralizes excess acid that caused pain. It consisted of a four-stage progression from a milk–cream hourly feeding to a three- to six-feeding, low-fiber diet. Current practice is to allow the person to eat anything that does not cause distress. (Refer to Chapter 13.)

TABLES

TABLE 71-1. Foods That Produce an Acid Ash Residue

Breads, cakes and cookies, cereals, crackers
Cheese, eggs, fish, meats, poultry
Corn and lentils
Cranberries, plums, prunes
Macaroni, noodles, and spaghetti
Some nuts (Brazil, filberts, peanuts, walnuts)

Diet manual. 1972. 9th ed. Ann Arbor: University Hospital, University of Michigan.

TABLE 71-2. Foods That Produce an Alkaline Ash Residue

Milk and cream
Molasses
Most fruits
Most vegetables
Some nuts (almonds, coconut, chestnuts)

Diet manual. 1972. 9th ed. Ann Arbor: University Hospital, University of Michigan.

TABLE 71-3. Foods High in Purine

Alcohol beverages
Grains: bran, oatmeal, wheat germ
Meat: anchovies, sardines
Meat extracts
Organ meats: brains, heart, kidney, liver, sweetbreads
Vegetables: spinach, dried beans and peas, lentils

Diet manual. 1972. 9th ed. Ann Arbor: University Hospital, University of Michigan.

REFERENCES

ACID ASH DIET

MATTICE, M. R. 1950. *Bridges' food and beverage analysis,* pp. 201–232. 3rd ed. Philadelphia: Lea & Febiger.

WILLIAMS, H. E. 1944. Nephrolithiasis. *N. Eng. J. Med.* 290:33.

ZINSSER, H. H.; SENECA, H.; LIGHT, I.; MAYER, G.; KARP, F.; MCGROY, G.; and TARRASOLI, H. 1968. Management of infected stones with acidifying agents. *New York State J. Med.* 68:3001.

ALKALINE ASH DIET

DEVRIES, A.; WEINBURGER, A.; and FRANK, M. 1973. Treatment of uric acid lithiasis, observations of 658 patients. In *Urinary Calculi. Int. Symp. Renal Stone Res.,* ed., S. Karger, Madrid 1972; Basil 1973.

FORBES, A. P., and DEMPSY, E. 1963. Nephrolithiasis. In *Diseases of the kidney,* eds. M. B. Strauss and L. G. Welt, pp. 712–719. Boston: Little, Brown.

MATTICE, M. R. 1950. *Bridges' food and beverage analysis,* pp. 201–232. 3rd ed. Philadelphia: Lea & Febiger.

ZINSSER, H. 1960. Urinary calculi. *JAMA* 174:2062.

GIOVANNETTI – MAGGIORE DIET

GIOVANNETTI, S., and MAGGIORE, Q. 1964. A low-nitrogen diet with proteins of high biological value for severe chronic uraemia. *Lancet* 1:1000.

KEMPNER SEMISTARVATION DIET

KEMPNER, W. 1944. Treatment of kidney disease and hypertensive disease with rice diet. *N. Card. Med. J.* 5:125.

PURINE-RESTRICTED DIET

1. FOX, I. H., and KELLEY, W. N. 1979. Management of gout. *JAMA* 242:361.
2. FOX, I. H. 1977. Hypouricaemic agents in the treatment of gout. *Clinics Rheumatic Dis.* 3:145.
3. TREADWELL, B. 1964. The treatment of gout. *N. Zealand Med. J.* 63:567.
4. SORENSEN, L. B. 1963. Current concepts of gout and its treatment. *Med. Clinics N. Am.* 47:169.
5. COE, F. L. 1978. Hyperuricosuric calcium oxalate nephrolithiasis. *Kidney Inter.* 13:418.
6. ARNOLD, W. J., and KELLEY, W. N. 1973. Hypoxanthine-guanine phosphoribosyl transferase (HGPRT) deficiency: Effect of dietary purines on enzyme activity. *Adv. Exp. Med. Biol.* 41:203.
7. ARNOLD, W. J., and KELLEY, W. N. 1973. Dietary-induced variation of hypoxanthine-guanine phosphoribosyl transferase activity in patients with Lesch–Nyhan syndrome. *J. Clin. Invest.* 54:970.
8. SIMMONDS, H. A.; VAN ACKER, K. J.; CAMERON, J. S.; and MCBURNEY, A. 1977. Purine excretion in complete adenine phosphoribosyltransferase deficiency: Effect of diet and allopurinol therapy. *Adv. Exp. Med. Biol.* 76(B):304.

SIPPY DIET

SIPPY, B. W. 1915. Gastric and duodenal ulcers. Medical care by efficient removal of gastric juice corrosion. *JAMA* 64:1625.

Appendices

TABLE A.1-1. Recommended Daily Dietary Allowances,[1] Revised 1980 (designed for the maintenance of good nutrition of practically all healthy people in the United States)

	Age (years)	Weight (kg)	Weight (lbs)	Height (cm)	Height (in)	Protein (g)	Fat-Soluble Vitamins: Vitamin A (μg RE)[3]	Vitamin D (μg)[4]	Vitamin E (mg α TE)[5]	Vitamin C (mg)	Thiamin (mg)
Infants	0.0–0.5	6	13	60	24	kg × 2.2	420	10	3	35	0.3
	0.5–1.0	9	20	71	28	kg × 2.0	400	10	4	35	0.5
Children	1–3	13	29	90	35	23	400	10	5	45	0.7
	4–6	20	44	112	44	30	500	10	6	45	0.9
	7–10	28	62	132	52	34	700	10	7	45	1.2
Males	11–14	45	99	157	62	45	1000	10	8	50	1.4
	15–18	66	145	176	69	56	1000	10	10	60	1.4
	19–22	70	154	177	70	56	1000	7.5	10	60	1.5
	23–50	70	154	178	70	56	1000	5	10	60	1.4
	51+	70	154	178	70	56	1000	5	10	60	1.2
Females	11–14	46	101	157	62	46	800	10	8	50	1.1
	15–18	55	120	163	64	46	800	10	8	60	1.1
	19–22	55	120	163	64	44	800	7.5	8	60	1.1
	23–50	55	120	163	64	44	800	5	8	60	1.0
	51+	55	120	163	64	44	800	5	8	60	1.0
Pregnant						+30	+200	+5	+2	+20	+0.4
Lactating						+20	+400	+5	+3	+40	+0.5

Food and Nutrition Board. 1980. *Recommended dietary allowances,* p. 187. 9th ed. Washington, D.C.: National Academy of Sciences.

[1] The allowances are intended to provide for individual variations among most normal persons as they live in the United States under usual environmental stresses. Diets should be based on a variety of common foods to provide other nutrients for which human requirements have been less well defined

[2] The folacin allowances refer to dietary sources as determined by *Lactobacillus caséi* assay after treatment with enzymes ("conjugates") to make polyglutanyl forms of the vitamin available to the test organism.

[3] Retinol equivalents. 1 Retinol equivalent = 1 μg retinol or 6μg carotene.

[4] As cholecalciferol. 10 μg cholecalciferol = 400 IU vitamin D.

[5] α tocopherol equivalents. 1 μg d-α-tocopherol = 1 α T.E.

[6] 1 NE (niacin equivalent) is equal to 1 mg of niacin or 60 μg of dietary tryptophan.

[a] The RDA for vitamin B_{12} in infants is based on average concentration of the vitamin in human milk. The allowances after weaning are based on energy intake (as recommended by the American Academy of Pediatrics) and consideration of other factors such as intestinal absorption.

[b] The increased requirement during pregnancy cannot be met by the iron content of habitual American diets or by the existing iron stores of many women; therefore the use of 30–60 mg of supplemental iron is recommended. Iron needs during lactation are not substantially different from those of nonpregnant women, but continued supplementation of the mother for 2–3 months after parturition is advisable to replenish stores depleted by pregnancy.

TABLE A.1-2. Estimated Safe and Adequate Daily Dietary Intakes of Additional Selected Vitamins and Minerals[1]

	Age (years)	Vitamins: Vitamin K (μg)	Biotin (μg)	Pantothenic Acid (mg)	Copper (mg)	Manganese (mg)
Infants	0–0.5	12	35	2	0.5–0.7	0.5–0.7
	0.5–1	10– 20	50	3	0.7–1.0	0.7–1.0
Children and adolescents	1–3	15– 30	65	3	1.0–1.5	1.0–1.5
	4–6	20– 40	85	3–4	1.5–2.0	1.5–2.0
	7–10	30– 60	120	4–5	2.0–2.5	2.0–3.0
	11+	50–100	100–200	4–7	2.0–3.0	2.5–5.0
Adults		70–140	100–200	4–7	2.0–3.0	2.5–5.0

Food and Nutrition Board. 1980. *Recommended dietary allowances,* p. 178. 9th ed. Washington, D.C.: National Academy of Sciences.

[1] Because there is less information on which to base allowances, these figures are provided here in the form of ranges of recommended intakes.

[2] Since the toxic levels for many trace elements may be only several times usual intakes, the upper levels for the trace elements given in this table should not be habitually exceeded.

Water-Soluble Vitamins					Minerals						
Riboflavin (mg)	Niacin (mg NE)[6]	Vitamin B_6 (mg)	Folacin[2] (μg)	Vitamin B_{12} (μg)	Calcium (mg)	Phosphorus (mg)	Magnesium (mg)	Iron (mg)	Zinc (mg)	Iodine (μg)	
0.4	6	0.3	30	0.5[a]	360	240	50	10	3	40	Infants
0.6	8	0.6	45	1.5	540	360	70	15	5	50	
0.8	9	0.9	100	2.0	800	800	150	15	10	70	Children
1.0	11	1.3	200	2.5	800	800	200	10	10	90	
1.4	16	1.6	300	3.0	800	800	250	10	10	120	
1.6	18	1.8	400	3.0	1200	1200	350	18	15	150	Males
1.7	18	2.0	400	3.0	1200	1200	400	18	15	150	
1.7	19	2.2	400	3.0	800	800	350	10	15	150	
1.6	18	2.2	400	3.0	800	800	350	10	15	150	
1.4	16	3.2	400	3.0	800	800	350	10	15	150	
1.3	15	1.8	400	3.0	1200	1200	300	18	15	150	Females
1.3	14	2.0	400	3.0	1200	1200	300	18	15	150	
1.3	14	2.0	400	3.0	800	800	300	18	15	150	
1.2	13	2.0	400	3.0	800	800	300	18	15	150	
1.2	13	2.0	400	3.0	800	800	300	10	15	150	
+0.3	+2	+0.6	+400	+1.0	+400	+400	+150	[b]	+5	+25	Pregnant
+0.5	+5	+0.5	+100	+1.0	+400	+400	+150	[b]	+10	+50	Lactating

Trace Elements[2]				Electrolytes			
Fluoride (mg)	Chromium (mg)	Selenium (mg)	Molybdenum (mg)	Sodium (mg)	Potassium (mg)	Chloride (mg)	
0.1–0.5	0.01–0.04	0.01–0.04	0.03–0.06	115– 350	350– 925	275– 700	Infants
0.2–1.0	0.02–0.06	0.02–0.06	0.04–0.08	250– 750	425–1275	400–1200	
0.5–1.5	0.02–0.08	0.02–0.08	0.05–0.1	325– 975	550–1650	500–1500	Children and adolescents
1.0–2.5	0.03–0.12	0.03–0.12	0.06–0.15	450–1350	775–2325	700–2100	
1.5–2.5	0.05–0.2	0.05–0.2	0.1–0.3	600–1800	1000–3000	925–2775	
1.5–2.5	0.05–0.2	0.05–0.2	0.15–0.5	900–2700	1525–4575	1400–4200	
1.5–4.0	0.05–0.2	0.05–0.2	0.15–0.5	1100–3300	1875–5625	1700–5100	Adults

TABLE A.1-3. Mean Heights and Weights and Recommended Energy Intake*

Category	Age (years)	Weight		Height		Energy Needs (with range)	
		(kg)	(lb)	(cm)	(in.)	(kcal)	(MJ)
Infants	0.0–0.5	6	13	60	24	kg × 115 (95–145)	kg × .48
	0.5–1.0	9	20	71	28	kg × 105 (80–135)	kg × .44
Children	1– 3	13	29	90	35	1300 (900–1800)	5.5
	4– 6	20	44	112	44	1700 (1300–2300)	7.1
	7–10	28	62	132	52	2400 (1650–3300)	10.1
Males	11–14	45	99	157	62	2700 (2000–3700)	11.3
	15–18	66	145	176	69	2800 (2100–3900)	11.8
	19–22	70	154	177	70	2900 (2500–3300)	12.2
	23–50	70	154	178	70	2700 (2300–3100)	11.3
	51–75	70	154	178	70	2400 (2000–2800)	10.1
	76+	70	154	178	70	2050 (1650–2450)	8.6
Females	11–14	46	101	157	62	2200 (1500–3000)	9.2
	15–18	55	120	163	64	2100 (1200–3000)	8.8
	19–22	55	120	163	64	2100 (1700–2500)	8.8
	23–50	55	120	163	64	2000 (1600–2400)	8.4
	51–75	55	120	163	64	1800 (1400–2200)	7.6
	76+	55	120	163	64	1600 (1200–2000)	6.7
Pregnancy						+300	
Lactation						+500	

*Footnotes on facing page

TABLE A.1-4. Dietary Standard for Canada—Recommended Daily Nutrient Intake

Age	Sex	Weight (kg)	Height (cm)	Energy[1]		Protein (g)	Water-Soluble Vitamins				
				(kcal)	(MJ)[2]		Thiamin (mg)	Niacin (NE)[3]	Riboflavin (mg)	Vitamin B_6[4] (mg)	Folate[5] (μg)
0–6 mo	Both	6	—	kg × 117	kg × 0.49	kg × 2.2(2.0)[a]	0.3	5	0.4	0.3	40
7–11 mo	Both	9	—	kg × 108	kg × 0.45	kg × 1.4	0.5	6	0.6	0.4	60
1–3 yrs	Both	13	90	1400	5.9	22	0.7	9	0.8	0.8	100
4–6 yrs	Both	19	110	1800	7.5	27	0.9	12	1.1	1.3	100
7–9 yrs	M	27	129	2200	9.2	33	1.1	14	1.3	1.6	100
	F	27	128	2000	8.4	33	1.0	13	1.2	1.4	100
10–12 yrs	M	36	144	2500	10.5	41	1.2	17	1.5	1.8	100
	F	38	145	2300	9.6	40	1.1	15	1.4	1.5	100
13–15 yrs	M	51	162	2800	11.7	52	1.4	19	1.7	2.0	200
	F	49	159	2200	9.2	43	1.1	15	1.4	1.5	200
16–18 yrs	M	64	172	3200	13.4	54	1.6	21	2.0	2.0	200
	F	54	161	2100	8.8	43	1.1	14	1.3	1.5	200
19–35 yrs	M	70	176	3000	12.6	56	1.5	20	1.8	2.0	200
	F	56	161	2100	8.8	41	1.1	14	1.3	1.5	200
36–50 yrs	M	70	176	2700	11.3	56	1.4	18	1.7	2.0	200
	F	56	161	1900	7.9	41	1.0	13	1.2	1.5	200
51+ yrs	M	70	176	2300[e]	9.6[e]	56	1.4	18	1.7	2.0	200
	F	56	161	1800[e]	7.5[e]	41	1.0	13	1.2	1.5	200
Pregnancy				+300[f]	1.3[f]	+20	+0.2	+2	+0.3	+0.5	+50
Lactation				+500	2.1	+24	+0.4	+7	+0.6	+0.6	+50

Dietary Standards for Canada, (1979), pp. 70 and 71, with the permission of the Minister of Supply and Service Canada.

[1] Recommendations assume characteristic activity pattern for each age group.
[2] Megajoules (10^6 joules). Calculated from the relation 1 kcal = 4.184 Kj and rounded to one decimal place.
[3] 1 NE (niacin equivalent) is equal to 1 mg of niacin or 60 mg of tryptophan.
[4] Recommendations are based on estimated average daily protein intake of Canadians.
[5] Recommendation given in terms of free folate.
[6] One RE (retinol equivalent) corresponds to a biological activity in humans equal to 1 μg retinol (3.33 IU) or 6 μg β-carotene (10 IU).
[7] One μg cholecalciferol is equivalent to 1 μg ergocalciferol (40 IU vitamin D activity).
[a] Recommended protein intake of 2.2 g/kg body weight for infants age 0–2 months and 2.0 g/kg body weight for those age 3–5 months. Protein recommendation for infants 0–11 months assumes consumption of breast milk or protein of equivalent quality.

Food and Nutrition Board. 1980. *Recommended dietary allowances*, p. 23. 9th ed. Washington, D.C.: National Academy of Sciences.

The energy allowances for the young adults are for men and women doing light work. The allowances for the two older age groups represent mean energy needs over these age spans, allowing for a 2% decrease in basal (resting) metabolic rate per decade and a reduction in activity of 200 kcal/day for men and women between 51 and 75 years, 500 kcal for men over 75 years and 400 kcal for women over 75. The customary range of daily energy output is shown for adults in parentheses, and is based on a variation in energy needs of ±400 kcal at any one age, emphasizing the wide range of energy intakes appropriate for any group of people.

Energy allowances for children through age 18 are based on median energy intakes of children these ages followed in longitudinal growth studies. The values in parentheses are 10th and 90th percentiles of energy intake, to indicate the range of energy consumption among children of these ages.

		Fat-Soluble Vitamins			Minerals						
Vitamin B_{12} (μg)	Vitamin C (mg)	Vitamin A (RE)[6]	Vitamin D (μg cholecal-ciferol)[7]	Vitamin E (mg d α-toco-pherol	Calcium (mg)	Phosphorus (mg)	Magnesium (mg)	Iodine (μg)	Iron (mg)	Zinc (mg)	Age
0.3	20[b]	400	10	3	500[c]	250[c]	50[c]	35[c]	7[c]	4[c]	0–6 mo
0.3	20	400	10	3	500	400	50	50	7	5	7–11 mo
0.9	20	400	10	4	500	500	75	70	8	5	1–3 yrs
1.5	20	500	5	5	500	500	100	90	9	6	4–6 yrs
1.5	30	700	2.5[d]	6	700	700	150	110	10	7	7–9 yrs
1.5	30	700	2.5[d]	6	700	700	150	100	10	7	
3.0	30	800	2.5[d]	7	900	900	175	130	11	8	10–12 yrs
3.0	30	800	2.5[d]	7	1000	1000	200	120	11	9	
3.0	30	1000	2.5[d]	9	1200	1200	250	140	13	10	13–15 yrs
3.0	30	800	2.5[d]	7	800	800	250	110	14	10	
3.0	30	1000	2.5[d]	10	1000	1000	300	160	14	12	16–18 yrs
3.0	30	800	2.5[d]	6	700	700	250	110	14	11	
3.0	30	1000	2.5[d]	9	800	800	300	150	10	10	19–35 yrs
3.0	30	800	2.5[d]	6	700	700	250	110	14	9	
3.0	30	1000	2.5[d]	8	800	800	300	140	10	10	36–50 yrs
3.0	30	800	2.5[d]	6	700	700	250	100	14	9	
3.0	30	1000	2.5[d]	8	800	800	300	140	10	10	51+ yrs
3.0	30	800	2.5[d]	6	700	700	250	100	9	9	
+1.0	+20	+100	+2.5[d]	+1	+500	+500	+25	+15	+1[g]	+3	Pregnancy
+0.5	+30	+400	+2.5[d]	+2	+500	+500	+75	+25	+1[g]	+7	Lactation

[b] Considerably higher levels may be prudent for infants during the first week of life to guard against neonatal tyrosinemia.
[c] The intake of breast-fed infants may be less than the recommendation but is considered to be adequate.
[d] Most older children and adults receive vitamin D from irradiation but 2.5 μg daily is recommended. This intake should be increased to 5.0 μg daily during pregnancy and lactation and for those confined indoors or otherwise deprived of sunlight for extended periods.
[e] Recommended energy intake for age 66+ years reduced to 2000 kcal (8.4 mj) for men and 1500 kcal (6.3 mj) for women.
[f] Increased energy intake recommended during second and third trimesters. An increase of 100 kcal (418.4 kj) per day is recommended during the first trimester.
[g] A recommended total intake of 15 mg daily during pregnancy and lactation assumes the presence of adequate stores of iron. If stores are suspected of being inadequate, additional iron as a supplement is recommended.

U.S. Dietary Goals

In 1977, the U.S. Senate Select Committee on Nutrition and Human Needs was organized by Senator George McGovern to propose dietary goals for the United States.

The goals focus on the prevention of diet-related diseases such as obesity, cardiovascular diseases, diabetes, and dental disease.

The dietary goals are to (1)

- Avoid overweight; consume only as much energy as is expended. If overweight, decrease energy intake and increase energy expenditure.
- Increase the consumption of complex carbohydrates and "naturally occurring" sugars from about 28% of energy intake to about 48% of energy intake.
- Reduce the consumption of refined and other processed sugars by about 45% to account for about 10% of total energy intake.
- Reduce overall fat consumption from approximately 40% to about 30% of energy intake.
- Reduce saturated fat consumption to account for about 10% of total energy intake and balance with polyunsaturated and mono-unsaturated fats, which should account for about 10% of energy intake each.
- Reduce cholesterol consumption to about 300 mg per day.
- Limit the intake of sodium by reducing the intake of salt (sodium chloride) to about 5 g per day (approximately 2 g sodium).

The U.S. dietary goals have been both supported and criticized. Statements supporting the U.S. dietary goals are as follows:

1. To achieve further major health gains in the United States, emphasis must be placed on the prevention of disease. The health of many Americans is at risk from excessive intakes of calories, fat, saturated fat, cholesterol, salt, and sugar. (2)
2. The recommended changes are moderate; they do not eliminate any foods from the diet. These recommendations are without nutritional risk for a large proportion of the population. (3)

Statements criticizing the U.S. dietary goals are as follows:

1. The dietary goals do not allow for individual requirements based on age, sex, activity level, or degree of health. Some investigators state that conclusive evidence is unavailable indicating that adherence to the recommendations will improve the future health of Americans. (4)
2. Composition of the diet is only one of many factors that contribute to the probability of disease. Other factors include smoking, exercise and rest habits, alcohol consumption, obesity, age, sex, life-style, income, genetics, dental and medical care. (6)

REFERENCES CITED

1. U.S. Senate Select Committee on Nutrition and Human Needs. 1977. *Dietary goals for the United States.* 2nd ed. Washington, D.C.: GPO, December 1977.
2. Hegsted, D. M. 1978. Dietary goals—A progressive view. *Am. J. Clin. Nutr.* 31:1504.
3. Hegsted, D. M. 1978. Rationale for change in the American diet. *Food Tech.* 32:44.
4. Harper, A. E. 1978. What are appropriate dietary guidelines? *Food Tech.* 32:48.
5. Harper, A. E. 1978. Dietary goals–A skeptical view. *Am. J. Clin. Nutr.* 31:310.
6. American Dietetic Association. 1978. *A reaction statement by the American Dietetic Association to dietary goals for the United States.* Statement No. 0002. Chicago. September 1978.

OTHER REFERENCES

Peterkin, B. L.; Shore, C. J., and Kerr, R. L. 1979. Some diets that meet the dietary goals for the United States. *J. Am. Dietet. A.* 74:423.

A3

Dietary Guidelines for Healthy Americans—Nutrition and Your Health

The U.S. Department of Agriculture and the U.S. Department of Health and Human Services have jointly prepared a booklet "Nutrition and Your Health" (1980). The audience is most healthy Americans who would like to establish "good" eating habits to maintain and improve health.[1] The guidelines are to

- Eat a variety of foods
- Maintain ideal weight
- Avoid too much fat, saturated fat, and cholesterol
- Eat foods with adequate starch and fiber
- Avoid too much sugar
- Avoid too much sodium
- If you drink alcohol, do so in moderation

REFERENCES

Nutrition and your health, dietary guidelines for Americans. 1980. *Nutr. Today* 15:14.

GREENBERG, D. S. 1980. A long wait for a little advice. *Nutr. Today* 15:20.

HARPER, A. E. 1980. Dear secretary—. *Nutr. Today* 15:19.

[1] Individuals can order one copy free from Consumer Information Center, #656-H, Pueblo, Colorado 81009.

A4

Fluid Requirements

Total body water represents 44–73% of the weight for adults and 70–83% of the weight for newborn infants. Obese individuals have more fat and less water as a percentage of total body weight than do lean individuals. Women have less water and more fat than do men. With advancing age (over age 60), total body water decreases 5–8%. Body fluids participate in cellular metabolism, transportation, chemical reactions, temperature regulation, elimination, and acid–base balance. Body fluid volume, electrolyte composition, and osmolarity are maintained by parathyroid and pulmonary regulatory mechanisms. (1, 2)

FLUID BALANCE

Fluid balance in the healthy individual depends upon absorption of water from the gastrointestinal tract, the water produced by metabolic processes, and the loss through respiration, urination, defecation, and perspiration. In the normal individual, water intake and output balance closely with daily body weight, which usually fluctuates less than 2%. (3)

$$\text{Fluid balance} = \text{Intake} - \text{output}$$

Intake. Fluid intake is derived from (1) water and other fluids ingested and (2) solid food ingested. The fluid in solid food includes water content of the ingested food, which may be as much as 90%, and water of oxidation, which is derived from the combustion of foods within the body. Table A.4-1 lists the approximate yield of water of oxidation per 100 g of major nutrients.

The average intake of fluid varies with habit and climate. Table A.4-2 lists the average daily fluid intake of adults in a temperate climate.

When calculating fluid intake for a fluid-restricted diet, only water and other items that are fluid at body temperature are considered in the calculations. Fluid intake from solid foods and from the oxidation of foodstuffs approximately equals fluid lost from extrarenal losses and is not calculated.

Output. Fluid is lost from the body from (1) measurable output (urine and fecal) and (2) insensible losses (evaporation from respiration and skin). The average loss of fluid varies with input and climate. Table A.4-3 lists the average daily fluid output of adults in a temperate climate.

FLUID REQUIREMENTS

Requirements for fluid are based upon the amount necessary to replace that lost daily. Calculation of the fluid requirement is based upon urinary volume and estimated extrarenal losses. The following factors increase fluid requirements (3–5):

fever (7 ml/kg/day/°F)
sweating
hyperpnea
failure of renal conservation
vomiting or gastric suctioning

intestinal losses via diarrhea, colostomy, or fistula
high environmental temperature (500 ml for every 5° above 85°F)

humidity
diabetes in poor control
denuded body surface

Under normal conditions, daily water maintenance requirements for children, adolescents, and adults are 100 ml/100 kcal consumed or 30–45 ml water per kilogram ideal body weight for adolescents and adults. (1, 3, 4) Individuals over the age of 55 years with no major cardiac or renal disease need approximately 30 ml water per kilogram body weight. (3) For hospitalized children, water requirements are based on expected caloric expenditure. (5) Table A.4-4 lists a method for estimating calorie expenditure of hospitalized children.

FLUID IMBALANCE

Fluid imbalance occurs in the form of dehydration or overhydration.

Dehydration results from loss of total body fluid. Extracellular fluid accounts for the majority of the fluid lost. A loss of 2% causes thirst and oliguria. A loss of 4% may lead to oliguria, tachycardia, and postural hypotension. A loss of 6% of body fluid is life threatening. When this occurs, interstitial fluid and plasma volume are reduced by 30%, affecting both blood pressure and renal function. (3) Dehydration may be caused by increased output–vomiting, diarrhea, open wounds, fistulas, diabetes insipidus, diabetic ketoacidosis, fever, or hyperthyroidism–and/or by decreased intake.

Treatment of mild dehydration is accomplished by increasing oral intake of fluids. More severe cases are treated by appropriate intravenous fluid replacement. Intravenous fluid therapy is given to replace previous losses, to provide maintenance requirements, and to replace concurrent losses. The amount and type of fluid replacement therapy is determined by evaluating and monitoring the following:

serum electrolyte values
weight changes
fluid intake and output records
urine pH
sweating

diarrhea
drug therapy
pre- and postoperative fasting
renal function
cardiac function

suction of bronchial secretions
fluid loss from wounds, fistulas, etc.

Overhydration results from retention of excessive fluid. Hyponatremia and hyperkalemia often occur in overhydration. Treatment is by restriction of total fluid intake. The amount of restriction is determined by the severity of the situation. The amount of urinary output is a good indicator of the level of restriction required. The following conditions may require fluid restrictions:

inappropriate antidiuretic hormone secretion
cardiac disease
renal disease

liver disease
neurosurgery or head injury

bacterial meningitis
chronic bronchitis

individuals on positive pressure ventilators
Goodpasture's syndrome (pulmonary/kidney disease)
asphyxia

TABLES

TABLE A.4-1. Water of Oxidation of Ingested Nutrients (per 100 g) (1)

Nutrients	Water of Oxidation (g)
Protein	41
Fat	107
Carbohydrate	55

TABLE A.4-2. Average Daily Fluid Intake, Healthy Adults (3)

Source of Fluid	Range (ml)
Water and other fluid	1000–2500
Water in semisolid and solid food	1000–1500
Water of oxidation	200– 400
Total	2200–4400

TABLE A.4-3. Average Daily Fluid Loss, Healthy Adults (3)

Source of Fluid	Range (ml)
Urine	1000–2500
Feces	100– 200
Respiratory insensible loss	300– 750
Surface evaporation, sweat	400– 600
Total	1800–4050+

TABLE A.4-4. Method of Estimating Daily Caloric Expenditure of Hospitalized Children (5)

Weight (kg)	Calorie Expenditure
0–10	100 kcal/kg
10–20	(100 kcal/kg − 10)(50)
Over 20	(150 kcal/kg − 20)(50)

REFERENCES CITED

1. Goodhart, R. S., and Shils, E. 1980. *Modern nutrition in health and disease,* pp. 355–394. 6th ed. Philadelphia: Lea & Febiger.
2. Wilkinson, A. W. 1973. *Body fluids in surgery.* Edinburgh: Churchill and Livingston.
3. Harper, H. A. 1973. *Review of physiological chemistry.* Los Altos, Calif.: Lange Medical Publications.
4. Schneider, H. A.; Anderson, C. E.; and Coursin, D. B. 1977. *Nutritional support of medical practice.* New York: Harper & Row.
5. Faculty and Department of Pediatrics and Communicable Diseases. 1978. *Pediatric syllabus.* 4th ed. Ann Arbor: University of Michigan, July 1978 (update).
6. Feigin, R. D., and Kaplan, S. 1977. Inappropriate secretion of antidiuretic hormone in children with bacterial meningitis. *Am. J. Clin. Nutr.* 30:76.

Food–Drug Interactions

DRUG INTERACTION WITH NUTRITIONAL STATUS

An insidious side effect of drug therapy is alteration of nutrient metabolism. A drug usually interacts with more than one nutrient and may act on one nutrient in several ways. Table A.5-1 lists the mechanisms of drug interference with nutritional status. Susceptibility to drug-induced nutritional deficiencies is greatest in the elderly, the chronically ill, anyone with a history of marginal or inadequate nutritional intake, or anyone who is receiving multidrug therapy. (2)

Table A.5-2 lists drug categories capable of interfering with nutritional status. For more detailed information concerning specific drugs, their effect on nutritional status, the mechanism involved, and the significance, refer to an appropriate reference. Prevention of a deficiency or minimization of the effect may be achieved by consuming an adequate nutritional intake prior to drug therapy and by supplementation with the nutrient involved in the drug interaction in amounts greater than the normal requirement. (9)

FOOD INTERACTION WITH DRUG THERAPY

The mechanism of drug therapy can be altered by specific foods and the timing of meals. Table A.5-3 lists the mechanisms in which food interferes with drug therapy. Recommendations for the administration of drugs in relation to timing of meals or intake of specific foods is provided in Table A.5-4. An example of this is when the ingestion of tyramine-containing foods causes a hypertensive crisis in people taking monoamine oxidase inhibitors. (11) Use of a monoamine oxidase inhibitor inhibits the body's ability to oxidize monoamines. Tyramine, a pressoramine, which normally undergoes oxidative deamination by monoamine oxidase, is contained in some foods. Table A.5-5 lists known tyramine-containing foods.

TABLES

TABLE A.5-1. Mechanisms of Drug Interference with Nutritional Status (1)

- Suppression or stimulation of appetite
- Alteration of nutrient absorption
    - Alteration of gastrointestinal transit time
    - Alteration of gastrointestinal pH
    - Alteration of bile acid activity
    - Alteration of peristalsis
    - Inactivation of absorptive enzyme systems
    - Competitive inhibition at nutrient's site of absorption
    - Damaging of absorptive mucosal cells of gastrointestinal tract
    - Complexation of nutrient by drug
- Alteration of nutrient's metabolism and utilization
- Alteration of nutrient's excretion

TABLE A.5-2. Drug Categories Capable of Interfering with Nutritional Status

Drug	Effect	Reference
Alcohol	Increase of magnesium	3, 4
	Malabsorption of folic acid, B_{12}	3, 4
Analgesics	Gastrointestinal disturbances	5
Anorexiants	Growth suppression in young children	3,5
	Insomnia	6
	Hypertension	6
	Dry mouth	6
	Constipation	6
Antacids	Destruction of thiamin may lead to a deficiency (chronic use)	5, 4, 7, 8
Anticoagulants	Increased uptake of vitamin K may alter prothombin time	5
Anticonvulsants	Gastrointestinal irritant	5, 7
	B_{12} deficiency with large doses	3, 5, 7
	Impairment and utilization of folic acid, B_{12} and D-xylose	4
Antidepressants	Stimulation of appetite	3
Anti-infectives	Decreased folic acid utilization	4
	B_{12} malabsorption	4
	Decreased bacterial synthesis of vitamin K	4
	Impaired absorption of calcium, magnesium; pyridoxine inactivation	4
	Gastrointestinal disturbances	7
Antimicrobials	Appetite suppression	3, 1
	Diarrhea	3, 1
	Decreased nutrient absorption	3, 1
Antineoplastics	Gastrointestinal disturbances	7
	Anorexia	7
Autonomics	Decreased peristalsis	3
	Gastrointestinal disturbances	7
Cathartics	Potassium and calcium loss and steatorrhea with chronic use	4, 7
Chelating agents	Decreased absorption of metals	8
Corticosteroids	Decreased glucose tolerance	3, 1
	Decreased muscle protein	3, 1
	Increased liver fat	3, 1
	Increased retention of sodium	3, 1
	Decreased calcium and iron absorption	3
Diuretics	Hypokalemia	4, 7
	Hypomagnesemia	7
	Increased urinary thiamin, pyridoxine, calcium	7
Hypocholesterol-emics	Malabsorption of B_{12}, D-xylose, carotene, MCT, electrolytes, iron, and sugar absorption	4
Laxatives	Loss of electrolytes	11
	Decreased intestinal uptake of glucose	11
Oral contraceptives	Increased blood lipids	3
	Increased intestinal absorption of iron	3
	Impairment of folic acid absorption and utilization	3, 4
	Increased turnover of B_6	3

TABLE A.5-2. Drug Categories Capable of Interfering with Nutritional Status [*Concluded*]

Drug	Effect	Reference
Potassium chloride	Decreased absorption of B_{12}	3
Sedative-hypnotics	Multivitamin deficiency	3
	Gastrointestinal disturbances	7
Surfactants	Alteration of nutrient absorption	3
Tranquilizers	Stimulation of appetite	3, 7
	Hypercholesterolemia	3, 7

TABLE A.5-3. Mechanisms of Food Interferences with Drug Therapy (1)

- Alteration of absorption of orally administered drugs
  - Alteration of gastrointestinal transit time and motility
  - Alteration of gastrointestinal secretions and pH
  - Alteration of osmolality of gastrointestinal tract
  - Alteration of ionization of drug
  - Alteration of stability of drug
  - Alteration of solubility of drug
  - Complexation of drug by dietary component
- Alteration of drug's distribution
- Alteration of drug's metabolism
- Alteration of drug's excretion
- Exertion of agonistic of antagonistic pharmacologic response by active substance in food

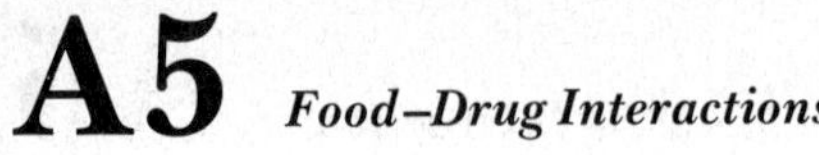

TABLE A.5-4. Drug Administration in Relation to Meals

		Timing of Meals[1]					
Drug Trade Name (Generic Name)	Classification	1	2	3	4	5	6
Acetylsalicylic acid (APC)	Mild pain reliever	—	—	X	—	—	—
(aminophylline)	Bronchial asthma and pulmonary emphysema	—	—	X	—	—	—
(ampicillin)	Anti-infective	—	—	—	—	X	—
(antidiabetic)		—	—	X	—	—	—
(antihistamine)		—	—	—	—	—	X
Antivert (meclizine hydrochloride)		—	—	—	—	—	X
Artane (trihexyphenidyl hydrochloride)		—	—	X	—	—	—
(belladonna) and its alkaloids	Anticholinergic drug	—	X	—	—	—	—
(benzathine penicillin G)		X	—	—	—	X	—
(chloral hydrate)	Sedative	—	—	—	—	—	X
DBI (pheniformin hydrochloride)	Antidiabetic agent	—	—	—	—	—	X
Diabinese (chlorpropamide)	Antidiabetic agent	—	—	—	—	—	X
Dilantin (diphenylhydantain)	Anticonvulsant drug	—	—	X	—	—	—
Divril (chlorothiazide)	Diuretic	—	—	X	—	—	—
Donnatal (hyoscyamine sulfate)		—	X	—	—	—	—
Dulcolax (bisacodyl)	Cathartic	—	—	—	X	—	—
Dymelor (acetohexamide)	Antidiabetic agent	—	—	—	—	—	X
Dyrenium (triamterene)	Diuretic, potassium sparing	—	—	X	—	—	—
(erythromycin)	Anti-infective agent	X	—	—	—	X	—
Flagyl (metronidazole)	Anti-infective agent	—	—	X	—	—	X
Furadantin (nitrofurantoin)	Urinary germicide	—	—	X	—	—	—
Librax (chlordiazepoxide hydrochloride)		—	X	—	—	—	—
Librium (chlordiazepoxide)	Anti-anxiety agent	—	—	—	—	—	X
Lincocin (lincomycin)	Antibiotic	X	—	—	—	—	—
Lomotil (diphenoxylate hydrochloride)	Antidiarrhea	—	—	—	—	—	X
Macrodantin (nitrofurantoin)	Urinary germicide	—	—	X	—	—	—
Monoamine oxidase (MAO) inhibitors	Psychotic drugs	—	—	—	—	—	?
Mydrodiuril (chlorothiazide)	Antidepressive	—	—	X	—	—	—
Nacrotics	Pain reliever	—	—	—	—	—	X
Orinase (tolbutamide)	Antidiabetic	—	—	—	—	—	X
Penicillin V (phenyoxymethyl penicillin)	Anti-infective agent	X	—	—	—	—	—
Ponstel (mefenamic acid)	Analgesic	—	—	X	—	—	—
(potassium chloride)	Mineral electrolyte	—	—	—	X	—	—
(potassium iodide)		—	—	—	X	—	—
(prednisone)	Anti-inflammatory agent Corticosteroid	—	—	X	—	—	—
(prednisolone)	Anti-inflammatory agent Corticosteroid	—	—	X	—	—	—
Preludin (phenmetrazine hydrochloride)	Anorexic	—	X	—	—	—	—
Pro-banthine (propantheline bromide)	Anticholinergic	—	X	—	—	—	—
Pyridium (phenazopyridine)		—	X	—	—	—	—
Quaalude (methaqualone)	Sedative	—	—	—	—	—	X
(rauwolfia) and its alkaloids		—	—	X	—	—	—
Ritalin (methylphenidate)	Respiratory and cerebral stimulant	—	X	—	—	—	—

Lambert, M. L., Jr. 1975. Drug and diet interactions. *Am. J. Nursing* 75:3.

[1] Key to the numbering system:
1–Take on an empty stomach.
2–Take one half hour before meals.
3–Take with meals or food.
4–Do not take with milk.
5–Do not take with fruit juice.
6–Do not drink alcohol while taking.

Table A.5-4. Drug Administration in Relation to Meals [*Concluded*]

Drug Trade Name (Generic Name)	Classification	Timing of Meals[1]					
		1	2	3	4	5	6
Rondomycin (methacycline)		X	—	—	—	—	—
Serpasil (reserpine)	Cardiovascular	—	—	X	—	—	—
Tegapen (cloxacillin)	preparation treatment of hypertension	X	—	—	—	—	—
Temaril (trimeprazine tartrate)		—	—	X	—	—	—
(tetracyclines) except Declomycin (demethylchlor-tetracycline), which can easily upset the stomach	Antibiotic	X	—	—	—	—	—
(tetracyclines) except Vibramycin (doxycycline)	Antibiotic	—	—	X	—	—	—

Table A.5-5. Tyramine-Containing Foods[1] (12–24)

Banana skins
Beer and wine
Cheese, pickled herring, sausage, and other aged animal protein-containing foods except cottage, ricotta, and cream cheese[2]
Meat extracts
Millet hulls
Pods of broad beans (fava beans)[3]
Soy sauce
Yeast extracts (Barmene, Befit, Bovril, Marmite, Yeastral, Yex)

[1] Tyramine-containing foods may need to be avoided 24 hours prior to use of monoamine oxidase inhibitors and up to 2 weeks after the end of drug therapy to avoid a hypertensive crisis.
[2] The proteolytic action by various aerobic bacteria during aging, fermentation, or spoilage of high-quality proteins (animal) releases tyramine. (12–14)
[3] Some vegetables contain tryamine; however, their contribution is small and has little risk of precipitating a hypertensive crisis. (23)

REFERENCES CITED

1. Hethcox, J. M., and Stanaszek, W. F. 1974. Interactions of drugs and diet. *Hosp. Pharm.* 9:373.
2. March, D. 1978. *Handbook: Interactions of selected drugs with nutritional status in man.* Chicago: American Dietetic Association.
3. Meredith, O., and Lukert, B. 1977. *Clinical nutrition, a physiologic approach in man.* Chicago: Year Book Medical Publishers, Inc.
4. Pierpaoli, P. G. 1972. Drug therapy and diet. *Drug Intelligence and Clin. Pharm.* 6:89.
5. Grant, A. 1979. *Handbook of nutritional assessment.* Seattle.
6. Thiel, V. F. 1976. *Clinical nutrition,* p. 36. Saint Louis, Mo.: C. V. Mosby.
7. March, D. C. 1979. *Handbook: Interactions of selected drugs with nutritional status in man.* Chicago: American Dietetic Association.
8. Christakis, G., and Miridjanian, A. 1968. Diets, drugs and their interrelationships. *J. Am. Dietet. A.* 52:21.
9. Roe, D. 1971. Drug induced deficiencies of B vitamins. *N.Y. State J. Med.* 71:2770.
10. Lambert, M. L., Jr. 1975. Drug and diet interactions. *Am. J. Nursing* 75:402.
11. Blackwell, B.; Marley, E.; Price, J.; and Taylor, D. 1967. Hypertensive interactions between monoamine oxidase inhibitors and foodstuffs. *Brit. J. Psychiat.* 113:349.
12. Rice, S. L.; Eitenmiller, R. R.; and Koehler, P. E. 1975. Histamine and tyramine content of meat products. *J. Milk Food Tech.* 38:256.
13. Rice, S. L., and Koehler, P. E. 1976. Tyrosine and histidine decarboxylase activities of *Pediococcus cerevisiae* and *Lactobacillus* species and the production of tyramine in fermented sausages. *J. Milk Food Tech.* 39:166.
14. Vandekerckhove, P. 1977. A research note. Amines in dry fermented sausage. *J. Food Sci.* 42:283.
15. Blackwell, B., and Mabbitt, L. A. 1965. Tyramine in cheese related to hypertensive crises after monoamine oxidase inhibition. *Lancet* 1:938.
16. Horwitz, D.; Lovenberg, W.; Engelman, K.; and Sjoerdsma, A. 1964. Monoamine oxidase inhibitors, tyramine, and cheese. *JAMA* 188:1108.
17. Kaplan, E. R.; Sapeika, N.; and Moodie, I. M. 1974. Determination of the tyramine content of South African cheeses by gas–liquid chromatography. *Analyst.* 99:565.
18. Kayaalp, S. O.; Renda, N.; Kaymakcalan, S.; and Özer, A. 1970. Tyramine content of some cheeses. *Toxicol. Appl. Pharmacol.* 16:459.
19. Sapeika, N.; Moodie, I. M.; and Sapeika, N. 1975. Tyramine content of South African cheeses. *South African Med. J.* 49:637.
20. Lovenberg, W. 1973. Some vaso- and psychoactive substances in food: Amines, stimulants, depressants, and hallucinogens. In *Toxicants occurring naturally in foods,* pp. 170–188. Washington, D.C.: National Academy of Sciences.
21. Rice, S. L.; Eitenmiller, R. R.; and Koehler, P. E. 1976. Biologically active amines in food: A review. *J. Milk Food Tech.* 39:353.
22. Sen, N. P. 1969. Analysis and significance of tyramine in foods. *J. Food Sci.* 34:22.
23. Udenfriend, S.; Lovenberg, W.; and Sjoerdsma, A. 1959. Physiologically active amines in common fruits and vegetables. *Arch. Biochem. Biophys.* 85:487.
24. Blackwell, B.; Mabbitt, L. A.; and Marley, E. 1969. Histamine and tyramine content of yeast products. *J. Food Sci.* 34:47.

OTHER REFERENCES

Berman, H. A., and Weinstein, L. 1971. Antibiotics and nutrition. *Am. J. Clin. Nutr.* 24:260.

Bosso, J. A., and Pearson, R. E. 1973. Sugar content of selected liquid medicinals. *Diabetes* 22:776.

Butterworth, C. E. 1973. Interactions of nutrients with oral contraceptives and other drugs. *J. Am. Dietet. A.* 62:510.

LAMY, P. P. 1975 (October). OTC drug and the ambulant patient. II. The problems of analgesics, antacids and cold preparations. *Hospital Formulary.* 449.

ROE, D. A. 1976. *Drug-induced nutritional deficiencies.* Westport, Conn.: Avi Publishers.

REFERENCES FOR THE LAY PUBLIC

Consumer Information Center. *FDA consumer: Food and drug interactions.* Pueblo, CO 81009.

Weights and Measures

TABLE A.6-1. U.S. to Metric Conversions

Symbol	If Measure Is in	Multiply by	To Find	Symbol
Length				
in.	inches	25.4	millimeters	mm
in.	inches	2.54	centimeters	cm
ft	feet	30.48	centimeters	cm
ft	feet	0.305	meters	m
cm	centimeters	0.394	inches	in.
m	meters	3.281	feet	ft
Weight (mass)				
gr	grains	64.799	milligrams	mg
oz	ounces	29.35	grams	g
lb	pounds	454	grams	g
lb	pounds	0.454	kilograms	kg
g	grams	15.432	grains	gr
g	grams	0.035	ounces	oz
g	grams	0.0022	pounds	lb
kg	kilograms	2.205	pounds	lb
Capacity (volume)				
tsp	teaspoons	4.7	milliliters	ml
tbsp	tablespoons	14.1	milliliters	ml
fl oz	fluid ounces	29.573	milliliters	ml
c	cups (8 oz)	238	milliliters	ml
pt	pints	0.473	liters	l
qt	quarts	0.946	liters	l
ml	milliliters	0.034	fluid ounces	fl oz
l	liters	1.057	quarts	qt
Energy				
kcal	kilocalories	4.184	kilojoules	kj
kj	kilojoules	0.239	kilocalories	kcal
Temperature				
°F	Fahrenheit	subtract 32; then multiply by $\frac{5}{9}$	Celsius (Centigrade)	°C
°C	Celsius (Centigrade)	multiply by $\frac{9}{5}$ then add 32	Fahrenheit	°F

TABLE A.6-2. Metric Measures

Metric equivalents
- 1 kilogram (kg) = 1000 grams
- 1 gram (g) = 1000 milligrams
- 1 milligram (mg) = 1000 micrograms
- 1 microgram (mcg, μg, γ) = 1000 nanograms
- 1 nanogram (ng) = 1000 picograms (pg)

Multiples
- deca- = 10
- hecto- = 10^2 (100)
- kilo- = 10^3 (1000)
- mega- = 10^6 (1,000,000)

Submultiples

deca-	= one tenth	10^{-1} (0.1)
centi-	= one hundredth	10^{-2} (0.01)
milli-	= one thousandth	10^{-3} (0.001)
micro-	= one millionth	10^{-6} (0.000,001)
nano-	= one billionth	10^{-9} (0.000,000,001)
pico-	= one trillionth	10^{-12} (0.000,000,000,001)

TABLE A.6-3. Some Common Household Measure Equivalents

Measure (Liquid)		Equivalent
3 teaspoons	=	1 tablespoon
1 tablespoon	=	½ fluid ounce
16 tablespoons	=	1 cup
1 cup	=	8 fluid ounces
2 cups	=	1 pint
2 pints	=	1 quart
4 quarts	=	1 gallon
1 jigger	=	3 tablespoons (1½ fluid ounces)

TABLE A.6-4. Milliequivalent/Milligram Conversions

Definition

Milliequivalent (mEq) is an expression of concentration of a substance per liter of solution, calculated by dividing the concentration in milligrams (mg) by the molecular weight.

Conversions

Milligrams to milliequivalents. Divide milligrams by the atomic weight of the element being converted. Multiply the result by the valence.

$$\frac{\text{Weight of element (mg)}}{\text{Atomic weight}} \times \text{Valence} = \text{Milliequivalents}$$

Example: Convert 300 mg calcium to milliequivalents:

$$\frac{300 \text{ mg } Ca^{++}}{40} \times 2 = 15 \text{ mEq calcium}$$

Milliequivalents to milligrams. Multiply the milliequivalents by the atomic weight. Divide the result by the valence.

$$\frac{\text{Milliequivalents} \times \text{atomic weight}}{\text{Valence}} = \text{Weight of element (mg)}$$

Example: Convert 70 mEq of sodium to milligrams:

$$\frac{70 \text{ mEq } Na^{+} \times 23}{1} = 1610 \text{ mg sodium}$$

TABLE A.6-5. Atomic Weight and Valence of Five Elements

Element	Atomic Weight	Valence
Calcium	40	2
Chlorine	35	1
Magnesium	24	2
Potassium	39	1
Sodium	23	1

A7

Nutrient Conversions

Table A.7-1. Approximate Physiologic Fuel Value of Major Nutrients (per 1 g)

Nutrient	Fuel Value (kcal)[1]
Carbohydrate	4
Protein	4
Fat	9
Alcohol	7

[1] Kilocalorie is the amount of heat necessary to raise 1 kg of water 1° Celsius.

Table A.7-2. Protein/Nitrogen Conversions[1]

Convert protein (g) to nitrogen (g):

$$\frac{\text{Protein (g)}}{6.25} = \text{Nitrogen (g)}$$

Convert nitrogen (g) to protein (g):

$$\text{Nitrogen (g)} \times 6.25 = \text{Protein (g)}$$

[1] It would appear that these simple conversions could be used either to recommend absolute amounts of extra daily protein intake needed to replace nitrogen lost or to estimate absolute amounts of lean body mass (protein) lost from the daily output of nitrogen. This assumption is subject to technical error. All proteins are not utilized equally. The quality of protein and exercise influence the ability of the body to lay down lean body mass as does the total calorie intake in relationship to dietary requirements.

A8 Nutrient Composition Tables

TABLE A.8-1. Food Composition Tables Cited

The listing is by order of how they were used to develop food exchange systems or groups throughout the manual. When other tables or manufacturer's data were used, they are so identified.

LIST OF FOOD COMPOSITION TABLES

(1) Composition of Foods
Watt, B. K., and Merrill, A. L. 1963. *Agriculture handbook no. 8.* Washington, D. C.: USDA.

The original reference from which most other United States food composition tables are derived. Contains 2500 foods listed in alphabetical order.

The following six titles are the first installments of revision of *Handbook no. 8.*

(2) Posati, L., and Orr, M. 1976. *Agriculture handbook no. 8-1. Dairy and egg products.* Washington, D. C.: USDA.

(3) Marsh, A.; Moss, M.; and Murphy, E. 1977. *Agriculture handbook no. 8-2. Spices and herbs.* Washington, D. C.: USDA.

(4) Gebhardt, S.; Cutrufelli, R.; and Matthews, R. 1978. *Agriculture handbook no. 8-3. Baby foods.* Washington, D. C.: USDA.

(5) Reeves, J. B., and Weihrauch, J. L. 1979. *Agriculture handbook no. 8-4. Fats and oils.* Washington, D. C.: USDA.

(6) Posati, L. P. 1979. *Agriculture handbook no. 8-5. Poultry.* Washington, D. C.: USDA.

(7) March, A. C. 1980. *Agriculture handbook no. 8-6. Soups, sauces, and gravies.* Washington, D. C.: USDA.

Future installments: Sausage and luncheon meats, Pork products.

(8) Nutritive Value of American Foods
Adams, C. 1975. *Agriculture handbook no. 456.* Washington, D. C.: USDA.

Tables of nutritive value of 1500 foods. Data derived from *Handbook no. 8.*

(9) Food Values of Portions Commonly Used
Pennington, J. A. T., and Church, H. N. 1975. *Bowes and Church.* 13th ed. Philadelphia: J. B. Lippincott.

Tables of nutritive value of foods. Data compiled from many sources. Foods listed alphabetically in food groups.

(10) Nutritive Value of Foods
Consumer and Food Economics Research Division. 1970. *Home and garden bulletin no. 72.* Washington, D. C.: USDA.

Table of nutritive value of 615 foods commonly used in the United States. Data derived from *Handbook no. 8.*

(11) Paul, A. A., and Southgate, D. A. T. 1978. *McCance and Widdowson's the composition of foods.* 4th ed. London: Her Majesty's Stationery Office.

Tables of nutritive value of foods. Data compiled from many sources. Foods are listed alphabetically in food groups.

TABLE A.8-1. Food Composition Tables Cited [*Concluded*]

PORTIONS DESCRIBED

1 100 gram
2 1 pound
3 Household measure

Composition	(1) 8	(2) 8-1	(3) 8-2	(4) 8-3	(5) 8-4	(6) 8-5	(7) 8-6	(8) 456	(9) P&C	(10) 72	(11) P&S
Portion described	1 2 3	1 2 3	1 2 3	1 2 3	1 2 3	1 2 3	1 2 3	3	1 3	3	1
Water	x	x	x	x	x	x	x	x	–	–	x
Fiber, crude	x	x	x	x	x	x	x	x	x	–	–
Fiber, dietary	–	–	–	–	–	–	–	–	–	–	x
Energy	x	x	x	x	x	x	x	x	x	x	x
Protein	x	x	x	x	x	x	x	x	x	x	x
Amino acids	–	–	x	x	x	x	x	–	x	–	x
Carbohydrate	x	x	x	x	x	x	x	x	x	x	x
Fat (total)	x	x	x	x	x	x	x	x	x	x	x
Saturated fat	x	x	x	x	x	x	x	x	–	x	x
Polyunsaturated fat	–	x	x	x	x	x	x	–	x	–	x
Oleic acid	x	x	x	x	x	x	x	x	–	x	x
Linoleic acid	x	x	x	x	x	x	x	x	–	x	x
Cholesterol	x	x	x	x	x	x	x	–	–	–	x
Vitamin A	x	x	x	x	x	x	x	x	x	x	x
Thiamin	x	x	x	x	x	x	x	x	x	x	x
Riboflavin	x	x	x	x	x	x	x	x	x	x	x
Pyridoxine	–	x	x	x	x	x	x	–	–	–	x
Niacin	x	x	x	x	x	x	x	x	x	x	x
Vitamin B_{12}	–	x	x	x	x	x	x	–	–	–	x
Folic acid	–	x	x	x	x	x	x	–	–	–	x
Pantothenic acid	–	x	x	x	x	x	x	–	–	–	x
Biotin	–	–	–	–	–	–	–	–	–	–	x
Vitamin C	x	x	x	x	x	x	x	x	x	x	x
Vitamin D	–	–	–	–	–	–	–	–	x	–	x
Vitamin E	–	–	–	–	x	–	–	–	–	–	x
Calcium	x	x	x	x	x	x	x	x	x	x	x
Copper	–	–	–	x	–	x	x	–	–	–	x
Iron	x	x	x	x	x	x	x	x	x	x	x
Magnesium	x	x	x	x	x	x	x	–	x	–	x
Phosphorus	x	x	x	x	x	x	x	x	x	–	x
Potassium	x	x	x	x	x	x	x	x	x	–	x
Sodium	x	x	x	x	x	x	x	x	x	–	x
Zinc	–	x	x	x	x	x	x	x	–	–	x
Sulfur	–	–	–	–	–	–	–	–	–	–	x
Chlorine	–	–	–	–	–	–	–	–	–	–	x
Alcohol	–	–	–	–	–	–	–	–	x	–	x

TABLE A.8-2. References Listing Other Food Composition Tables

Nutrition Policy and Programmed Service, Food Policy and Nutrition Division. 1975. *Food composition tables, updated, annotated bibliography.* Rome: Food and Agriculture Organization of the United Nations.

A review of the contents of the most current food composition tables from all countries that have published such tables. For countries for which food composition tables do not exist, the principal publications on food composition have been reviewed.

The review includes
- reference
- background
- portion analyzed
- nutrients covered
- presentation and grouping
- additional information

Nutrient composition of foods: Selected references and tables. Boston Area Research Dietitians, Special Practice Group. 1978. Boston: Massachusetts Dietetic Association.

A compilation of references of general food composition tables and of food tables for individual nutrients. Reference for food tables of the following nutrients are included:

arsenic	nickel	tin
cadmium	niobium	vitamin B_6
calcium	oxalic acid	vitamin B_{12}
chromium	pantothenic acid	vitamin E
copper	phosphorus	zinc
folic acid		amino acids
iodine		carbohydrate
lead		cholesterol
magnesium		fatty acids
manganese		fiber

TABLE A.8-3. Nutrient Composition and Food Exchange Value of Some Alcoholic Beverages

Beverage	Volume (fl oz)	Alcohol[1] (g)	Carbohydrate (g)	(kcal)	Diabetic Food Exchange Value[2]		Hyperlipidemia Food Exchange Value[3]	
					Fat	Bread	Fruit	Bread
Beer								
regular	12	13	14	147	2	1	2	1
light[4]	12	12	2	92	2	—	—	1
Liquor								
Gin, rum, scotch, vodka, whiskey								
80 proof	1.5	14	Trace	98	2	—	1	1
90 proof	1.5	16	Trace	112	3	—	1	1
100 proof	1.5	18	Trace	126	3	—	1	1
Wine								
Dry, table	3.5	10	4	86	2	—	1	1
Sweet, dessert	3.5	16	8	144	Use not recommended		2	1

[1] Alcohol content determined by weight.

[2] The hyperlipidemia alcohol exchange list is appropriate for use with those individuals who only consume alcohol occasionally. When an individual consumes alcohol on a daily basis, alcohol should be calculated into the diet, not to exceed 5% of total calories (Chapter 32).

[3] Explanation of variance of food exchange group values between the diabetic and the hyperlipidemia is

The diabetic exchanges identify alcohol primarily as fat. Alcohol has a hypoglycemic effect; substituting alcohol for carbohydrate-containing foods such as fruit and bread would further potentiate the hypoglycemic effect. The omission of fat exchanges appears to have little immediate effect on blood glucose levels while maintaining caloric balance of the diet.

The hyperlipidemia exchanges identify alcohol primarily as carbohydrate or fruit and bread exchanges. In hyperlipidemia, the hypoglycemic effect of alcohol is not of primary concern. If fat were exchanged for alcohol, it would be difficult to achieve a desirable polyunsaturated-to-saturated fat ratio.

[4] The nutrient content of light beers varies widely from brand to brand. Values for calories and diabetic food exchange values are from the American Diabetes Association, Inc. and the American Dietetic Association. 1977. *A guide for professionals: The effective application of "exchange lists for meal planning."*

TABLE A.8-4. Caffeine Content of Common Beverages (per 8 fl oz)[1]

Beverage	Caffeine (mg)
Carbonated beverages	
Coca Cola	43
Diet Dr Pepper	36
Diet RC	22
Diet-Rite	22
Dr Pepper	40
Mountain Dew	37
Pepsi-Cola	29
RC Cola	23
Tab	33
Cocoa, instant	13
Coffee	
Dripolated	223
Instant	101
Percolated	168
Tea, bagged	
Black, 1 min brew	46
Black, 5 min brew	76
Tea, loose	
Black, 5 min brew	67
Green, 5 min brew	58
Green, Japan, 5 min brew	34
Tea,	
Iced, instant, made according to package directions	96

Adapted from Bunker, M. L., and McWilliams, M. 1979. Caffeine content of common beverages. *J. Am. Dietet. A.* 74:28, and Groisser, D. S. 1978. A study of caffeine in tea. II. Concentration of caffeine in various strengths, brands, blends, and types of tea. *Am. J. Clin. Nutr.* 31:1727.

[1] The pharmacologic effect of caffeine-containing foods or beverages is related to the amount consumed relative to body weight. When two individuals of greatly different weights consume the same amount of a caffeine-containing beverage, the effect will be greater on the smaller individual.

A9

Nutrition Position Papers

A nutrition position paper is a formal statement by a professional health organization stating, identifying, or defining their official view on nutrition-related subjects. The following is a list of nutrition papers and includes the professional organization source and literature reference for papers that have been published in professional journals. Copies of those listed may be obtained directly from the professional group that authored the paper. Addresses of professional health organizations are listed in Table A.9-1.

DIET AND CORONARY HEART DISEASE

American Heart Association. 1978. *Diet and coronary heart disease.*

American Heart Association. 1978. The value and safety of diet modification to control hyperlipidemia in childhood and adolescence. *Circulation* 58:381A.

American Medical Association; Council on Foods and Nutrition; Food and Nutrition Board, National Academy of Sciences, National Research Council. 1972. Diet and coronary heart disease. Joint policy statement. *JAMA* 222:1647.

American Medical Association. 1977. *Dietary goals for the United States.* Statement submitted to the U.S. Senate Select Committee on Nutrition and Human Needs. April 18, 1977.

DIET AND GASTROINTESTINAL DISEASE

American Dietetic Association. 1971. Bland diet in the treatment of chronic duodenal ulcer disease. *J. Am. Dietet. A.* 59:244.

FOOD LABELING

American Dietetic Association. 1977. ADA statement on labeling of fats and oils. *J. Am. Dietet. A.* 70:402.

American Dietetic Association. 1978. Food labeling: ADA comments to the Food and Drug Administration. *J. Am. Dietet. A.* 73:664.

American Medical Association. 1978. *Food labeling.* Comments submitted to the Food and Drug Administration, U.S. Department of Agriculture, Federal Trade Commission, November 10, 1978.

American Medical Association. 1979. *Food labeling.* Statement submitted to the Subcommittee on Nutrition, Committee on Agriculture, Nutrition, and Forestry, United States Senate, February 28, 1979.

FOOD SENSITIVITY

Food and Nutrition Board, National Research Council. 1972. *Background information on lactose and milk intolerance.* Washington, D.C.: National Academy of Sciences, May 1972.

INFANT/CHILD FEEDING

Collected reprints 1967–1977. 1977. American Academy of Pediatrics, Committee on Nutrition.

American Dental Association. 1978. National Task Force for the prohibition of the sale of confections in schools position statement. November 1978.

American Dietetic Association. 1974. Position paper on child nutrition programs. *J. Am. Dietet. A.* 64:520.

Food and Nutrition Section, American Public Health Association. 1980. Position paper on infant feeding in the United States.

NUTRITION AND EXERCISE

American Dietetic Association. 1980. Nutrition and physical fitness, a statement. *J. Am. Dietet. A.* 76:437.

Food and Nutrition Board, National Research Council. 1974. *Water deprivation and performance of athletes.* Washington, D.C.: National Academy of Sciences, May 1974.

NUTRITION SERVICES

American Dietetic Association. 1971. Food and nutrition services in day care centers. *J. Am. Dietet. A.* 59:47.

American Dietetic Association. 1971. The nutrition component of health services delivery systems. *J. Am. Dietet. A.* 58:538.

American Dietetic Association. 1972. Position paper on nutrition services in health maintenance organizations. *J. Am. Dietet. A.* 60:317.

American Dietetic Association. 1973. Position paper on nutrition education for the public. *J. Am. Dietet. A.* 62:429.

American Dietetic Association. 1974. Position paper on nutrition education and fast food service. *J. Am. Dietet. A.* 65:54.

American Dietetic Association. 1977. ADA statement on nutritional care in long-term care facilities. *J. Am. Dietet. A.* 70:301.

American Dietetic Association. 1977. ADA statement to federal government regarding major gaps in nutritional knowledge. *J. Am. Dietet. A.* 70:294.

American Dietetic Association. 1977. The dietitian in primary health care. *J. Am. Dietet. A.* 70:587.

American Dietetic Association. 1978. Position paper on the scope and thrust of nutrition education. *J. Am. Dietet. A.* 72:302.

American Heart Association. 1977. *Guidelines for the development of nutrition programs.*

NUTRITION MISINFORMATION

American Dietetic Association. 1975. Position paper on food and nutrition misinformation on selected topics. *J. Am. Dietet. A.* 66:277.

National Nutrition Consortium. 1977. Laetrile (vitamin B_{17})—A statement. *J. Am. Dietet. A.* 70:354.

NUTRITIVE VALUE OF FOODS

Council on Foods and Nutrition, American Medical Association. 1973. Improvement of the nutritive quality of foods. General policies. *JAMA* 225:1116.

Food and Nutrition Board, National Research Council. 1973. *General policies in regard to improvement of nutritive quality of foods.* Washington, D.C.: National Academy of Sciences.

Food and Nutrition Board, National Research Council. 1976. *Soil fertility and the nutritive value of crops.* Washington, D.C.: National Academy of Sciences, September 1976.

PARENTERAL NUTRITION

American Medical Association. 1972. Guidelines for total parenteral nutrition. *JAMA* 220:1721.

Department of Foods and Nutrition, American Medical Association. 1975. Guidelines for multivitamin preparations for parenteral use. December 1975.

Department of Foods and Nutrition, American Medical Association. 1979. Guidelines for essential trace element preparations for parenteral use. *JAMA* 241:2051.

POSITION PAPERS

American Dietetic Association. 1975. ADA position paper on position papers. *J. Am. Dietet. A.* 66:54.

VEGETARIAN DIETS

American Dietetic Association. 1980. Position paper on vegetarian approach to eating. *J. Am. Dietet. A.* 77:61.

Council on Foods and Nutrition, American Medical Association. 1971. Zen macrobiotic diets. *JAMA* 218:397.

Food and Nutrition Board, National Research Council. 1974. *Vegetarian diets.* Washington, D.C.: National Academy of Sciences, May 1974.

VITAMINS AND TRACE ELEMENTS

Fluoride

American Dietetic Association. 1974. Policy statement on fluoridation. *J. Am. Dietet. A.* 64:68.

National Nutrition Consortium. 1977. Fluoridation endorsed. *J. Am. Dietet. A.* 70:354.

Selenium

Food and Nutrition Board, National Research Council. 1977. Are selenium supplements needed (by the general public)? *J. Am. Dietet. A.* 70:249.

Vitamin D

Food and Nutrition Board, National Research Council. 1974. *Hazards of overuse of vitamin D.* Washington, D.C.: National Academy of Sciences, November 1974.

Vitamin E

Food and Nutrition Board, National Research Council. 1973. *Supplementation of human diets with vitamin E.* Washington, D.C.: National Academy of Sciences, June 1973.

Institute of Food Technologists' Expert Panel on Food Safety and Nutrition and the Committee on Public Information. 1977. Vitamin E. A scientific status summary. *Food Tech.* 31:77.

WEIGHT REDUCTION DIETS

American Dietetic Association. 1976. ADA supports FTC proposal on protein supplement marketing. *J. Am. Dietet. A.* 68:162.

American Dietetic Association. 1978. Statement by the American Dietetic Association on diet protein products. *J. Am. Dietet. A.* 73:547.

Council on Foods and Nutrition, American Medical Association. 1973. A critique of low-carbohydrate ketogenic weight reduction regimens. A review of Dr. Atkins' diet revolution. *JAMA* 224:1415.

TABLES

TABLE A.9-1. Addresses of Professional Health Associations

American Academy of Family Physicians 1740 North 92nd Street Kansas City, Mo. 64114	American Heart Association 7320 Greenville Avenue Dallas, Tex. 75231
American Academy of Pediatrics 1801 Hinman Avenue Evanston, Ill. 60201	American Hospital Association 840 North Lake Shore Drive Chicago, Ill. 60611
American Cancer Society, Inc. 777 Third Avenue New York, N.Y. 10017	American Medical Association 535 North Dearborn Street Chicago, Ill. 60610
American College of Cardiology Heart House 9111 Old Georgetown Road Bethesda, Md. 20014	American Nurses Association 2420 Pershing Road Kansas City, Mo. 64108
American College of Obstetricians and Gynecologists 1 East Wacker Drive Chicago, Ill. 60601	American Public Health Association 1015 18th Street, N.W. Washington, D.C. 20036
American Dental Association 211 East Chicago Avenue Suite 1804 Chicago, Ill. 60611	Food and Nutrition Board National Research Council National Academy of Sciences 2101 Constitution Avenue, N.W. Washington, D.C. 20418
American Dietetic Association 430 North Michigan Ave. Chicago, Ill. 60611	

Index

Index

I

K

L

M

N

O

P

R

S

T

U

V

W